Clinical Simulations in Nursing Education:
Advanced Concepts, Trends, and Opportunities

Clinical Simulations in Nursing Education: Advanced Concepts, Trends, and Opportunities

Edited by:
Pamela R. Jeffries, PhD, RN, FAAN, ANEF

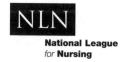

National League
for **Nursing**

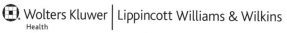 Wolters Kluwer | Lippincott Williams & Wilkins
Health

Philadelphia · Baltimore · New York · London
Buenos Aires · Hong Kong · Sydney · Tokyo

Acquisitions Editor: Christina Burns
Product Development Editor: Eve Malakoff-Klein
Production Project Manager: Marian Bellus
Designer: Stephen Druding
Illustration: Jennifer Clements
Manufacturing Coordinator: Karin Duffield
Composition: Aptara, Inc.
Printer: DRC

351 West Camden Street   Two Commerce Square/2001 Market Street
Baltimore, MD 21201   Philadelphia, PA 19103

Printed in the United States

Library of Congress Cataloging-in-Publication Data

Clinical simulations in nursing education : advanced concepts, trends, and opportunities/edited by Pamela R. Jeffries ; National League for Nursing.
  p. ; cm.
Includes bibliographical references.
ISBN 978-1-934758-19-9 (alk. paper)
I. Jeffries, Pamela R., editor of compilation.   II. National League for Nursing.
[DNLM: 1. Education, Nursing–methods.   2. Patient Simulation.   3. Problem-Based Learning–methods. WY 18]
RT84.5
610.7301′1–dc23
                                              2013038999

Disclaimer
Care has been taken to confirm the accuracy of the information presented and to describe generally accepted practices. However, the authors, editors, and publisher are not responsible for errors or omissions or for any consequences from application of the information in this book and make no warranty, expressed or implied, with respect to the currency, completeness, or accuracy of the contents of the publication. Application of this information in a particular situation remains the professional responsibility of the practitioner; the clinical treatments described and recommended may not be considered absolute and universal recommendations.

The authors, editors, and publisher have exerted every effort to ensure that drug selection and dosages set forth in this text are in accordance with the current recommendations and practice at the time of publication. However, in view of ongoing research, changes in government regulations, and the constant flow of information relating to drug therapy and drug reactions, the reader is urged to check the package insert for each drug for any change in indications and dosage and for added warnings and precautions. This is particularly important when the recommended agent is a new or infrequently employed drug.

Some drugs and medical devices presented in this publication have Food and Drug Administration (FDA) clearance for limited use in restricted research settings. It is the responsibility of the health care provider to ascertain the FDA status of each drug or device planned for use in his or her clinical practice.

To purchase additional copies of this book, call our customer service department at (800) 638-3030 or fax orders to (301) 223-2320. International customers should call (301) 223-2300. Visit Wolters Kluwer Health | Lippincott Williams & Wilkins online at www.lww.com. Visit the National League for Nursing online at www.nln.org.

This book is dedicated to our colleagues in health care education and practice who work to prepare health professionals to deliver quality, safe care to our clients, families, and the community.

It is also dedicated to the health professional students who desire to learn and practice the delivery of patient care to be the best practitioners they can be, and also to our students who expect educators to be innovative, creative, and explorers of emerging technologies and new teaching strategies to promote student engagement and experiential activity, with all facilitating optimal learning outcomes.

Finally, the book is dedicated to my husband, Joe, and our four children, Josie Elizabeth, Jayne Kristen, Jerrod Allen, and Jaclyn Anne, who make all things possible through their unending support.

About the Editor

Dr. Pamela R. Jeffries, PhD, RN, FAAN, ANEF, professor and associate dean for academic affairs at Johns Hopkins University School of Nursing, is nationally known for her research and work in developing simulations and online teaching and learning. At the Johns Hopkins University School of Nursing and throughout the academic community, she is well regarded for her expertise in experiential learning, innovative teaching strategies, new pedagogies, and the delivery of content using technology in nursing education. Dr. Jeffries has served as principal investigator on grants with national organizations such as the National League for Nursing (NLN), has provided research leadership and mentorship on national projects with the 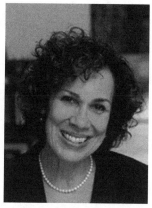 National Council State Board of Nursing, and has served as a consultant for health care organizations, corporations, and publishers, providing expertise in clinical education, simulations, and other emerging technologies.

Dr. Jeffries is a fellow of the American Academy of Nursing (FAAN), an American Nurse Educator Fellow (ANEF), and most recently, a Robert Wood Johnson Foundation Executive Nurse Fellow (ENF). She also serves as a member of the Institute of Medicine's Global, Intraprofessional Education (IPE) forum and has just been appointed as president-elect to the interprofessional, international Society for Simulation in Healthcare (SSH) by her health professional colleagues.

Dr. Jeffries has numerous publications, is sought to deliver presentations nationally and internationally, and has just edited two books: *Simulations in Nursing Education: From Conceptualization to Evaluation,* 2nd edition, and *Developing Simulation Centers Using the Consortium Model.* She has received federal and state grant funding to support her research focus in nursing education and the science of innovation and learning. Jeffries has been inducted into the prestigious Sigma Theta Tau Research Hall of Fame and is the recipient of several teaching and research awards from the Midwest Nursing Research Society and the International Nursing Association of Clinical Simulations and Learning (INACSL) and teaching awards from the NLN and Sigma Theta Tau International.

About the Contributors

Juriah Abdullah, MBBS, MEd. Juriah Abdullah is an Assistant Professor and Director of the Clinical Skills Unit at the Perdana University Graduate School of Medicine. She was previously the Head of the Clinical Sciences Division as well as the Head of the Skills Centre in IMU. She was intricately involved in the planning and delivery of the clinical skills curriculum as well as the planning and management of the Skills Centre. She developed the Simulated Patient Program and was instrumental in the recruitment and training of simulated patients in the early years of the program. In addition, she has long experience in organizing and planning clinical examinations in particular the Objective Structured Clinical Examinations (OSCE). Her research interest involves the use of simulated patients in skills training for students and she has conducted conference workshops on simulated patient training.

Katie A. Adamson, PhD, RN. Katie Adamson earned her PhD in nursing at Washington State University and is an assistant professor at the University of Washington–Tacoma. Her dissertation research, "Assessing the reliability of simulation evaluation instruments used in nursing education," provided a foundation for her continued research in the areas of simulation and evaluation instrument development. In her multidisciplinary teaching roles, Dr. Adamson emphasizes the importance of validity and reliability in evaluation.

Diane S. Aschenbrenner, MS, RN. Diane S. Aschenbrenner is an undergraduate faculty member and a course coordinator at the Johns Hopkins University School of Nursing. She is an award-winning educator, most recently the recipient of the Maryland Nursing Association Nursing Educator of the Year 2011 award and ranked number one on the 2012 online list by CNAthrive.com of "75 Nursing Professors You Would Be Lucky to Have Teach Your Classes." She has over 25 years of classroom and clinical teaching experience and creates modern, active learning experiences for students 20 to 60 years of age. She established and is now the faculty coordinator for the Simulation and Nursing Practice Labs. In this role she is responsible for integrating simulation into the school of nursing's undergraduate and graduate curriculum. Numerous national and international nursing educators have visited and consulted with her at the Johns Hopkins University Simulation and Nursing Practice Labs. Her areas of scholarly expertise and interest include clinical simulations; teaching strategies; pharmacology; medication administration techniques and preventing errors; medical-surgical nursing, adults; and teaching clinical skills. She has presented at 18 international and 35 domestic conference presentations related to simulation, teaching strategies, and skills acquisition. She has provided international consulting related to teaching nursing skills (Egypt, 2006), nursing documentation (China, 2008), and simulation (Switzerland, 2012).

Jim Battin, BS. Jim Battin is currently president of Strategic Consulting Group, Inc., located in Columbus, Indiana. For the past 15 years, Jim has consulted with over 50 clients in strategic planning and project management assignments. Most recently,

Jim partnered with Dr. Pam Jeffries, Johns Hopkins University School of Nursing, to form a regional Simulation Consortium of multiple academe and clinical partners in southeast Indiana. They worked together for four years in planning and implementing simulation development within the region. Based on their experience in that development, they coauthored *Developing Successful Health Care Educational Simulation Centers*, which was published in 2011.

Eric B. Bauman, PhD, RN. Dr. Eric B. Bauman received his PhD from the University of Wisconsin–Madison School of Education, Department of Curriculum and Instruction in 2007. He was one of the early Games+Learning+Society (GLS) students and was advised by Professors Betty Hayes and Kurt Squire, both renowned scholars in the game-based learning movement. Dr. Bauman is also a registered nurse, fire chief, and paramedic with more than 20 years of clinical, research, teaching, and command experience. He is the founder and managing member of Clinical Playground, LLC, a consulting group dedicated to integrating game-based learning and simulation throughout health care and public safety education. Dr. Bauman continues to work in higher education in a variety of roles and is dedicated to educational processes that focus on clinical expertise and patient safety.

Teri K. Boese, MSN, BSN, RN. Teri Boese is currently an associate professor, clinical at the University of Texas Health Science Center at San Antonio. She serves as the director of the Center for Simulation Innovation in the school of nursing. Teri is one of the cofounders of the International Nursing Association for Clinical Simulation and Learning and remains an active member of the board of directors.

Mary L. Cato, EdD, RN. Mary Cato is currently on the faculty of the School of Nursing at Oregon Health and Science University. Mary has been a nurse educator for over 15 years and has been using simulation in nursing education for almost 10 years. As a course developer for the NLN Simulation Innovation Resource Center (SIRC), Mary has been involved in the creation of three faculty development courses, which are offered online through the NLN. Mary has also been involved in the development of the NLN Advancing Care Excellence for Seniors (ACES) resources.

Jeanne Cleary, BSN, MAN, RN. Jeanne Cleary is the director of simulation at Ridgewater College in Willmar and Hutchinson, Minnesota. She began teaching and using simulation at Ridgewater in 2003 and became its director in 2006. She has 25 years of critical care nursing experience. Jeanne has been using simulation and unfolding cases in the classroom and simulation labs. She has been involved with several NLN initiatives and pilot studies. She was selected to be a HITS scholar and was involved in the NLN Advancing Care Excellence for Seniors (ACES) project as a simulation expert.

Helen B. Connors, PhD, RN, DrPS (HON), FAAN. Helen B. Connors currently is the University of Kansas School of Nursing's associate dean for integrated technologies and the executive director of the KU Center for Health Informatics. Dr. Connors strives to expand the use of advanced information technologies for education and practice, to establish policy for health information technology and telehealth, and to promote the image of nursing nationally and internationally. She has a strong history of grant funding and her work has been disseminated nationally and internationally through numerous publications and presentations.

Sharon I. Decker, PhD, RN, ANEF, FAAN. Sharon Decker is a professor and the Covenant Health System Endowed Chair in Simulation and Nursing Education in the Anita Thigpen Perry School of Nursing at the Texas Tech University Health Sciences Center (TTUHSC) in Lubbock. She is the director of the F. Marie Hall SimLife Center and the director of the Health Sciences Center's Quality Enhancement Program (QEP): Interprofessional Team. As a member of international, interprofessional simulation organizations, Dr. Decker has promoted the development of the science and pedagogy of simulation. Dr. Decker's scholarship focuses on the pedagogy of simulation. Her educational research, supported by multiple grants, is related to how simulation can be used to improve learning and promote professional competencies. She presents nationally and internationally on topics related to simulation and interprofessional teamwork and serves as a national and international consultant to assist nurse educators in the integration of simulation into curricula and competency assessments. Dr. Decker received her BSN from Baylor University, her MSN from the University of Texas at Arlington, and her PhD from Texas Woman's University. She is a fellow in the National League for Nursing's Academy of Nursing Education and a fellow in the American Academy of Nursing.

Thomas Dongilli, AT. With over 20 years in the health care simulation industry, Tom Dongilli is director of operations for the WISER Institute. WISER has maintained its presence as a proven leader in the health care simulation industry since 1994. To date, Tom has assisted many hundreds of programs with facility design and implementation and run thousands of simulation-based training sessions. Currently he is the director of operations for a 12,000-square foot simulation center and seven additional simulation centers. He has designed simulation centers in the United States and around the world in addition to authoring book chapters on simulation center design and management. Tom has authored many courses including Simulation Center Design as well as Operational Best Practices. Tom's area of clinical interest is in the field of in situ simulation and patient safety and he has created simulation-based programs for mock codes, clinical site assessments, and most recently authored a course called "The First 5 Minutes, What to Do Until the Code Team Arrives." He also contributes expert knowledge and experience in the practical design, implementation, operation, and monitoring of simulation-based facilities and medical learning systems. Tom has been appointed the 2014 International Meeting for Simulation in Healthcare meeting chair. He has been an active member of the Society for Simulation in Healthcare since its inception. He was the lead author on the creation of the Society for Simulation in Healthcare's Policy and Procedure manual.

Kristina Thomas Dreifuerst, PhD, RN, ACNS-BC, CNE. Kristina Thomas Dreifuerst is an assistant professor at Indiana University School of Nursing in Indianapolis, Indiana. Dr. Dreifuerst received her BA in nursing from Luther College, Decorah, Iowa, her MS in nursing from University of Wisconsin–Madison, and her PhD in nursing from Indiana University. Dr. Dreifuerst has taught undergraduate and graduate nurses for many years in Wisconsin and Michigan. She currently teaches graduate students in nursing education at Indiana University. She is a 2011 NLN-Jonas Scholar for Excellence in

Nursing Education Research, and her program of research focuses on the development of clinical reasoning in prelicensure nurses. Dr. Dreifuerst is the author of the "Debriefing for Meaningful Learning" method for clinical and simulation debriefing.

Jennifer Dwyer, MSN, RN-BC, CNRN, FNP-BC. Jennifer Dwyer is currently an education specialist at Indiana University (IU) Health in Indianapolis, Indiana. For over 35 years, Jennifer has served in the roles of preceptor, charge nurse, school of nursing faculty, clinical nurse specialist, and as a staff development educator at three institutions in Indiana. Jennifer was actively involved in the design and build of a 31,000-square foot, 21-room simulation center at IU Health. She serves as a liaison and simulation grant recipient for the center, which is a partnership between IU Health, Indiana University School of Medicine, and Indiana University School of Nursing. Her most recent accomplishment has been the curriculum integration of an electronic medical record with new hire didactic-facilitated education of nurses.

Scott Alan Engum, MD, FACS. Dr. Scott Engum is currently the director of the Simulation Center at Fairbanks Hall, Indianapolis, Indiana, which is a collaborative facility between Indiana University Health and the Indiana University's schools of medicine and nursing. Scott is a practicing pediatric surgeon at the James Whitcomb Riley Hospital for Children and has devoted the past 17 years to advancing skills of medical students, residents, and fellows and continues to be involved in national organizations that advance the use, training, and assessment of simulation.

Jennifer W. Geers, MHA. Jennifer Geers is currently the simulation coordinator for the Southeast Indiana Simulation Consortium. In this role, she has facilitated the growth and development of the 14-member consortium and supported its research, data tracking, and continuing education activities. She received her master's of health administration from Xavier University in Cincinnati, Ohio, and has managed projects and operations in both the inpatient and medical office environments.

Henry Henao, MSN, RN, ARNP, FNP-BC, CHSE. Henry Henao is clinical assistant professor of nursing and founding director of the Simulation Teaching and Research (STAR) Center at Florida International University (FIU), Miami, Florida. Mr. Henao served as FIU's principal investigator for the National Simulation Study of the National Council of State Boards of Nursing (NCSBN) and was among the first in the nation to become a certified health care simulation educator through the Society for Simulation in Healthcare. He served as a contributor and as a subject matter expert reviewing standards published by the International Nursing Association for Clinical Simulation and Learning (INACSL) and was selected to participate in the inaugural class of the NLN's Leadership Development Program for Simulation Educators. Mr. Henao is currently pursuing his PhD in nursing science at the Indiana University in Indianapolis.

Desiree Hensel, PhD, RN, PCNS-BC, CNE. Desiree Hensel is an assistant professor at Indiana University School of Nursing. Desiree is an award-winning teacher who has given national presentations and authored several publications related to the use of simulation in the field of maternal-child nursing. Desiree was an original participant in the NLN and HRSA Health Information Technology Scholar project and now uses her expertise in simulation to develop simulation scenarios and train faculty.

Sara L. Horton-Deutsch, PhD, CNS, RN. Sara L. Horton-Deutsch is currently a full professor at the Indiana University School of Nursing and coordinator of the graduate psychiatric mental health nurse practitioner program. The program is based on a reflection-centered framework that facilitates students through ongoing reflection on the quality of their interactions and learning through time. She coedited her first book on reflective practice in 2012. As a senior faculty member, she teaches nursing leadership, psychiatric mental health nursing, and interprofessional education courses in the areas of mental health and illness. A member of the original 2008 cohort in the Johnson & Johnson and NLN Faculty Leadership and Mentoring Program, she continues to partake in collaborative research on becoming a nurse faculty leader.

Suzan Kardong-Edgren, PhD, RN, ANEF, CHSE. Suzan (Suzie) Kardong-Edgren is currently a research associate professor and the Jody De Meyer Endowed Chair in Nursing at Boise State University, in Boise, Idaho. She is a recognized thought leader in simulation and simulation research. Suzie is the editor-in-chief of *Clinical Simulation in Nursing*, the flagship journal for the International Association of Clinical Simulation and Learning (INACSL), and is widely published in simulation. She is also an active member of the Society for Simulation in Healthcare, serving in numerous capacities for the organization.

Sarah Knapfel, RN, BSN, CCRN. Sarah Knapfel is currently the project coordinator for the iTEAM Grant Program in the College of Nursing at the University of Colorado–Denver. Sarah has several years of clinical intensive care experience, most specifically in the neurosurgical setting. She is currently working on her master's in science degree with a health care informatics focus.

Joseph O. Lopreiato, MD, MPH. Joseph O. Lopreiato is currently the Associate Dean for Simulation Education and Professor of Pediatrics at the Uniformed Services University of the Health Sciences in Bethesda, MD. He is also the medical director of the National Capital Area Medical Simulation Center, a 30,000-square foot facility that uses standardized patients, human patient simulators, task trainers and virtual reality simulations to train 165 medical students, 45 advanced practice nurses and several residency and fellowship programs in the Washington, DC area. His current interests include the use of simulation technologies to teach and assess a variety of learners from medical students to faculty. He recently completed a 31-year career in the United States Navy Medical Corps and is now a federal employee of the U.S. Department of Defense.

Mary Elizabeth Mancini, PhD, RN, NE-BC, FAHA, ANEF, FAAN. Dr. Beth Mancini is professor, associate dean, and chair for undergraduate nursing programs at the University of Texas at Arlington College of Nursing. She holds the Baylor Health Care System Professorship for Healthcare Research. Dr. Mancini received a BSN from Rhode Island College, a master's in nursing administration from the University of Rhode Island, and a PhD in public and urban affairs from the University of Texas at Arlington. In 1994, Dr. Mancini was inducted as a fellow in the American Academy of Nursing. In 2009, she was inducted as a fellow of the American Heart Association. In 2011, she was inducted as a fellow in the National League for Nursing's Academy of Nurse Educators. Dr. Mancini is active in the area of simulation in health care including serving as president of the Society for Simulation in Healthcare; member of the Royal College of Physicians and

Surgeons of Canada's Simulation Task Force, Sigma Theta Tau International's Simulation and Emerging Technologies Content Advisory Group, and the World Health Organization's Initiative on Training and Simulation and Patient Safety.

E. LaVerne Manos, DNP, RN-BC. E. LaVerne Manos is currently faculty and the director of the master of science in informatics program, director of nursing informatics, and director of the academic electronic health record at the University of Kansas School of Nursing and Center for Health Informatics. LaVerne also serves as principal investigator for an HRSA-funded project-collaborative agreement with focus on interprofessional collaborative practice and interprofessional education. LaVerne has a long history in clinical nursing, informatics practice, and organizational and global business strategic leadership.

Marjorie A. Miller, MA, RN. With over 25 years of experience in academic and clinical settings, Marjorie is lead faculty and curriculum specialist for the California Simulation Alliance (CSA) and coordinates the simulation program at Cabrillo College School of Nursing. She develops and facilitates both academic and clinical interprofessional simulations. Marjorie coauthored courses for the "Train the Trainer Model" of the CSA. She is the cocreator of the GRASP Model for clinical decision-making. Marjorie has been a podium and workshop presenter on clinical decision-making, simulation faculty development, and simulation scenario development and debriefing at international, national, and statewide conferences.

Gina Moore, PharmD, MBA. Gina Moore is director of clinical affairs and assistant professor at the University of Colorado's Skaggs School of Pharmacy and Pharmaceutical Science. In her role there, she is responsible for a variety of contracts and projects, including medication therapy management and drug utilization review for the State of Colorado. Her practice interests are in pharmacy informatics and medication safety. She earned her doctorate in pharmacy from the University of the Pacific and her master's in business administration from the University of Colorado.

Janice C. Palaganas, PhD, RN, NP, CEN. Janice Palaganas is currently the associate director for the Institute for Medical Simulation and principal faculty for the Center for Medical Simulation. Dr. Palaganas has a long history of emergency nursing and nurse practitioner experience, as well as 10 years of hospital and university management experience. She earned her doctorate studying health care simulation as a platform for interprofessional education and has been a simulationist and social scientist studying interprofessional education for the past seven years.

Mary D. Patterson, MD, MEd. Mary Patterson is medical director of simulation services for Akron Children's Hospital. In addition to overseeing simulation services at Akron Children's, Dr. Patterson is also an attending physician in the Emergency department and has a special interest in the use of simulation in evaluating systems, medical education, staff training and improving quality and safety in health care. She serves on the board of directors and is the past president of the Society for Simulation in Health Care.

Penny Ralston-Berg, MS. Penny Ralston-Berg has been designing online courses since 1997. She has also served as a technology trainer and design consultant for K-12, community college, higher education, and non-profit groups. Penny is currently a telecommuting instructional designer for the Penn State World Campus. Her primary research interests are games and simulations for education and how student perspectives of quality impact online course design.

Cynthia E. Reese, PhD, RN, CNE. Cynthia Reese is currently the associate dean of nursing at Lincoln Land Community College, Springfield, Illinois. Cynthia has 15 years of experience as a professor of nursing in baccalaureate and associate degree nursing programs. She has held her current administrative position for three years. Cynthia has expertise in clinical simulation, developing the "Student's Perception of Effective Teaching in Simulation" instrument during her doctoral studies. She has been a part of the NLN's Advancing Care Excellence for Seniors simulation workgroup since 2009, designing simulation-based unfolding case studies.

Deanna L. Reising, PhD, RN, ACNS-BC, ANEF. Deanna Reising is associate professor at Indiana University School of Nursing in Bloomington, Indiana, where she teaches research, critical care, and medical-surgical nursing. Dr. Reising is also the research clinical nurse specialist and Magnet Program codirector for Indiana University Health–Bloomington Hospital in Bloomington. She coleads the Falls Major Improvement team, which is aimed at infusing best practices and testing innovations to prevent falls. Dr. Reising leads research initiatives in both undergraduate nursing students at Indiana University and research fellows at Indiana University Health–Bloomington Hospital, resulting in numerous presentations and publications. She is also a magnet appraiser and a legal nurse consultant.

Mary Anne Rizzolo, EdD, RN, FAAN, ANEF. Dr. Rizzolo's career has focused on exploring new technologies, determining how they can educate and inform nurses, operationalizing cost-effective delivery, and disseminating their value for nursing education and practice. She pioneered the development of interactive videodisc programs, created one of the first websites in the world to offer continuing education, journal articles, and other educational and networking opportunities for nurses. She has delivered over 200 national and international presentations and served on many national committees and advisory boards. She is a fellow in the American Academy of Nursing and the Academy of Nursing Education. Dr. Rizzolo retired from the NLN in 2010 and now maintains an active consulting practice that includes managing several simulation projects.

April J. Roche, MBA, CPEHR. April J. Roche is the Assistant Director of the Clinical Learning Lab and Project Manager for the Academic Electronic Health Record (AEHR) implementation at University of Kansas School of Nursing. She provides guidance to faculty in developing simulations and developed the technical implementation that combines simulation with the AEHR. Ms. Roche works closely with faculty to identify and implement innovative uses of the AEHR in the classroom. She is also a Certified Professional in Electronic Health Records through Health IT Certification.

Joan Roche, PhD, RN, GCNS-BC. Joan Roche is an associate clinical professor at the University of Massachusetts–Amherst. She holds a joint appointment as a clinical nurse specialist at Baystate Medical Center. Dr. Roche is the senior partner in a 10-year clinical practice partnership focused on clinical research, professional development, and evidence-based practice in the clinical setting. Her program of research focuses on human patient simulation, health care systems, and patient safety. Her research is focused on the relationship between the health care system and patient outcomes and the use of human patient simulation in nursing education. She is a board-certified gerontologic clinical specialist, and her population of interest is the elder adult in all settings. She is currently working on a RWJ PIN (Partners in Nursing) project developing a curriculum on care transitions across all health care settings; a partnership between industrial engineers and nurses to use a computer model to improve patient placement in acute care; the implementation and evaluation of a delirium prevention program in acute care; empowerment within nursing organizations; and the relationship between relational coordination and adverse events within health care organizations.

Rhonda Savage, MPH. Rhonda Savage currently serves as the executive director of East Indiana AHEC (Area Health Education Center) in Batesville, Indiana. Dear to her heart are projects that improve health by engaging community and organizational leaders. Since completing her MPH degree from Tulane University, Ms. Savage has volunteered with the Peace Corps and held positions with Habitat for Humanity International and International Medical Corps. She also cofounded a nonprofit, Everyone's Child International.

Andrea Parsons Schram, DNP, CRNP, FNP-BC. Andrea Parsons Schram is an assistant professor of nursing at the Johns Hopkins University and actively practices as a family nurse practitioner. For the past decade, she has employed innovative teaching strategies, including simulation, to engage nurse practitioner students in active learning. Andrea is investigating the use of simulation in graduate nursing education to evaluate student nurse practitioner competencies.

Nicole Ann Shilkofski, MD, MEd. Dr. Shilkofski is currently the vice dean for education at Perdana University Graduate School of Medicine in Kuala Lumpur, Malaysia, as well as an assistant professor of pediatrics, anesthesiology, and critical care at Johns Hopkins University School of Medicine. Nicole was the associate director of the Simulation Center at Johns Hopkins from 2008 to 2011, where she ran the standardized patient program and many of the manikin-based simulation education programs for medical students, nursing students, and resident or fellow trainees. As a pediatric intensivist, Nicole's research interests have been in the use of simulation to teach pediatric resuscitation, particularly in resource-limited settings and developing countries. Her grant-funded initiatives include simulation programs in Myanmar, Malaysia, the Philippines, and Uganda to target reductions in neonatal and pediatric morbidity and mortality.

Diane J. Skiba, PhD, FAAN, FACMI. Dr. Diane J. Skiba is professor and coordinator of health care informatics at the University of Colorado College of Nursing. She is the project director for the Colorado Health Information Technology Education Collaborative, a $2.6 million university-based training grant funded by the Office of the National Coordinator of Health Information Technology to prepare health care professionals for highly specialized health information technology roles and the project director of the iTEAM (Interprofessional Technology Enhanced Advanced Practice Model) project focused on infusing technology throughout interprofessional education experiences on the Anschutz Medical Campus. A frequent speaker about informatics and use of emerging technologies to facilitate health care and education, she also writes a column on emerging technologies for NLN'S journal *Nursing Education Perspectives.*

K. T. Waxman, DNP, MBA, RN, CNL, CENP. Dr. K. T. Waxman is a nurse leader with nearly 30 years of experience in health care and corporate settings. She is a tenure-earning assistant professor at the University of San Francisco School of Nursing and Health Professions and chair of the Doctor of Nursing Practice (DNP) Department. She teaches in both the executive leader and traditional DNP program. Dr. Waxman is also the director of the California Simulation Alliance (CSA) at the California Institute for Nursing and Health Care (CINHC). An internationally known speaker and author, Dr. Waxman is also a past president of the Association of California Nurse Leaders (ACNL) and recently elected to treasurer of the American Organization of Nurse Executives (AONE). She is currently serving as cochair of the International Meeting on Simulation in Healthcare for the Society for Simulation in Healthcare (SSH).

Janet Willhaus, PhD, RN. Janet Willhaus is a recent PhD graduate of Washington State University–Spokane and a new assistant professor at Boise State University, Boise, Idaho. In 2011, Janet was selected as the first NLN simulation scholar in residence and spent a year working on NLN simulation initiatives with nursing faculty across the nation. Janet has been a scholar of simulation pedagogy since 2003. Her current research focuses on the impact of psychological and physiologic stress on performance during simulation.

Foreword

Of all the changes in nursing education over the past decade, the most significant and widespread has been the use of simulation. Clinical simulations allow learners to experience a situation and think through possible decisions and actions, developing their higher-level cognitive skills and clinical judgment. Students can analyze complex scenarios, assess clinical situations, make decisions about priorities and interventions, implement those interventions, and evaluate outcomes. In clinical simulations, they can learn to use technologies, develop their skills, and practice to maintain them. Simulation also allows students to experience the challenges of providing care in a stressful clinical environment with multiple distractions and interruptions.

Practice with other health profession students and providers in simulated settings is critical for understanding one another's roles, learning to work together and communicate as a team, and ultimately improving quality of care and patient safety. With simulation-based education, students can identify potential errors and experience situations that lead to poor quality and unsafe care. Teachers need to know how to develop these types of simulations for nursing students, for interprofessional education, and for nurses and other providers in the practice setting.

These outcomes, however, can be achieved only if educators understand the pedagogy of using simulations in teaching and key considerations in designing and implementing them. There are too many educators assigned to teach in simulation laboratories and centers who are not prepared for their role and have limited, if any, knowledge of the research findings and other evidence that should guide developing and using clinical simulations. One of the many strengths of this book is that it provides the essential concepts for using simulation in nursing and other health professions to achieve and evaluate the outcomes identified earlier. The chapters are based on the available evidence and are written by leading experts in each of the areas addressed in them. This book is what we need in nursing and other health professions for simulations to be of high quality and achieve their desired outcomes.

I remember teaching students in the skills laboratory with "Mrs. Chase," a manikin for learning and practicing basic nursing skills. One only needs to look through the chapters in this book to gain a sense of how far we have progressed in this area—to three-dimensional virtual worlds where students can socialize and use their avatars to interact with patients and collaborate with other clinicians. Not all educators will be involved in developing these types of simulations, but all need to understand the trends and possibilities for their use in nursing.

Regardless of the type of simulation, the teacher should be prepared for developing simulations and implementing them in his or her own nursing programs. Simulations are not separate from the curriculum. They should be integrated carefully in courses based on the intended learning outcomes and competencies to be developed. They should not be an "add on" to the course without any rationale for doing so, and they should not be used in place of clinical practice without evidence of their effectiveness or at least a discussion among the faculty about their equivalency. There are best practices associated with simulation, and teachers need to understand these practices and their research base and to use them in their own teaching and interactions with students.

Simulations are effective not only for instruction in nursing but also for assessment *if* teachers are prepared for their role as evaluators, the outcomes or competencies to be assessed with simulation are identified, the simulations are developed to evaluate those designated outcomes, and the tools and process are valid and reliable. Teachers need to decide in advance if the assessment is for formative evaluation only (feedback to the learner) or for summative evaluation (grading and high-stakes evaluation such as verifying whether students have met the end-of-program outcomes). If used for summative evaluation, the teacher must ensure that the process for rating performance and the evaluation tool produce valid and reliable results. Chapters in this book, such as the ones on evaluation tools and developing a research focus, guide teachers in making these types of decisions.

This book is intended for nurse educators and others who envision expanded uses of clinical simulation in their programs and health care settings but are unsure of the next steps. With this reference, teachers across all settings can move beyond the basics of simulation design and implementation to learn new concepts, trends, and future possibilities. This is a must-read book for educators who teach or want to teach with simulation or those who manage simulation centers.

Marilyn H. Oermann, PhD, RN, ANEF, FAAN
*Director of Program Evaluation and
Educational Research*
Duke University School of Nursing
Durham, North Carolina

Preface

Nurse educators are facing great challenges today with health care transformation, changes in higher education, and faculty and clinical site shortages, all impacting the future of clinical education. These challenges bring new demands on education to prepare nursing graduates for the 21st-century health care practice. Health care environments have become more complex and high-tech, have higher patient acuity, and place more demands on health care professionals to treat patients quickly without facilitating long hospital stays and recovery times. Different revenue models, financial constraints, the explosion of advanced technologies, and the emphasis on interprofessional education and practice are additional challenges facing nursing education. Confronting many of these challenges, nurse educators are exploring new opportunities for innovative teaching and learning methods, new clinical models, and educational practices to provide high-quality education to promote optimal, quality patient care.

Clinical Simulations in Nursing Education: Advanced Concepts, Trends, and Opportunities contains 20 chapters that cover topics of interest for the current intermediate and advanced simulation educators and users. Expert simulation researchers, educators, and users were selected as chapter authors to provide the latest information in their content area. The content in these chapters is practical, of value to your practice and education in simulations, and timely because many of the topics are just surfacing as health care professionals embrace the simulation pedagogy.

With today's health care reform and changing health care needs, new skill competencies are needed by our nursing graduates to care for all types of patients in diverse health care settings. Nurse educators are responsible for preparing nursing graduates for the transition to practice, whether it is in acute care, primary care, or within the community, so ultimately the new practitioners can provide safe, quality, competent care. Clinical simulations can provide health care educators one approach to create student-centered, experiential environments that engage and prepare the learner for real-world practice. National reports, such as the *Future of Nursing: Leading Change, Advancing Health* (2011) and other landmark reports, have focused on nursing education and practice, highlighting critical roles of nurse educators, practitioners, and the delivery of nursing care in complex health care environments. Critical messages from these national reports require health care educators to consider different, innovative teaching strategies and experiences to better prepare our graduates. Once the exception, now incorporation of clinical simulations in a nursing curriculum is commonplace. This book provides content on how to take the simulation pedagogy to the next level; content is directed toward other concepts, such as taking simulations globally, serious gaming, and others to name a few. We are at a new phase of incorporating simulations into the health care curriculum; therefore, new concepts demand attention and evaluation.

To use clinical simulations, faculty members are required to learn the new pedagogy in order to obtain optimal outcomes expected from using this methodology. This edition of *Clinical Simulations in Nursing Education: Advanced Concepts, Trends, and Opportunities* has been developed to better prepare nurse educators and superusers for their role in developing, implementing, and conducting the research when using clinical simulations in education and practice. When incorporating simulations into health care education, educators need to consider the following:

- Utilizing the science of learning correlated to the simulation pedagogy
- Identifying best practices that are emerging in the field of clinical simulations
- Promoting a student-centered approach used in simulations versus a teacher-centered approach seen in traditional clinical models
- Providing a safe, nonthreatening environment for health care professionals to practice their scope of practice and to work in teams, all toward learning their roles and responsibilities better
- Having an orientation and being developed to use the simulation pedagogy to facilitate an efficient and effective manner to optimize learning outcomes
- Facilitating clinical simulations that faculty are prepared for, with the focus on their clinical expertise and practice
- Promoting the concept of collaborative practice, partnerships, and consortiums to work more efficiently, share resources, and to learn from one another
- Providing a faculty development program for educators integrating simulations into the teaching-learning environment
- Developing a comprehensive evaluation plan or process to measure learning outcomes and competencies required of the health care professional learner
- Developing a plan of research to study the clinical simulation pedagogy to identify best practices and to contribute to the science of nursing education

This book has been written to take the educators and superusers to the next level and to learn more about simulation concepts that have been discussed sparsely in the literature. Readers will learn about using simulations to enhance interprofessional education and practice, how to conduct meaningful debriefing, how to consider taking clinical simulations global, and how to understand the information needed to develop a good business plan and consider the economic model of a simulation center. More research and evaluation of clinical simulations are needed and in chapters 11 and 12, the reader will learn more about these approaches and strategies, as well as the instruments to consider when conducting research. New on the forefront is certification of the educator in simulation, the possibility of high-stakes simulation, and how simulation leaders can get their simulation center accredited. The goal of this book is to provide the simulation educators more in-depth information and best practices in existing concepts in addition to new information on simulation topics that are emerging.

Education in health care is in revolution—new approaches, considerations, and a movement toward interprofessional education and practice are just a few directions moving to a new clinical redesign to prepare our health care professionals in a better, more meaningful manner. Let's embrace the change and challenges ahead of us; the time is now to explore new possibilities and opportunities in health care education. The content in this book will help educators move forward to the next level of educating the health care professionals, creating, implementing, integrating, and evaluating this amazing experiential pedagogy that has begun a new model of education to prepare better, more competent quality health care professionals.

ACKNOWLEDGMENTS

Without the support, expertise, and contributions from my health professional colleagues and simulations experts, this book would not have been possible. Many thanks go to the National League for Nursing for their unwavering support of this new book written for the intermediate to advanced simulations users and experienced simulation educators. Without your resources and guidance, the book would have been only a dream.

A big thank you to the Lippincott team who provided support, had confidence in the authoring team, and published the book, all integral to make this endeavor become reality! Also thanks to Marie Brown for all her hard work and expertise in organizing and editing the book chapters from the outset.

Also thanks to my family and colleagues for their continued love, support, patience, and encouragement throughout this undertaking. A special thanks to Eileen Tagliareni, chief program officer of the National League for Nursing, for her continued encouragement, positive attitude, and support for faculty development in clinical simulations and the use of this pedagogy. Finally, I wish to thank the many students and faculty who used, explored, and immersed themselves in simulations to bring the content to life in this book.

Pamela R. Jeffries, PhD, RN, FAAN, ANEF
Professor
Associate Dean for Academic Affairs
RWJF Executive Nurse Fellow (ENF)
Johns Hopkins University School of Nursing
Baltimore, Maryland

Contents

List of Figures and Tables

History and Evolution of Simulations:
From Oranges to Avatars

Mary Anne Rizzolo, EdD, RN, FAAN, ANEF

■ Learning Objectives

1. Trace the evolution of the use of simulation in schools of nursing from the early 1900s.
2. Describe early computer-based simulations, patient case study interactive video-disc programs, and web-based applications for nursing education.
3. Discuss how the emergence of technology-rich learning resource centers laid the groundwork for the simulation centers of today.
4. Explain factors that led to the extraordinary growth in use of simulation, particularly manikin-based simulations, in the past decade.
5. Speculate about the future of simulation and simulators in nursing education.

■ Key Terms

- Avatar
- Haptic device
- Manikin
- Partial trainer

EARLY MANIKINS AND COMPUTERS: MRS. CHASE, SimOne, AND PLATO

I remember the first time I went into the skills lab as a nursing student. I was so excited to see all of the equipment and so eager to learn how to manipulate such wondrous tools as sphygmomanometers and syringes. I can't remember how many times I injected an orange. I wanted to feel comfortable with my skills so my patients would not be

1

concerned over having a 17-year-old take care of them. Even making beds "like a nurse" was something I approached with enthusiasm, especially making a bed with a person in it! And there was Mrs. Chase, a simple **manikin** created over 100 years ago, to help. I am sure many of you have memories of Mrs. Chase. She inspired poems and tributes that can be viewed in several articles that praise her contribution to nursing education (Grypma, 2012; Herrmann, 1981, 2008; Jamme, 1923; Price, 1939; Schlosser, 1947).

My experiences in the skills lab were in the 1960s, and we certainly have come a long way since then. But the first computerized manikin was actually built during that same time period. SimOne (Denson & Abrahamson, 1969), the first full-body computerized manikin designed for anesthesia training, could breathe, blink his eyes, and respond to the administration of gases. Amazing! But it was an idea before its time, and a SimTwo was never built (Cooper & Taqueti, 2004). However, another simulator, although not computer driven, did survive and moved us along to the manikins of today. Resusci Anne®, developed by Laerdal in 1960, led us into the current era. But more about her later.

A milestone in the use of computers for learning also occurred in the 1960s. The PLATO (Programmed Logic for Automatic Teaching Operations) system, which ran on a mainframe computer, was created in 1960 at the University of Illinois. Maryann Bitzer began using it to teach nursing and pharmacology, incorporating slides of patients into the lessons and using a self-directed inquiry teaching strategy. Her evaluative research was published in prestigious journals, including *Nursing Research* (Bitzer, 1966; Bitzer & Bitzer, 1973; Bitzer & Boudreaux, 1969). But mainframes were too expensive for most schools, and it was not until personal computers became available and affordable that screen-based simulations began to have an impact on nursing education.

EVOLUTION OF LEARNING RESOURCE CENTERS

In the mid-1970s, there was a philosophical shift in higher education, which recognized that students can learn on their own when they have clear learning objectives and with the help of emerging instructional technologies. At the same time, technology such as cameras, audio cassettes, and videotapes were dropping in price and could be operated by anyone. This shift in thinking and technology economics paved the way for the development of robust, media-rich learning resource centers.

Among the first nurse educators who saw the potential for these new teaching and learning environments in schools of nursing were Charlene Clark and Dr. Kathleen Mikan. Both of these pioneers were influenced by the work of Dr. Samuel Postlethwait from Purdue University (personal communications: K. Mikan, April 5, 2013, and C. Clark, April 17, 2013). In 1961, Dr. Postlethwait began using an audio tutorial system that allowed students to learn at their own pace in his biology labs (Postlethwait, Novak, & Murray, 1969). Kathleen Mikan, a faculty member and doctoral student at Michigan State University, established an "Independent Study Laboratory" where nursing students used audiotapes, slides, and film loops in study carrels. Dr. Mikan's dissertation, "Development of a Classification Scheme of Pupil Questions Asked by Nursing Students within a Self-Instructional Learning Environment" (1972), examined the effectiveness of some of her instructional units. In 1973, Dr. Mikan was hired as the first director of the recently constructed Learning Resource Center (LRC) at the University of Alabama, Birmingham

(UAB). This state-of-the-art facility was the vision of Dr. Marie O'Koren, dean of the UAB School of Nursing, and was one of the first LRCs located in a school of nursing building.

Meanwhile, Charlene Clark started developing independent study modules for her students at the Intercollegiate Center for Nursing Education (ICNE). Students viewed instructional media and other activities, practiced skills with an RN preceptor who was available for assistance, and were held accountable to be prepared to practice the skills in the clinical setting. Demonstrations in the skills lab by faculty, with return demonstrations by students, were eliminated. In 1974, impressed by Charlene's work and the response of students to her approach, the dean at ICNE asked Charlene to take leadership in developing a learning lab that would be different from the traditional skills lab. She began by using existing media, but finding them inadequate, she assembled a team to produce their own videotapes. A new building at ICNE opened in 1980, complete with a state-of-the-art television studio, so Charlene and her group could produce, and sell, higher quality videos.

Charlene Clark, Kathleen Mikan, and Joanne Crow from the University of Texas, San Antonio, all attended the Health Education Media Association conference in 1976 and began to discuss the need for a conference focusing on LRCs in schools of nursing. Dr. Mikan held the First National Learning Resource Center conference, titled "A New Challenge for Nursing Education," in December 1978 at the UAB with over 100 attendees. A monograph, "Learning Resources Center Conference: Proceedings and Evaluation" (Mikan, 1980), based on data from the conference participants, offers a picture of a variety of models for LRCs that were emerging in schools of nursing.

Shortly thereafter, other creative early adopters began moving forward with the establishment of LRCs. Schools in the forefront, many of which received federal funding, included the University of Wisconsin, Milwaukee, and the University of Maryland. Dr. Betty Skaggs at the University of Texas, Austin, Dr. Diane Billings, at Indiana University, and Dr. Kay Hodson at Ball State presented at a variety of national conferences for nurse educators across the country, talking about the new learning experiences they were designing for students in their centers. All of these innovators also worked collaboratively to offer nine more LRC conferences hosted by state-of-the-art LRCs in the United States and Canada. The 10th and final conference was held in June 2004 at the ICNE. By then, the International Nursing Association for Clinical Simulation and Learning (INACSL) had been established and began offering their own educational events. The history page on the INACSL website (INACSL, 2013) traces the origin of the organization back to the early LRC conferences.

Dr. Susan Sparks also played a role in advancing the growth of LRCs and the use of media. She earned her PhD in instructional technology and was hired as a technology specialist at the National Audiovisual Center in Atlanta. Dr. Sparks was the keynote speaker at the first LRC conference in 1978. She continued to champion the use of quality media at national and international nursing conferences, raised awareness about the National Library of Medicine's AVLINE database, which was designed to aid in the selection, use, and sharing of quality audiovisual material in the education of health care professionals (Sparks & Kudrick, 1979), and managed the Educational Technology Network, ET Net; (Sparks, 1994), an early discussion board on various media, hardware, and software.

In many schools, the skills laboratory was integrated into the LRC, so when students were learning how to perform skills, they could move from viewing media in study carrels into a clinical lab space for hands-on practice. In the 1980s, more simulator

---

BOX 1.1 AN HONORABLE MENTION

On health science campuses, the simulation centers often service many health care disciplines, and simulation-based interprofessional education is finally getting off the ground. It is fitting to mention one person who was internationally recognized for her leadership in the evolution of simulation centers, Deborah L. Spunt, DNP, RN, FAAN, who was responsible for the design, administration and management of the 28 clinical simulation laboratories at the University of Maryland School of Nursing. She co-founded the International Nursing Association for Clinical Simulation and Learning, serving as its first president, and worked tirelessly to encourage the integration of simulation into the curricula of nursing programs. Dr. Spunt passed away in 2007, but her contributions to simulation are recognized each year at the NLN Summit via a lectureship established in her honor and funded by the Laerdal Foundation.

---

models with increasingly realistic properties were produced. I remember how excited I was to see the first manikin that weighed as much as a real person from Medical Plastics Laboratory, a company that was eventually bought by Laerdal Medical. Pelvic models for practicing catheterization and ostomy care, breast and testicular examination models with interchangeable nodules, and more were purchased and well used by students. The LRCs grew into robust environments for self-directed learning and laid the groundwork for the journey toward the sophisticated simulation centers of today (Box 1.1).

FROM PERSONAL COMPUTERS TO INTERACTIVE MULTIMEDIA

In the early 1980s, when personal computers began to arrive on the scene, they were extremely limited in computing power and memory. Despite those limitations, a few creative people developed some wonderful simulations and games. "Eliminating Medication Errors," developed in 1987 and requiring only 512 K of memory (Bolwell, 1993), was one example. Opening the program took you to a hospital unit, represented by little squares framing the screen. Each square signified a patient's room, and the challenge to the student was to dispense medications to all the patients in those rooms within 60 minutes. In each room, there was a "problem." A patient might be in the shower, for example. Multiple choice questions tested the learner's knowledge about how to handle that situation. As the little medicine cart clicked around the screen, the dilemmas increased in complexity. If you made a medication error, you had to fill out an incident report. Meanwhile, the clock in the corner of the screen ticked the minutes away. Then came a "ring, ring, ring." There was a phone call and the student needed to go to the desk and answer it. How can you ever get your meds passed out with all these interruptions!

But those early personal computers had limitations in terms of what they could display on the screen, so some of the educational technology pioneers connected videotape players to the computer to provide a more engaging and visually interesting program. Early screen-based patient case study programs ran on an Apple 2 computer connected to a Sony Betamax videotape player (Rizzolo, 1984), but they were shortly replaced by interactive videodisc systems that portrayed screen-based patient care situations and challenged learners to make appropriate nursing care decisions (Rizzolo, 1994). The 1990s was a decade when technology was advancing rapidly, and soon the capacity of computers and CD-ROMs increased, enabling program development on platforms that were less complicated to set up and run. Space in rapidly expanding LRCs made room for computers to replace older media in study carrels. A survey by Childs (2002) documents the equipment that was present in LRCs when we crossed into the new millennium, along with those that were most and least used.

Federal grants, many from the Division of Nursing, Department of Health and Human Services (Rizzolo, 1994), supported the early development of innovative multimedia. More and more sessions on computer-based learning and multimedia appeared on conference schedules. The National League for Nursing (NLN) created the Council on Nursing Informatics, and the American Nurses Association created the Council on Computer Applications in Nursing. Conferences devoted to only technology-mediated teaching and learning emerged. Publishers began developing products and exhibited them at conferences. The fifth edition of Bolwell's *Directory of Educational Software for Nursing* (1993), which was a formidable 719 pages in length, described a mix of tutorials and patient case study simulations. And the LRCs in schools of nursing became more media-rich environments with each passing decade as filmstrips and slides were replaced with computers and multimedia.

MANIKINS AND TASK TRAINERS

The origin of SimOne was an early technological marvel, but it was Resusci Anne that led us into the modern era of full-body manikins. Created in 1960 by Asmund Laerdal (Tjomsland, 2005), it was soon recognized as a well-built and practical tool for learners to develop skills in the newly developed practice of cardiopulmonary resuscitation. By 1982, David Hon (1982) had embedded sensors into Resusci Anne and hooked her up to a videodisc player. Learners received immediate feedback from the expert on the video monitor as they practiced. The system was further developed and sold by Actronics Inc. and was approved by the American Heart Association and the American Red Cross.

The 1990s heralded serious work in the development of computerized manikins. Louis Oberndorf founded Medical Education Technologies (METI), Inc. and built a high-fidelity Human Patient Simulator™ (HPS) with cardiovascular, respiratory, neurological and pharmacological modeling. It was adopted mainly for training in anesthesia management; the high cost of the HPS was prohibitive for most other purposes. In 2000, SimMan® was introduced to the market by Laerdal Medical. The affordability of this product and the VitalSim® product line opened up the new world of teaching with simulation. More companies began producing manikins at prices that were affordable for nursing schools. Gaumard developed the NOELLE® birthing simulator and METI (acquired by CAE Healthcare in 2011) produced new models that were significantly less expensive than their HPS. And each new product released had improved functionality and realism. In 2000, only 3 percent of nursing schools had purchased manikins (personal communication, R. Fuqua, Laerdal Medical, April 17, 2010), but by 2010, that number had grown to 87 percent (Hayden, 2010). Affordable pricing coupled with pedagogical frameworks and research on simulation in nursing education (Jeffries & Rizzolo, 2006) created the tipping point for this phenomenal growth in 10 short years.

Partial trainers and **haptic devices** evolved along a similar path. Harvey®, the cardiology patient simulator, was developed in the 1960s (Gordon, 1974). Although it was mainly used to teach medical students, sales to schools of nursing have increased in recent years, particularly in those schools with advanced practitioner programs. The first intravenous arm was a collaboration between the State University of New York, Plattsburgh School of Nursing, and HT Medical (formerly High Techsplanations) (Hodson-Carlton, 1996). The initial price was about $35,000, a hefty expense in 1995. But like manikins, partial trainers also decreased in price, and an increase in sales shortly followed.

THEN ALONG CAME THE WEB

Concomitant to the development of the manikins we use today was the rise of the Internet and the World Wide Web. Again, creative individuals seized the new medium for developing simulations. The "Interactive Patient" (Hayes & Lehmann, 1996), developed at Marshall University, was a multimedia encounter with a patient. Users typed in questions to take a history, and a click of the mouse on various body parts generated sounds and images. Fast forward to 2003 and the birth of "Second Life," the online virtual world with millions of folks milling about as **avatars**, where you will find many environments and experiences designed for nursing students. We have only scratched the surface of possibilities for educating students in immersive environments and through the growing number of serious games (Bauman, 2013; Beard, Wilson, Morra, & Keelan, 2009; Skiba, 2007, 2009).

THE FUTURE OF SIMULATION

What will simulation look like in the future? Holograms? Holodecks? Programmable humanoids? It is anyone's guess. New technologies seem to burst on the scene daily. Most are not really new, but rather a new way of conceptualizing what we already have, using it in new ways. And technologies are merging. Our communication devices keep us "connected," and computers are mobile and wearable. What applications can you envision emerging from Google Glass (http://www.google.com/glass/start/) or Google Now (http://www.google.com/landing/now/) that could have an impact on nursing education?

The history of simulation is dotted with remarkable inventions that were ideas ahead of their time. It is also marked with genuine creativity that motivated others and led to the development of truly useful products that survived and thrived in the marketplace. Of course, simulation is not defined by technological inventions. It is a pedagogy that encompasses many modalities. Certainly standardized or simulated patients can provide some of the most meaningful learning experiences for learners. New simulation methods and modalities will succeed if they are engaging, feel "real," provide learning experiences that have not been possible before, and most of all, if the learning they provide has significant potential for a positive impact on the care of our patients.

■ Key Concepts

- Some early simulation products were ideas before their time.
- The 1980s and 1990s saw rapid advances in computer technology and creative screen-based simulations on personal computers, interactive videodisc systems, and web-based programs, many supported by federal grants.
- The emergence of media-rich learning resource centers laid the groundwork for the sophisticated simulation centers of today.
- Affordable manikins and emerging simulation pedagogy and research spurred phenomenal growth of the use of simulation in schools of nursing in the past decade.
- Simulation modalities of the future will be successful if they are engaging, feel "real," provide learning experiences that have not been possible before, and if the learning they provide has significant potential for a positive impact on the care of our patients.

References

Bauman E. B. (Ed.). (2013). *Game-based teaching and simulation in nursing and healthcare.* New York: Springer.

Beard, L., Wilson, K., Morra, D., & Keelan, J. (2009). A survey of health-related activities on second life. *Journal of Medical Internet Research, 11*(2), e17.

Bitzer, M. (1966). Clinical nursing instruction via the PLATO simulated laboratory. *Nursing Research, 15*(2), 144–150.

Bitzer, M. D., & Bitzer, D. L. (1973). Teaching nursing by computer: An evaluative study. *Computers in Biology and Medicine, 3*(3), 187–204.

Bitzer, M. D., & Boudreaux, M. C. (1969). Using a computer to teach nursing. *Nursing Forum, 8*(3), 234–254.

Bolwell, C. (1993). *Directory of educational software for nursing* (5th ed.). New York: National League for Nursing.

Childs, J. C. (2002). Clinical resource centers in nursing programs. *Nurse Educator, 27*(5), 232–235.

Cooper, J. B., & Taqueti, V. R. (2004). A brief history of the development of mannequin simulators for clinical education and training. *Quality and Safety in Health Care, 13*(Suppl 1), i11–i18.

Denson, J. S., & Abrahamson, S. (1969). A computer-controlled patient simulator. *Journal of the American Medical Association, 208*(3), 504–508.

Gordon, M. S. (1974). Cardiology patient simulator: Development of an automated manikin to teach cardiovascular disease. *American Journal of Cardiology, 34,* 350–355.

Grypma, S. (2012). In retrospect: Regarding Mrs. Chase. *Journal of Christian Nursing, 29*(3), 181.

Hayden, J. (2010). Use of simulation in nursing education: National survey results. *Journal of Nursing Regulation, 1*(3), 52–57.

Hayes, K. A., & Lehmann, C. U. (1996). The interactive patient: A multimedia interactive educational tool on the World Wide Web. *M.D. Computing: Computers in Medical Practice, 13*(4), 330–334.

Herrmann, E. K. (1981). Mrs. Chase: A noble and enduring figure. *American Journal of Nursing, 81*(10), 1836.

Herrmann, E. K. (2008). Remembering Mrs. Chase. *Imprint, 55*(2), 52–55.

Hodson Carlton, K. E. (1996). Implications for nursing education: A virtual Mrs. Chase and cyberspace. *CIN: Computers, Informatics, Nursing, 14*(3), 148–149.

Hon, D. (1982). Interactive training in cardiopulmonary resuscitation. *Byte, 7*(6), 108.

International Nursing Association for Clinical Simulation and Learning (INACSL).

History of INACSL. Retrieved from https://inacsl.org/about/history

Jamme, A. C. (1923). Nursing education in China. *American Journal of Nursing, 23*(8), 666–675.

Jeffries, P. R. & Rizzolo, M. A. (2007) Designing and implementing models for the innovative use of simulation to teach nursing care of ill adults and children: a national, multi-site, multi-method study. Retrieved from http://www.nln.org/research/LaerdalReport.pdf.

Mikan, K. J. (1972). *Development of a classification scheme of pupil questions asked by nursing students within a self-instructional learning environment.* (Unpublished doctoral dissertation). Michigan State University, East Lansing.

Mikan, K. J. (1980). Learning Resources Center Conference: Proceedings and Evaluation [monograph], ED222180.

Postlethwait, S. N., Novak, J. D., & Murray, H. T. (1969). *The audio-tutorial approach to learning, through independent study and integrated experiences.* Minneapolis: Burgess.

Price, A. L. (1939). The autobiography of Sally Chase. *American Journal of Nursing, 39*(1), 25–27.

Rizzolo, M. A. (1984). Development of a CATI program for basic nursing students. *Proceedings of the 8th Annual Symposium on Computer Applications in Medical Care.* Washington, DC: IEEE Computer Press, 941–944.

Rizzolo, M. A. (Ed.) (1994). *Interactive video: Expanding horizons in nursing.* New York: American Journal of Nursing Company.

Skiba, D. J. (2007). Nursing education 2.0: Second life. *Nursing Education Perspectives, 28*(3), 156–157.

Skiba, D. J. (2009). Nursing education 2.0: A second look at second life. *Nursing Education Perspectives, 30*(2), 129–131.

Sparks, S. M., & Kudrick, L. W. (1979). An audiovisual information retrieval system: Avline. *Journal of Nursing Education, 18*(7), 47–55.

Sparks, S. M. (1994). The Educational Technology Network (E.T.NET). *Nursing and Health Care, 3,* 134–141.

Schlosser, F. E. (1947). Rebirth of a school of nursing: The rehabilitation of a nursing school and hospital in central China. *American Journal of Nursing, 47*(8), 532–534.

Tjomsland, N. (2005). *Saving more lives— together.* Stavanger, Norway: Laerdal Medical.

Faculty Development to Implement Simulations:
Strategies and Possibilities

K. T. Waxman, DNP, MBA, RN, CNL, CENP
Marjorie A. Miller, MA, RN

■ Learning Objectives

1. Identify the essential components and teaching methodologies to include in an effective curriculum to develop faculty for roles as simulation program educators.
2. Identify and apply key educational theories that support simulation faculty development.
3. Describe elements of successful faculty development programs.

■ Key Terms

- Adult learning theory
- Constructivism
- Educational frameworks
- Educational theory
- Experiential learning
- Faculty development
- Learning strategy

Faculty development is critical to a successful and sustainable simulation program. Although health care professionals often focus on the technology of simulation, we need to change that paradigm of thinking and focus on the methodology of simulation. This chapter will discuss the importance of faculty development and ongoing education, as well as curriculum development and the educational theory that supports it. Finally, this chapter will describe successful models and simulation alliances that promote and foster collaboration, learning, and partnerships.

BACKGROUND

Picture this scenario: Your hospital or school purchases simulation equipment and tells you that you are now in charge of developing a program with no additional budget. Or, you are the administrator of a facility that houses a simulation center with expensive equipment, and you have no remaining budget to train staff to use it! This is a common theme with simulation. Equipment is purchased, the budget has been blown, and faculties are not adequately trained. Improper training can lead to not only student frustration but also to staff pushback. When institutions venture into the world of simulation, a solid faculty development plan should be developed that includes the background, numbers, levels, and anticipated roles of the learners; the depth, breadth, and frequency of the training; and logistical considerations such as space, equipment, and budget. Fundamental to this faculty development plan is a comprehensive curriculum for those staff who will be facilitating the learning process through the use of simulation. Because this chapter focuses on the faculty development piece of the equation, it will discuss the rationale for standardized faculty development, review supporting **educational frameworks** with application to simulation faculty development, examine the critical elements in curriculum development, and highlight examples of successful programs.

RATIONALE FOR FACULTY DEVELOPMENT

With the rapid pace of change in health care professional education internationally, various types of simulation have emerged, evolved, and infiltrated health professional education (Waxman, Nichols, O'Leary-Kelley, & Miller, 2011). This is not only evident at the undergraduate level but it is also an important component of ongoing professional development. The dynamic nature of health care provision requires the health care professional to participate in ongoing training and assessment to continually refine and update their clinical practices (Gaba, 2004).

With the emergence of simulation as an educational strategy and the opportunity to purchase high-technology equipment and manikins at affordable grant-funded rates, there has been a rapid proliferation of equipment at educational sites, yet minimal attention has been paid to faculty development. Faculty development ensures that simulation users—nurse educators, faculty, instructors, or anyone else who uses simulation in the workplace—acquire the training and knowledge to develop, implement, and evaluate simulation scenarios (Jeffries & Battin, 2012). Traditionally, the skills lab faculty have assumed responsibility for simulation and the technical equipment. In some instances, clinical faculty were tasked with the extra duty of conducting simulation. Vendors quickly added simulation design to their technical training in an attempt to meet their consumers' needs. However, the technical aspects of simulation have been the focus rather than the educational methodology. Simulation should be about the methodology, not the technology (Gaba, 2004)!

Often faculty are reluctant to learn the technological piece because they are intimidated or merely have no interest. Additionally, technical training typically does not cover the educational strategy for the organization or department. Critical elements are missing: the foundational principles of learning in simulation, crucial elements of curriculum design, scenario development focusing on learning outcomes, strategies for facilitating a simulation scenario, roles of individuals in the simulation, approaches for successful debriefing, and evaluation processes. Therefore, faculty development curricula must be expanded beyond technology for faculty to be fully engaged in simulation.

EDUCATIONAL FRAMEWORKS

Health care education has traditionally relied on a structure that includes cognitive learning theory, behavioristic skill training, and the apprenticeship model, whereby practitioners attend didactic presentations, practice skills in linear fashion on static manikins, and then immediately train on real patients in a highly acute clinical setting. Although the clinical environment with actual patients is proven and appreciated, the current clinical opportunities afforded to the learner are highly complex and risky to the patient, the patient's family, and the learner. Moreover, in today's health care education environment, faculty who are new to teaching or simulation face a situation similar to that of novice students. Strong clinicians may be catapulted into their new roles without sufficient preparation or continuing mentorship, leading to the feeling of being overwhelmed as well as rapid burnout. Even with nurses who are already established in their role, there is a need for training the trainer.

The use of simulation as a **learning strategy** in education is based on current cognitive science and constructivist and adult learning theories, with a strong experiential and contextual slant. The strategy takes into consideration individual learning styles for processing information and engages learners through visual, kinesthetic, auditory, and other preferred modes of taking in and processing new information. Current literature describes the educational frameworks that support simulation as a learning strategy for health care professionals (Anderson, 2006; Lisko & O'Dell, 2010; Rutherford-Hemming, 2012; Waxman & Telles, 2009; Zigmont, Kappus, & Sudikoff, 2011), but few highlight the development of simulation faculty. The following sections briefly describe elemental theories and link crucial elements that are applicable to simulation faculty development.

Benner's (1984) phenomenological theory of skill acquisition is a fundamental theory that drives nursing education in the academic or clinical setting. It is evident that when taking on a teaching role, expert clinicians transition from the novice to expert milestones just as basic nursing students do. Clearly, the same process is required when expert educators and clinicians transition to simulation faculty.

Constructivism

The foundational learning theory that supports simulation as an effective tool for health care educators is **constructivism**, which views learning as a "process of constructing meaning; it is how people make sense of their experience" (Merriam, Caffarella, & Baumgartner, 2007, p. 291). Constructivism incorporates several learning theories, includes both behavioristic and cognitive ideals, and is the foundation of both experiential and **adult learning theory**. An elemental framework of constructivism holds that the learner generates knowledge, skill, and value from direct experiences. This movement shifted the focus in teaching from the teacher to the learner. In applying this theory, the teacher employs learner-centered strategies that modify the teacher's role to that of facilitator and moderator of learning rather than the dispenser of information (Huang, 2002).

For learning outcomes to be achieved in simulation, it is essential for the educational methodology to be learner focused rather than teacher or trainer focused. Nursing faculty often hear "we need to take advantage of that teaching moment" expressed by expert teachers who are new to simulation. Expert faculty are tempted to stop a simulation and step in with the "right answer" or to redirect the learners, taking advantage of what is called the "teaching moment." It is essential for faculty to reframe the concept of teaching moments into a more applicable concept of "learning moments." The role of the simulation faculty is not to tell, or be the fountain of all knowledge, but to create a scaffold of carefully crafted experiences that facilitate the learner to construct a new meaning or a new mental model. A pivotal concept in education—where learning resides within the learner and is enhanced by the educator—is at the core of constructivism theory and critical in the development of faculty for their roles in simulation.

Adult Learning Theory

Adult learning theory, with its roots in constructivism, differentiates the way adults learn (Knowles, 1970). An operational understanding of adult learning theory and the best practices that facilitate that learning is crucial for the simulation faculty (Zigmont et al., 2011). Best practices take into consideration the unique characteristics of adults as they engage in the learning process. Adults are characteristically self-motivated and self-regulated, and their readiness to learn is triggered by a *need to know* how to best perform in one's own life and work situation. Each adult comes to the learning encounter with prior knowledge and experience, as well as an ego that expects that knowledge and experience are recognized and valued.

Adults correspondingly present with a frame of reference or mental model that informs and directs their performance. Learning occurs when the adult experiences a situation that triggers the relevant portions of that frame of reference or mental model, provoking the exploration and construction of an updated and more expanded mental model. An understanding of adults' formation of mental models is crucial, as mental models are at the core of clinical decision making (Zigmont et al., 2011). Additionally, adults connect their previous mental models to new information, targets, or preferred mental models by using analogical reasoning, which allows the learner to form conclusions from prior events and can be used to respond to a newer event. When a conclusion is accurate, the learner forms a new mental model to guide practice in related situations. The purpose of simulation in health care education is to create new mental models based on current best practices. As such, it drives the health care team to promote and attain patient safety outcomes (Zigmont et al., 2011). In the development of faculty to become expert simulation faculty, a new mental model about teaching and learning must be created.

The design of faculty development courses, workshops, and apprenticeships must take into consideration the mental makeup of the participants and provide the opportunity for them to relate their prior knowledge, skills, attitudes, and experiences to simulation and the faculty role. Following the interactive initial discussion, the trainers can assess the learners' *need to know* and flex the basic framework of the course to meet those needs.

Experiential Learning

Experiential learning theory is rooted in constructivism and is also evident in adult learning theory. This theory holds that learning occurs when an individual engages in an experience, then processes and reflects upon that experience, constructing new meaning based on the individual's prior knowledge and experience. Dewey (1938), the originator of experiential learning theory, indicated that learning from experience is not limited to the experience itself, but requires continuity and interaction with the environment.

Kolb (1984), a principal theorist following Dewey in the development of experiential learning theory, believed that learning is a multidimensional process involving the way individuals take in and process new information. Learning occurs when an individual has a concrete experience in a relevant context, is able to reflect on that experience and formulate new ideas or new mental models as a result, and is then able to act on that new model in a similar context.

Rogers and Freiberg (1994) viewed experiential learning as equivalent to personal change and growth. They believed that learning was enhanced when the teacher created a positive climate for learning, clarified the purpose of the experience, made learning resources available, balanced both the intellectual and emotional components of the experience, and shared thoughts and feelings with the learners without taking over the responsibility for the learning. This notion is pivotal in the creation of a specialized learning program for the development of simulation faculty and requires that trainers model effective behaviors by *walking the walk* and not merely *talking the talk* (Curran, 2008).

For Rogers and Freiberg, the components of effective learning are directly related to the need for simulation faculty to create a positive learning environment and to scaffold the experience to optimize learning. Effective scaffolding for learning requires faculty to create an organized scenario focused on relevant learning outcomes and prepare a realistic environment to promote contextual learning and transfer. Another application of Rogers and Freiberg's theory is seen when performance expectations are balanced to include not only knowledge and skills but also the attitudes and human factors that arise in simulation. The originators of faculty development programs must design a curriculum and the learning environment to model these standards when interacting with their learners as they expand to encompass this new role. In addition, resources such as debriefing scripts (Cheng et al., 2011) or scenarios with clearly identified debriefing points (CSA Simulation template, 2011) support novice simulation faculty in what they perceive to be the most challenging part of their new role.

Two additional experiential learning theories, reflective practice and situated cognition or contextual learning, apply directly to faculty development in simulation. Schon (1983), followed by the more recent theorists Boud and Walker (1991), discussed the concepts of *reflection-in-action* and *reflection-on-action*. The necessary ability of the learner to reflect, analyze, and correct decision making while in a situation, or *thinking on one's feet,* is referred to as reflection-in-action. However, the learning is not complete until the learner has the opportunity to reflect after the experience to formulate new models of thinking (reflection-on-action). Lave and Wenger (1991) further supported the practice of structured reflection and contextualized learning, indicating that learning is enhanced when knowledge, skills, and attitudes to be learned are presented and practiced in real life. It is crucial for simulation faculty to guide participants in reflective practice following immersion in simulation and debriefing. Effective modeling of this strategy allows novice faculty to recognize instances in which they demonstrated reflection-in-action during their immersive experience. Consistent faculty feedback supports novice faculty to see where they facilitated reflection-on-action in debriefing sessions and is a significant element in learning from the experience.

Benner (1984), described experiential learning in nursing as "clinical learning that is accomplished by being open to having one's expectations refined, challenged, or disconfirmed by the unfolding (events)." Experiential learning is apparent in every situation in which preconceptions are challenged, clinical inquiry is demonstrated, and self-reflection is required (Benner, 1984). Benner's phenomenological theory explains how nurses, in the "transition from novice to expert, move from a rule-driven, concrete thinking approach in solving problems to an approach that applies abstract principles and evidence-based practice at the bedside" (Benner, 1984). Faculty development programs for simulation faculty must have an immersive, experiential component in which self-reflection is required and preconceptions can be challenged in a safe environment. In the context of simulation faculty development, *clinical inquiry* can be interpreted as the practice of exploring preconceptions about the teacher's role in learning and exploring strategies to modify the existing beliefs to one embracing the facilitator's role in the simulation environment. Table 2.1 presents a synthesis of key theories with application to simulation faculty development.

CURRICULUM DEVELOPMENT

Successful Models

There are a number of models for faculty development in simulation, whether internal to an organization or external such as through an alliance, collaborative, or consortium. One example of a structured faculty development plan based on Benner's novice-to-expert framework is the Bay Area Simulation Collaborative (BASC) faculty development plan.[1] The BASC is a group of more than 100 member schools and hospitals, totaling more than 600 faculty and hospital educators from both service and academia in the 10 counties of the San Francisco Bay Area. The California Institute for Nursing and Healthcare (CINHC) was funded to create the BASC through a grant from the Gordon and Betty Moore Foundation from 2006 to 2009. The three-year BASC project was designed to train and teach nursing faculty and hospital educators in the concepts of simulation. The BASC was also designed to develop clinical simulation scenarios for use among its members.

---

[1]http://www.bayareanrc.org/BayAreaSimulationCollaborative.aspx

TABLE 2.1

Synthesis of Key Theories, Frames, and Application to Development of Simulation Faculty

Theory and Theorists	Frames	Application to Development of Simulation Faculty
Constructivism: Piaget, Vygotsky, Bruner, Kolb	• Learning: process of constructing meaning and *making sense* of experience • Learning: process through which learner generates knowledge, skill, and value from direct experiences • Learner: builds on current and prior information to create ideas and make decisions	• Assess preexisting frames of faculty role in simulation • Check in with participants at strategic intervals as they *make sense* of the experience • Design content and activities that facilitate reconstruction and sharing of revised mental models (frames)
Adult Learning: Knowles	Andragogy: adult learner: • is self-motivated/directed • is motivated by "need to know" • holds prior mental models (frames) • expects to have a role in own learning	Design courses/workshops/ apprenticeships that: • Respect participants' prior knowledge, skills, attitudes, and experience • Focus on participants' *need to know* • Immerse participant in experience consistent with anticipated performance environment • Engage participant by role modeling, role practice, feedback, and coaching
Experiential: Dewey, Kolb, Rogers, Zigmont	Learning... • Experience requires continuity and interaction with the environment (Dewey) • Requires the learner to be open to new experience and possess reflective, analytical, and problem-solving skills (Kolb) • Is equal to personal change and growth (Rogers) • Involves creation of new mental models (Zigmont)	• Craft authentic situations that allow for challenge, inquiry, and self-reflection • Ensure safe immersive environment fostering participants' openness to challenge • Clarify purpose of immersive activities and provide necessary resources • Balance cognitive and affective components • Explore relevant current mental models and expand to simulation environment

(continued)

TABLE 2.1

Synthesis of Key Theories, Frames, and Application to Development of Simulation Faculty (*Continued*)

Theory and Theorists	Frames	Application to Development of Simulation Faculty
Reflective Practice: Schon, Boud, Walker	• Reflection in action: *"thinking on one's feet"* or self-correction during experience • Reflection on action: reflecting after experience with formation of new models	• Support participants through coaching during simulation, facilitating reflection-in-action • Debrief participants following simulation experience, fostering reflection-in-action
Situated Cognition: (Contextual Learning) Lave and Wenger	• Learning enhanced when knowledge, skills, and attitudes are presented in the context of *real life* • Structured reflection is key to making sense and learning from experience	• Immerse participants in all facets of an authentic simulation exercise
Novice to Expert: Benner	• Clinical learners progress through milestones from novice to expert • Clinician moves from rule-based approach and concrete thinking to application of abstract principles and evidence-based practice • Expert clinicians and faculty progress through the same milestones, progressing through novice to expert levels	• Support participants in reality that progression through novice to expert stages when taking on new role as simulation faculty is expected • Highlight clinician and faculty characteristics that transfer to simulation facilitator role • Provide tools and strategies designed to facilitate learning at each level in novice to expert continuum

The BASC designed the faculty development plan with the goal to train a large number of expert clinicians and nursing faculty in the San Francisco Bay Area, built on the novice-to-expert model, as shown in Figure 2.1.

In this plan, the faculty member in level 1 training (basic technical skills) is in the novice stage, level 2 (simulation methodology) is the advanced beginner stage, level 3 (apprenticeship) is the competent stage, and level 4 (train the trainer) is the proficient and expert stage. Ultimately, a train-the-trainer model allowed the BASC to have its own qualified instructors to teach others (Waxman & Telles, 2009). More than 600 health care educators were trained through the program over a three-year period. Because simulation was

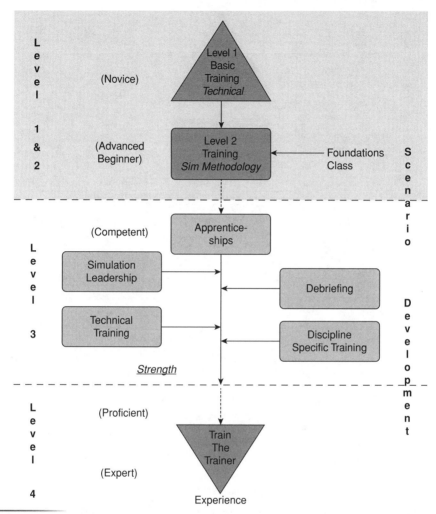

FIGURE 2.1 BASC Faculty Development Plan 2006–2009. (Reprinted with permission from the CSA.)

a new methodology for teaching, the design was to train a critical mass of faculty using standardized curriculum at the same level. The philosophy of the BASC was that all faculty and health care educators are novices when it comes to simulation, even if they have had decades of experience as a clinical faculty member.

The California Simulation Alliance

Leveraging the BASC funding and success, the California Simulation Alliance (CSA),[2] led by the CINHC, was developed in 2008 as a virtual alliance to benefit all simulation users

---

[2]www.californiasimulationalliance.org

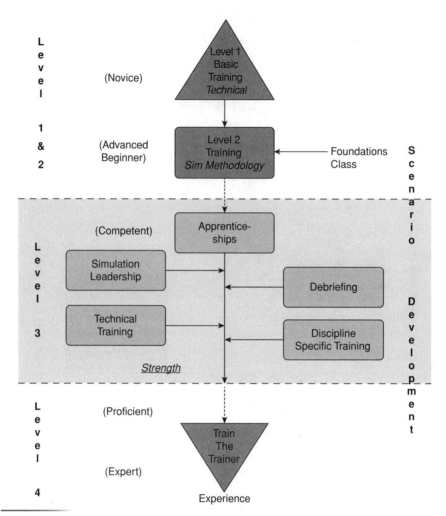

FIGURE 2.2 CSA Faculty Development Plan 2010–2012. (Reprinted with permission from the CSA.)

in California. The CSA Steering Committee adopted use of the BASC faculty development program to be implemented throughout the state. The first few years focused on moving faculty from the novice level (in simulation) to advanced beginner (Figure 2.1). Subsequently, the CSA continued implementing the model on a statewide basis and focused on building competency, as seen in Figure 2.2.

As Benner philosophized, competency comes with experience, which was the background for leveling the courses in the curriculum. This design encouraged learners to practice in their work environment before moving into the next level toward achieving competency. The statewide goals for 2013 to 2015 are to build expertise and create experts in each regional collaborative across the state, highlighted in level 4 of Figure 2.3.

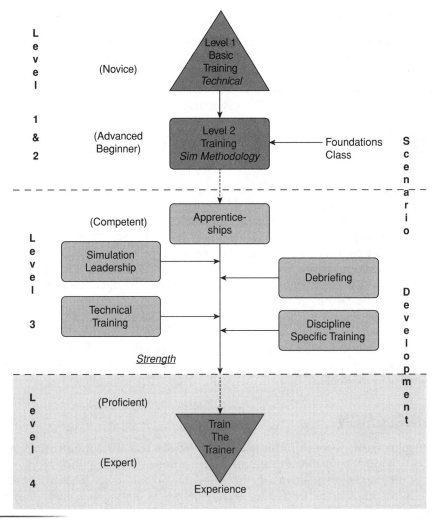

FIGURE 2.3 CSA Faculty Development Plan 2013–2015. (Reprinted with permission from the CSA.)

Since launching the CSA in 2008, initial grant-funded investments have been leveraged to build on and expand the resources available, with significant progress made in setting up and providing key programs as a foundation for simulation users in academic and service settings across California. More than 2,000 faculty, clinical educators, and providers have been trained through attending one or more of the novice-to-expert faculty development classes provided by the CSA. The CSA has identified and trained 16 individuals as CSA faculty, providing an average of 12 classes each year conducted in various locations across the state. Specialized simulation centers were identified around the state and prepared as apprentice sites to provide individualized coaching and mentoring of emerging simulation faculty, with 16 apprentice graduates having completed the program at the time of writing.

The Oregon Simulation Alliance

In 2002, the Oregon Simulation Alliance (OSA) began as an initiative from the State of Oregon's governor's office to improve health care delivery and increase the number of health care providers with the use of medical simulation technology statewide. The OSA worked under the umbrella of the Northwest Health Foundation until the OSA received its 501(c)(3) designation as a nonprofit organization in July 2010.

FACULTY DEVELOPMENT PROGRAM CHALLENGES

One obvious challenge in implementing a faculty development program is when learners feel that after they have completed just one or two courses, they are experts. As the literature reflects, competency is only achieved after two to three years (Benner, 1984; Dreyfus & Dreyfus, 1980). Competency as a simulation faculty member takes time and practice. A structured faculty development plan and institutional support are important to moving learners from novice to competent to proficient. Although expertise comes with experience, practice, and courses, courses alone do not teach learners to become experts. Because simulation is a fairly new industry, there are relatively few experts in the field worldwide.

Another challenge is funding faculty development. Budgeting and funding for this important line item are often overlooked. A solid plan to provide faculty release time from their current duties to participate in educational programs is crucial to the success of a simulation program. Articulating your needs to the financial leaders is something that cannot be overlooked.

CONCLUSION

Developing faculty—which includes all users, faculty, technicians, instructors, and anyone who uses simulation in their job (Jeffries & Battin, 2012)—is critical to the success of any simulation program, whether it is at the organizational, regional, or state level. Budgeting funding for faculty development is as important as budgeting for equipment.

■ Key Concepts

- The use of simulation as a learning strategy is based on current cognitive science and constructivist and adult learning theory, with a strong experiential and contextual slant.
- While developing curriculum for faculty development, it is important to focus on the methodology of simulation rather than the technology. Critical elements such as foundational principles in simulation, scenario development, debriefing, and evaluation need to be incorporated for a successful program.
- Educational theory supports the importance of ongoing education for faculty new to simulation.
- Rather than reinvent the wheel when developing a faculty development program, look to successful models to learn from their experience.

References

Anderson, J. (2006). Educational perspectives: Experiential learning: From theory to practice. *American Academy of Pediatrics, 7*(6), e287.

Bay Area Simulation Collaborative (BASC). Retrieved from www.bayareanrc.org/rsc on August 8, 2013.

Benner, P. (1984). *From novice to expert: Excellence and power in clinical nursing practice.* Menlo Park, CA: Addison-Wesley.

Boud, D., & Walker, D. (1991). *Experience and learning: Reflection at work.* Geelong, Australia: Deakin University Press.

Cheng, A., Hunt, E. A., Donoghue, A., Nelson, K., Leflore, J., Anderson, J., . . . EXPRESS Pediatric Simulation Research Investigators. (2011). EXPRESS—Examining pediatric resuscitation education using simulation and scripting: The birth of an international pediatric simulation research collaborative—from concept to reality. *Simulation in Healthcare, 6*(1), 34–41.

CSA Simulation template (2011). Retrieved from www.californiasimulationalliance.org on August 8, 2013.

Curran, I. (2008). Creating effective learning environments—Key educational concepts applied to simulation training. In R. Kyle & W. Bosseau Murray (Eds.), *Clinical simulation: Operations, engineering and management* (pp. 153–161). New York: Elsevier.

Dewey, J. (1938). *Experience and education.* New York: Macmillan.

Dreyfus, H., & Dreyfus, S. (1980). A five-stage model of the mental activities involved in directed skill acquisition. Unpublished study, University of California, Berkeley.

Gaba, D. (2004). The future vision of simulation in health care. *Quality and Safety in Health Care, 13*(Suppl 1), 2–10.

Huang, H. M. (2002). Toward constructivism for adult learners in online learning environments. *British Journal of Educational Technology, 33*, 27–37.

Jeffries, P., & Battin, J. (2012). *Developing successful healthcare education simulation centers: The consortium model.* New York: Springer.

Knowles, M. (1970). *Modern practice of adult education: From pedagogy to andragogy.* New York: Association Press.

Kolb, D. (1984). *Experiential learning.* Englewood Cliffs, NJ: Prentice-Hall.

Lave, J., & Wenger, E. (1991). *Situated learning: Legitimate peripheral participation.* Cambridge: Cambridge University Press.

Lisko, S., & O'Dell, V. (2010). Integration of theory and practice: experiential learning theory and nursing education. *Nursing Education Perspectives, 31*(2), 106–108.

Merriam, S. B., Caffarella, R. S., & Baumgartner, L. M. (2007). *Learning in adulthood: A comprehensive guide* (3rd ed.). San Francisco: Jossey-Bass.

Rogers, C., & Freiberg, H. J. (1994). *Freedom to Learn* (3rd ed.). New York: Pearson.

Rutherford-Hemming, T. (2012). Simulation methodology in nursing education and adult learning theory. *Adult Learning, 23*(3), 129–137.

Schon, D. A. (1983). *The reflective practitioner: How professionals think in action.* New York: Basic Books.

Waxman, K., Nichols, A., O'Leary-Kelley, C., & Miller, M. (2011). The evolution of a statewide network: The Bay Area Simulation Collaborative. *Simulation in Healthcare, 6*(6), 345–351.

Waxman, K., & Telles, C. (2009). The use of Benner's framework in high-fidelity simulation faculty development: The Bay Area Simulation Collaborative model. *Clinical Simulation in Nursing, 5*, e231–e235.

Zigmont, J. J., Kappus, L. J., & Sudikoff, S. N. (2011). Theoretical foundations of learning through simulation. *Seminars in Perinatology, 35*, 47–51.

3

Clinical Simulations Focused on Patient Safety

Deanna L. Reising, PhD, RN, ACNS-BC, ANEF
Desiree Hensel, PhD, RN, PCNS-BC, CNE

■ Learning Objectives

1. List safety competencies necessary for nursing practice.
2. Explain the professional and financial drivers to improve patient safety.
3. Identify the characteristics of a culture of safety.
4. Discuss ways simulation can be designed to teach safety competencies.
5. Describe the advantages of using simulation to improve teamwork and communication.
6. Explain how simulation can be used to teach about system vulnerability and safety threats.
7. Examine ways to use standardized patients and high-fidelity simulators in safety-focused simulations.

■ Key Terms

- Active failures or sharp-end failures
- Culture of safety, safety culture, and patient safety culture
- CUS words
- Failure modes and effect analysis
- In situ simulation
- Just culture
- Latent errors or blunt-end failures
- QSEN
- Serious reportable errors
- Stressors
- TeamSTEPPS®
- Value-based purchasing

CLINICAL SIMULATIONS FOCUSED ON PATIENT SAFETY

▍ *"Primum non nocere"* ("First, do no harm")

As nurses, we are familiar with this quote, which is grounded in the ethical principle of nonmaleficence. At first glance, "First, do no harm" implies a minimum requirement, which may be interpreted as passive in nature. With recent, and quite public, reports of patient safety issues, it has become clear that ensuring patient safety is far more than a passive act. Patient safety is the responsibility of each individual provider and the system, requiring *active* behaviors working in synergy to "do no harm." The American Nurses Association "Code of Ethics for Nurses with Interpretive Statements" emphasizes nursing's role in patient safety, including the nurse's responsibility to ensure patient safety in five of its nine provisions (ANA, 2001).

PROFESSIONAL ORGANIZATION DRIVERS TO IMPROVE PATIENT SAFETY

In November 1999, the Institute of Medicine (IOM) published the report "To Err Is Human." The report added to an already growing literature base on failure to rescue, which emerged in the early 1990s. Errors were categorized as diagnostic, treatment, preventative, and other (communication, equipment, and other) (IOM, 2000). The report shifts the emphasis from individual errors to systems that create an environment favorable to increased patient errors. The report does not exonerate individual providers from

---

BOX 3.1 QSEN ENTRY-LEVEL NURSE SAFETY COMPETENCIES IN THE "SKILLS" CATEGORY

1. Demonstrate effective use of technology and standardized practices that support safety and quality.
2. Demonstrate effective use of strategies to reduce the risk of harm to self or others.
3. Use appropriate strategies to reduce reliance on memory (such as forcing functions, checklists).
4. Communicate observations or concerns related to hazards and errors to patients, families, and the health care team.
5. Use organizational error reporting systems for near-miss and error reporting.
6. Participate appropriately in analyzing errors and designing system improvements.
7. Engage in root-cause analysis rather than blaming when errors or near-misses occur.
8. Use national patient safety resources for own professional development and to focus attention on safety in care settings.

SOURCE: Cronenwett et al., 2007, p. 128.

their individual responsibilities; rather, it emphasizes the impact of the lack of proactive checks and balances to prevent patient harm. The call to action from the IOM report highlighted the approaches needed to improve patient safety.

In 2007, work from the Quality and Safety Education in Nursing (**QSEN**) collaborative was published. The national initiative, funded by the Robert Wood Johnson Foundation, produced six QSEN competencies in knowledge, skills, and attitudes domains. Strategies for achieving QSEN competencies were developed that span the classroom, skills or simulation lab, and clinical environments (Cronenwett et al., 2007). Box 3.1 provides the key entry-level nurse safety competencies in the "skills" category.

In 2012, the American Association of Colleges of Nursing (AACN) developed QSEN competencies for graduate-level nurses as well. The skills domain competencies for graduate nurses are detailed in Box 3.2. Faculty resources and toolkits are available on the QSEN website (AACN, 2013).

In addition to the IOM and AACN, several national safety campaigns have been introduced in an effort to eliminate patient safety errors. One of the more prominent organizations leading the way in such campaigns is the National Patient Safety Foundation (NPSF, 2013). Some of the NPSF campaigns have included: "Ask Me 3," "Patient Safety

BOX 3.2 AACN QSEN SKILLS DOMAIN COMPETENCIES FOR GRADUATE NURSES

1. Use existing resources to design and implement improvements in practice (e.g., National Patient Safety Goals).
2. Use evidence and research-based strategies to promote a "just culture."
3. Integrate strategies and safety practices to reduce risk of harm to patients, self, and others (e.g., risk evaluation and mitigation strategy [REM]).
4. Demonstrate leadership skills in creating a culture in which safe design principles are developed and implemented.
5. Engage in systems focus when errors or near misses occur.
6. Promote systems that reduce reliance on memory.
7. Create high reliability organizations based on human factors research.
8. Report errors and support members of the health care team to be forthcoming about errors and near misses.
9. Anticipate/prevent systems failures/hazards.
10. Use evidenced-based best practices to create policies to respond to errors and "good catches."
11. Design and implement microsystem changes in response to identified hazards and errors.
12. Encourage a positive practice environment of high trust and high respect.
13. Develop a culture where a hostile work environment is not tolerated.
14. Use best practices and legal requirements to report and prevent harm.
15. Use national patient safety resources to design and implement improvements in practice.

SOURCE: AACN, 2012, pp. 7–8.

Awareness Week," and "Stand Up for Patient Safety." Other organizations launching patient safety campaigns include the Institute for Safe Medication Practices, the Agency for Healthcare Research and Quality (AHRQ), the National Quality Foundation (NQF), and the Joint Commission.

FINANCIAL DRIVERS TO IMPROVE PATIENT SAFETY

Although nurses know that any patient care error will most likely result in an increased cost related to increased length of the hospital stay, the need for more monitoring and additional patient treatments, and rehabilitation of patient disabilities, the most significant financial driver in our era is the 2010 Affordable Care Act and reimbursement schemas introduced by the Centers for Medicare and Medicaid Services (CMS). Since 2008, CMS has identified hospital-acquired conditions for which it would no longer reimburse health care facilities. Examples of such conditions include blood incompatibility, certain pressure ulcers, falls, and catheter-associated urinary tract infections (CMS, 2013b). **Value-based purchasing** is a "pay for performance" approach whereby CMS withholds a certain percentage of its upfront payments to acute care facilities and titrates the percentage of reimbursement of the withholding based on hospital performance benchmarked against other hospitals (CMS, 2013a). The measures include patient quality and safety indicators such as timely antibiotic administration for surgery and discharge instructions for heart failure patients, as well as patient experience survey scores (CMS, 2013c).

Safety information that affects every level of nurse provider can also be found on websites that display publicly reported data. One primary site is Hospital Compare, which is collated by CMS. Such websites allow the consumer to compare safety, quality, and patient experience data across multiple facilities. Although the data often lag behind, it is still powerful, allowing patients to drive the provider of choice. The ability of the patient to choose a provider based on comparative data has implications for nurses at every level of nurse and every level of provider.

THE ROLE OF SIMULATION

Simulation provides an *active* method in preparing individual nurses for the typical learning environment, where nurses are focused on skill management only. When nurses must learn proper procedures for implementing safe care in an isolated and controlled setting, simulation provides the ability to transition nurses to an environment that mimics a real clinical environment, with any number of distractions that could contribute to a patient error. Additionally, simulation provides the opportunity for nurses to practice skill sets repeatedly until they develop a routine and process for safe patient care. Another advantage to simulation is that it permits co-education and training of multiple professions, allowing each nurse to see the roles of other nurses and the complexity involved in ensuring safe patient care.

CULTURES OF SAFETY

Culture of safety, safety culture, and patient safety culture are all terms used to describe highly reliable organizations that strive to minimize errors in high-risk workplaces. These risks can be to patients, workers, or the environment. It is generally believed that the term *safety culture* became popular after investigators found the 1986 Chernobyl nuclear plant disaster was not solely caused by engineering design or equipment failure; rather, a lack of an organizational safety culture was found to be a major contributor to the accident. "To Err Is Human" was one of the earliest reports to call on health care organizations to create a culture of safety (IOM, 2000). Although the primary emphasis was patient safety, the report also suggested that systematic efforts to improve patient safety would also improve worker safety. A system's adoption of no-lift policies exemplifies such a worker–patient safety approach to reduce injuries to both parties.

Using Simulation to Build a Patient Safety Culture

Meta-analysis has identified seven subcultures of patient safety culture: (1) leadership, (2) just, (3) teamwork, (4) evidence-based, (5) communication, (6) learning, and (7) patient-centered (Sammer, Lykens, Singh, Mains, & Lackan, 2010). Simulation has potential value for assessing and improving aspects of each of these organizational subcultures.

Leadership

Safety cultures begin with leadership. Leaders are needed to acknowledge the high-risk nature of an organization's work and to align organizational resources with a vision to promote safety. Leaders also have the ability to devote resources to simulation training. Yet leadership is not exclusive to the executive level. Leadership with an emphasis on safety attitudes must permeate through all levels of an organization. Simulations can be designed to help improve leadership qualities. In scenarios used to teach emergency response, a common simulation debriefing question that is used is "Who was the leader?" Participants can then reflect on how a leader or lack thereof affected team functioning and patient outcomes.

Just Culture

Just culture is a term used to describe a balanced-scale approach to error prevention that includes both personal accountability and system effectiveness (Reason, 2000). Within a just culture, disclosure and nonpunitive error and near-miss reporting are the norms. Simulation can include situations that can lead to errors, such as delivering a wrong medication with a similar name (such as cefotaxime instead of cefoxitin). Another medication error scenario could involve a drug that is incompatible with the current intravenous (IV) solution. Consider a scenario in which a child has an IV of D5W ½ NS with no other orders and needs amphotericin B. A medication error would occur if the amphotericin was infused with the incompatible solution. In either of these scenarios, the debriefing could lead the participants through a root–cause analysis to what caused or could have prevented the error. The debriefing also offers the opportunity to discuss the concept of near misses and the importance of reporting these events just as they would report an actual error.

Teamwork and Communication

Teamwork and communication are unique but highly linked factors in patient safety. Teamwork involves open and respectful collaboration among all those who help in care delivery. Communication implies that all care providers have a voice in patient safety. Communications that are open and transparent promote patient safety. Simulation provides a vector for teamwork and communication. Just by including an incomplete handoff in almost any scenario, participants can begin to understand how missing information can compromise patient safety. Tools to measure teamwork, including the **TeamSTEPPS®** (Team Strategies and Tools to Enhance Performance and Patient Safety) Teamwork Perception Questionnaire and the TeamSTEPPS Teamwork Attitudes Questionnaire, can be used in conjunction with simulation and are freely available on the TeamSTEPPS website.[1]

Learning

The subculture of learning involves learning from mistakes. The Joint Commission (2012) specifically requires that institutions create action and monitoring plans following any sentinel event. Simulations geared toward future error prevention can be part of this action plan.

Evidence-Based Practice

Evidence-based practice includes using protocols and checklists to standardize care. Classic examples of simulations for evidence-based practice include those that require the use of American Heart Association's algorithms for pediatric or adult advanced life support or management of patients with ST-elevation myocardial infarction. Through simulation, team members have the opportunity to observe potential areas of unwanted variation that threaten patient safety.

Patient-Centered Approach

A patient-centered approach is one where patients are the source of control and full partners in their care. This includes empowering patients to question care and using patient stories to give a voice to errors. Effective patient teaching is crucial to prevent treatment failures and adverse reactions. Adding a patient teaching element to almost any scenario, where the provider must assess knowledge or modify a teaching plan, is one method to develop patient-centered skills.

Barriers to Cultures of Safety

Complex systems can produce many unintended consequences for patient safety. Barriers to safer systems include inadequate communication systems, lack of standardization, punitive reporting processes, tolerance for risk taking, and lack of ownership of patient

---

[1]http://TeamSTEPPS.ahrq.gov/abouttoolsmaterials.htm

safety (Barnsteiner, 2011). Just as leadership is central to creating a safety culture, a lack of leadership has been cited as a barrier to such cultures (Sammer et al., 2010). While leaders search for ways to maximize financial productivity, they must also be willing to acknowledge the potential for errors within a system and commit resources to closing the gaps.

Reason's (2000) "Swiss Cheese Model" is one of the most popular frameworks for explaining system errors. Every step in a process has a hole considered a potential for error. Each layer of cheese might be considered a defensive barrier, but if all holes align, catastrophic errors can occur. **Active failures**, also known as **sharp-end failures,** are those errors that are caused at the provider–patient interface. **Latent errors,** or **blunt-end failures,** are those contributory factors caused by the system.

Traditional patient safety efforts have focused on individual responsibilities with an underlying assumption that errors are caused by careless or perhaps morally deficient providers. Once a provider error has been determined, few efforts were devoted to look at how the system could have prevented the error. Reason (2000) challenged this approach, arguing that few active failures occur without contributory system factors. These factors can be related to factors such as organizational cultures, staffing, flawed protocols or processes, how knowledge is transferred, or external pressures. Consider the situation where a wrong dosage of heparin stocked incorrectly in an automated medication dispensing cabinet was administered in error to five infants, killing three (Roesler, Ward, & Short, 2009). Traditional approaches to future error prevention might have focused exclusively on the nurse's behavior, but working through the Unsafe Acts Algorithm (Reason, 1997), management was able to recognize the error had contributory factors. Similar packaging for different doses, lack of bar-coding practices, and even the fact that multidose vials of high-alert medication were available on the units all contributed to the error. Safety experts also revealed that automated medication dispensing cabinets are associated with operant conditioning and confirmation bias, making visual checks alone an insufficient process to prevent medication errors. The Unsafe Acts Algorithm remains a valuable tool facilitators might incorporate in any debriefing process to help learners understand blame-free errors.

Another barrier to safety cultures is that new providers often have received insufficient patient safety education and training during their prelicensure education. Traditional undergraduate nursing education has continued to emphasize care of individual patients with little emphasis on understanding complex systems (Barnsteiner, 2011). Curricula grounded in the QSEN competencies represent a paradigm shift to thinking about providing patient-centered care within systems. Simulation has served as an increasingly important strategy to bring about this shift. Although educators new to simulation may focus on scenarios that teach psychomotor skills or simple assessments, QSEN faculty development efforts have helped fuel the momentum to create scenarios focused on patient safety, including safety checks, procedural or medication errors, injury prevention, and disaster response (Barnsteiner et al., 2013).

SIMULATION TO TEACH SAFETY COMPETENCIES

In simulation, nurses are able to practice all eight QSEN safety competencies in the skill achievement domain (Box 3.1). Key areas of simulation activities might focus on safety checks, interruptions, stressors, adverse events, and handoffs. For each simulation event, it is important to determine who the target learner will be. After that step, two equally important types of simulations may be developed: (1) simulations that mimic the every-day environment for that nurse and (2) simulations that target low-volume but high-risk situations in which the nurse could benefit from experiential practice outside the clinical environment.

Safety Checks

There are multiple opportunities to practice and build competency in the area of safety checks. Specific examples include patient identification checks (i.e., medication administration, procedural "timeouts"), purposeful rounding, and behavioral health visual checks. The nurse's role in particular should be emphasized in creating an environment where routine safety checks are implemented by the individual nurse and enforced by the individual nurse working within a team. This approach creates an opportunity for practicing the skill as well as the communication to the patient and team that should accompany the skill. Reinforcing that technology (such as medication bar coding) does not replace the baseline safety checks, but rather enhances the technology and is a chance to develop key safety skill sets before less safe practices become entrenched in the nurse.

Interruptions

Interruptions have become a common occurrence as nurses learn to balance and manage their workloads. Although health care facilities have worked to implement such interventions as a "medication zone," which is a visual meant to prevent interruptions for a nurse in the process of preparing and giving medications, and quiet times, interruptions remain a fact of nurses' lives. Two situations are amenable to simulation with regard to interruptions: (1) nurses learn to be "mindful" of the impact that interruptions can have on their routines and patient safety; and (2) nurses learn to effectively communicate to peers that they should not interrupt certain patient care processes.

Interruptions can come from patients and families as well. Simulations can be built around the inevitable situation in which patients or family members have questions or need attention, which forces a deviation from the nurse's routine. Practicing the management of interruptions during a key patient care intervention is critical to develop a routine to safety checks. Having nurses practice reintegration in their safety routines after different kinds of interruptions during simulation hardwires the practice for consistent implementation at the point of patient care. This approach is also important when managing multiple patients, in which case the nurse might be interrupted by another patient emergency and then must return to provide care for the other patients or must assume care for patients when the primary nurse is attending to another patient's emergency.

Stressors

In addition to interruptions, **stressors** play a significant role in managing patient safety issues. Stressors may be self-imposed—for example, performance anxiety—or may be related to an emergent patient issue. Either situation can be simulated to improve the likelihood of a safe patient outcome.

Those of us who have watched and evaluated student nurse medication administration or other procedures know all too well how stress can cloud the ability to implement an otherwise sound routine. Although educators are more attentive to not interrupting student work unless an error is imminent, performance anxiety can exist in any nurse, whether new or expert. Simulating the environment consistent with how, when, and where nurses could encounter stressors during evaluation is key to embedding the behaviors critical to safe patient care. Providing simulated experiences with this approach will allow those who are being evaluated in the clinical environment to be able to anticipate their own stress responses and develop methods to manage those responses in a safe environment where the patient cannot be harmed.

Simulating patient stressors is also a valuable learning tool. Some common patient stressors used in simulations include asthma exacerbation, acute myocardial infarction, evolving stroke, hypoglycemia, and behavioral health manifestations. Nurses can learn how to manage their stress responses in order to act effectively during the patient stressor. Additionally, because patient stressors nearly always involve engaging other team members, nurses can practice using appropriate communication techniques that promote healthy teamwork and safe patient care.

Adverse Events

Although each adverse event is unique, some categories of adverse events are more common than others, and some are more dangerous than others. The NQF (2010) has recognized 29 **serious reportable errors** that they feel should be voluntarily disclosed to the public. These errors arise from seven broader event categories: (1) surgical or invasive procedures, (2) products or devices, (3) patient protection, (4) case management, (5) environmental, (6) radiologic, and (7) criminal. Simulation provides an opportunity to practice key prevention strategies as well as methods to manage an adverse event once it has occurred. The IOM (2000) identified treatment errors as a category of errors contributing to patient safety failures. Treatment errors include performance of a procedure, administering treatments, administering medications, responses to abnormal tests, and inappropriate care. This category of errors is highly impacted by the nursing care.

As you consider the range of possible errors, you might also consider the range of possible simulations that could impact the prevention of errors. Nurses might not encounter certain types of medications or administration routes commonly in their practice, but having simulation available to prepare them for the inevitability of a less common medication will assist nurses in maintaining a routine for safe practices aimed at reducing adverse events. Additionally, practices around medication administration change as we learn more about safe practices. One example is the change in the standard of care for intramuscular injections. Over a decade ago, giving intramuscular injections via the dorsogluteal route was no longer advocated in nursing procedure texts because evidence had mounted that this route was linked to sciatic nerve damage. At the same time, the ventrogluteal site emerged as a desired route to substitute for the dorsogluteal site. This change in practice and standard of care was slow to diffuse in some areas, partly because of a lack of knowledge around the change, but also partly because experienced nurses were comfortable with the dorsogluteal site and were not comfortable with, or had not been taught how to give, a ventrogluteal injection. This example lends itself to a simulation environment in which nurses can practice safely injecting the ventrogluteal site. In this situation, simulation prevents adverse events by eliminating the risk for sciatic nerve damage with the dorsogluteal site, while also building confidence and skill in nurses for administering medications via the ventrogluteal site.

There are many other opportunities related to preventing adverse events through simulations, including the following possible topics:

- Administering tube feedings to a neonate who is also on intravenous fluids (practice tube identification to prevent administration of feeding into wrong tubing).

- Assessment of heart rate or rhythm, blood pressure, and labs before administering furosemide (practice identification, location, attainment, and analysis of data to make a decision regarding whether it is safe to administer the medication).

- Setting up medications in the patient's home environment (practice designing safe medication practices in an environment outside the hospital environment).

- Administering a haloperidol injection to an agitated person (practice administering an injectable medication to a patient in an undesirable circumstance).

- Cross-checking compatibility of intravenous medication drips with a scheduled intravenous push medication (practice locating resources to safety combine medications).

- Display a critical platelet lab value for a patient who is in the oncology unit (practice communicating abnormalities in a timely manner, obtaining the proper order to resolve the lab, and implementing the appropriate nursing interventions to protect the patient).

A second area amenable to simulation is handling adverse events. What should the nurse do when an error is discovered and a potential adverse reaction could harm the patient? Simulated scenarios prime nurses to properly communicate the event, monitor for and detect early signs of a reaction, and administer the correct treatment for the reaction, including understanding the level of care a patient may need. For example, assume a patient received a double dosing of an opioid analgesic in a medication error. A simulation could be constructed that prompts nurses to marshal the resources needed to safety navigate the patient through an actual or potential adverse event. It is through this practice that nurses become familiar with and learn to navigate highly emotional situations, with the goal of reducing the uncertainty around managing such an important event. By practicing the management of a potential adverse event, nurses gain more experience for navigating the situation that will create an increased likelihood for an unfortunate event to have a better outcome.

A review of the literature, safety alerts, and events for the given area will guide the need for simulations regarding the prevention of adverse events. The number of simulations that can be created for this important patient safety issue is limitless.

Handoffs

Handoffs among health care providers have been linked to substantive patient safety failures. The AHRQ has identified handoff as a critical communication piece to safe patient care (AHRQ, 2013). Handoffs among providers can result in decreased quality and threats to safety. Consider a situation in which a nurse providing a change of shift report conveys the initial previous start-of-shift fall risk assessment but has since given the patient a large dose of diuretic. If the nurse fails to convey to the oncoming nurse the change in patient risk, the patient could fall and suffer harm. Practicing handoffs between nurses and among other providers such as physicians, pharmacists, and physical therapists provides the opportunity for closing a gap in patient safety. Tools have been developed to assist with a standardized, safe handoff such as Situation-Background-Assessment-Recommendation (SBAR) (Hohenhaus, Powell, & Hohenhaus, 2006). A sampling of handoff tools is available through the Association of periOperative Registered Nurses (AORN, 2012). Any number of simulations can be created that approximate the environment in which nurses work. Structuring simulations around the National Patient Safety Goals for improving staff communication is an excellent approach to ensure that nurses have an opportunity to practice safe and appropriate communication (The Joint Commission, 2013).

Simulation provides the ability to practice several skills in one situation or to isolate a particular skill. Handoff is one of those key skills that is possible to practice in any type of simulation. It is important to develop a standardized approach so that the practice is embedded in every method for patient handoff. Some of the simulation possibilities for handoff include:

1. Change of shift report for any type of patient (acute care, mental health, home care)
2. Report to and from charge nurses or other managers
3. Report to the physician or an advanced practice nurse (APN) on the initial assessment and needs for a patient
4. Report to a provider who will be conducting a procedure or test requiring the patient to leave the patient's primary site of care
5. Report to another receiving patient care facility

SIMULATION TO IMPROVE TEAMWORK AND COMMUNICATION

Communication has been highlighted in previous sections but deserves its own discussion. Poor communication has been linked to significant patient safety lapses including failure to rescue, handoffs, system vulnerabilities, and individual safety performances. The uncoordinated state of health care has promoted devastating patient errors and innumerable "near misses" (Mitchell et al., 2012). The IOM, which has been calling for increased teamwork and education among interprofessional teams for over a decade, identified working in interdisciplinary teams as a core health care professional competency. The action plan included education and socialization to the work of other disciplines toward preventing patient errors and improving overall patient outcomes (IOM, 2003).

In 2011, the Interprofessional Education Collaborative Expert Panel (IPEC), commissioned by leading health professional organizations from nursing, osteopathic medicine, pharmacy, dentistry, medicine, and public health, developed a set of competencies that would promote interprofessional competence. These competencies were centered in four domains: (1) values/ethics for interprofessional practice, (2) roles/responsibilities, (3) interprofessional communication, and (4) teams and teamwork (IPEC, 2011). The IPEC competencies provide a core set of behaviors and skills for interprofessional practice so that patient care errors can be minimized. Many nursing schools have adopted the competencies in their curricula, and accrediting bodies now include a provision for interprofessional education for all levels of nursing education.

Both practice and educational institutions have been working to improve interprofessional education and practice, with reports growing daily on opportunities to promote interprofessional communication. Simulation is a vector for developing interprofessional communication and teamwork.

Adverse Outcomes and Sentinel Events

Rarely does a health care provider work alone in the planning and implementation of care for patients. In addition, the patient can be missed as a critical component in the plan of care. Imagine a health care team operating in a code:

Physician: The patient is in a rapid atrial fibrillation, give atropine 6 mg IV push!

The drug is given by the nurse, and now the patient is in ventricular fibrillation without a pulse.

Physician: I don't understand. When the patient had this rhythm before, the adenosine always worked. We never even got the rhythm pause.

Nurse: But you ordered, and I gave, atropine.

Physician: But I didn't *mean* atropine!

One of the key prevention strategies implemented to prevent errors in a team is repeat or read back and verify (RBV) of orders. Many facilities include an RBV requirement in the transmission of a telephone or verbal order and have for the most part discouraged such orders. Replaying our scenario with RBV:

Physician: The patient is in a rapid atrial fibrillation, give atropine 6 mg IV push!

Nurse: You ordered atropine 6 mg IV for the patient who is in atrial fibrillation. Did you mean adenosine?

Physician: Thank you for catching my error. Yes, please give adenosine 6 mg IV push.

Nurse: Preparing adenosine 6 mg IV push.

One statement by the nurse saves the patient from a major error, yet that statement should be practiced in an environment that feels safe for the providers, and where they can learn the appropriate way to give and receive feedback. This practice prevents adverse and sentinel events, like the one in the first version of our scenario.

Organizations can use simulation to retrain health care professionals once an adverse or sentinel event has occurred. In the case of a medication or procedural error, practicing the procedure until the team is comfortable with both the procedure and expected communications is a ripe educational opportunity afforded by simulation. In the surgery area alone, timeouts are built around interprofessional efforts to prevent such sentinel events as wrong site surgery and retained foreign objects. Simulations can be built so that attention is paid to a scenario where any type of potential sentinel event is present, allowing participants to address the situation at hand and to communicate and follow proper procedures.

Improving Communication

Improving communication for safe care within a single site and across the continuum of care is critical to safe patient passage. What health care professionals assume a patient will do, just because they tell the patient to do so, often falls short of the desired goal.

Take, for example, the case of an older man who is hypertensive and requires extensive medication management. In talking with his primary care provider and the nurses, he is prescribed clonidine as an additional medication for management of his escalating hypertension. However, the patient has a new partner and desires to maintain intimacy with that partner, information that was captured on his intake assessment by the nurse. The new regimen of clonidine prevented him from meeting that need. The patient stops taking his clonidine abruptly and is seen later in the emergency department for a hemorrhagic stroke. This event is clearly a failure of the health care team to assess the patient and communicate with one another, but it is also a failure of the health care team to *complete* the team process by involving the patient in the rationale for the drug selection and discussing the drug's side effects.

Simulated situations that allow for health care providers to collect and analyze data, then sorting the data based on priority patient issues, can be constructed on various levels, including inpatient, outpatient, transitional care, and home environments. Practicing communication skills cannot be underestimated.

TeamSTEPPS

An innovative, standardized program was developed by AHRQ and the U.S. Defense Department to improve teamwork and communication among health care providers. TeamSTEPPS provides a network of experts, tools, and materials to support health care professionals in a "train-the-trainer" methodology for improving patient safety and quality (AHRQ, n.d.). One of the key issues toward preventing errors is that a provider could see there might be an error but lacked the words, and felt a lack of authority, to address the potential error. TeamSTEPPS provides a culture of safety training, but just as importantly, it provides the words a provider can use to stop an error.

To set the culture, TeamSTEPPS participants are trained that *anyone can* and *anyone should* feel obligated to "stop the line" when a patient safety issue is at stake. Included in this obligation is the skill of the "two-challenge rule" whereby the first challenge is in the form of a question, and the second challenge provides the rationale for the concern, which is always stated in terms of the patient safety issue.

TeamSTEPPS provides words and phrases to assist in the management of patient safety issues. These words are called **CUS words,** with the acronym derived from the points:

1. State your concern. "I am concerned that we are raising the patient's head of bed."

2. State why you are uncomfortable. "The patient's mean arterial pressure is 58, and if we continue to raise the head of the bed, we will further compromise the patient's perfusion."

3. If unresolved, state that there is a safety issue. "This is a safety issue because we will cause harm to the patient if the head of the bed remains elevated."

If the issue is not resolved, a supervisor is notified. Additionally, other suggested phrases, such as "I would like some clarity about..." and "Would you like some assistance?," are provided (AHRQ, n.d.).

Other strategies promoted by TeamSTEPPS include: SBAR, callout (clearly communicating a piece of information in the patient room so that everyone can benefit from the information and plan the next steps), check-back (closed-loop communication to verify and validate information, often used with a callout). For example:

Nurse: The patient is in SVT. Would you like me to give adenosine 6 mg IV push?

APN: Yes, please give adenosine 6 mg IV push.

Nurse: Preparing adenosine 6 mg IV push.

Nurse: Adenosine 6 mg IV push given.

APN: Thank you.

A critical piece to TeamSTEPPS training is that all members hold one another accountable for appropriate communications and actions, with full focus on the best patient outcome. The program prepares the team and individuals to be accountable and to hold one another accountable (AHRQ, n.d.).

TeamSTEPPS provides a framework for the educator to structure simulations around teamwork and communication. Simulations that prompt a situation where group think is desired, which is true for almost all patient care scenarios, will sharpen individuals on their communication skills while also promoting teamwork toward managing a positive patient outcome. Any number of clinical scenarios can be built that allow the incorporation and practice of TeamSTEPPS skills. Clinical scenarios can range from low-risk, high-volume situations to high-risk, low-volume situations. Often, building a stressor into a clinical situation will heighten the development of team communication and teamwork skills. Scenarios that require the "brain power" of all disciplines are ideal opportunities to practice drawing out the skill set of all involved to get to the best and safest patient outcome. A TeamSTEPPS scenario is provided as an exemplar near the end of this chapter.

Error Disclosure

Simulation can be used to foster communication to the patient and family in the occurrence of an adverse or sentinel event. Disclosing errors to patients is a stressful experience for health care providers. Proper use of the team during error disclosure promotes a caring approach when informing a patient and the family about the error, which in turn can decrease malpractice claims and create the appropriate relationship among care providers and the patient. The team approach and learning the suitable words to use in a nonthreatening environment are critical to being able to navigate the disclosure.

Because error disclosure is a highly personal event, simulations involving standardized patients and families are a key approach to this sensitive topic. Like other simulation scenarios, error disclosure using standardized patients can be designed using a novice-to-expert stepped methodology. From beginning students to expert practitioners, practicing error disclosure promotes empathy and caring for patients and allows the practitioner to "walk in the patient's shoes."

Many cultural and professional beliefs may need to be overcome during these scenarios, including addressing the legal ramifications of error disclosure. State-by-state malpractice laws are not comparable, so practitioners should be coached on different methods of disclosure based on whether their disclosure can be used as evidence in litigation. Nonetheless, from an ethical perspective, promoting error disclosure in a humane manner is critical to the team cohesiveness, patient trust, and patient safety. An error disclosure scenario is provided as an exemplar later near the end of this chapter.

SIMULATIONS TO TEACH SYSTEM VULNERABILITY AND SAFETY THREATS

Well-designed simulations test system processes. The more a simulation setting replicates actual workflow, the more likely it is to reveal system vulnerabilities. **In situ simulations**, or those done in the actual clinical environment as opposed to a simulation lab, can be particularly diagnostic (Patterson, Blike, & Nadkarni, 2008). Simulations of this type focus on skill rehearsal and problem solving and are ideal to "crash test" provider competencies and identify latent system errors. They can identify if actual equipment is present and working, if emergency medications are available, and if all emergency team members know their role and can quickly assemble and work efficiently within a defined space. When Patterson, Geis, Falcone, LeMaster, and Wears (2013) conducted 90 simulations in a pediatric emergency department over a one-year period, they found 73 latent safety threats at a rate of one threat per every 1.2 simulations.

There are some disadvantages to in situ simulations. Portability varies by simulator type, methods to pay for consumable supplies have to be addressed, filming for debriefing may or may not be possible, and planned simulations may have to be canceled during times of high census or acuity (Patterson et al., 2008). These simulations are also most likely to not be canceled if they are quite short with a limited debriefing. If system problems are found, a detailed analysis is unlikely to immediately occur. Thus facilitators must be prepared to schedule follow-up sessions to address such issues.

ACTIVE AND LATENT FAILURES

As previously discussed, active failures are easy to identify during simulation. A provider gives a wrong medication or fails to recognize early signs of respiratory failure, leading to an arrest. Although a simple debriefing might focus only on the general human fallibility aspect of those errors, a better debriefing would address contributory system factors as well as the three levels of human fallibility of a just culture: human error that involves unintentional behaviors, at-risk behavior that involves taking shortcuts, and reckless behavior that involves disregard for standard procedures (Roesler et al., 2009).

Consider a scenario in which a nurse is called in midshift because another nurse left urgently with an incomplete handoff. Upon review of a medication administration record, the nurse finds digoxin was due over two hours ago but was not charted. The nurse must decide whether or not to give the medication. If the nurse makes the assumption the drug was not given and administers the medication, the patient would develop signs of toxicity with dizziness that could lead to a fall. Here the Unsafe Acts Algorithm (Reason, 1997) could be used to help guide the debriefing. The first question would be: Was the act intended? Here the answer is no, the nurse did not intend to give a second dose of digoxin. The next question examines: Did illicit drugs or substances influence the nurse's decision? Again, the answer is no. The next question is: Did the nurse knowingly violate safety procedures? At this point, the system's safety procedures for incomplete handoffs or for verifying whether uncharted medications have been given enter into the discussion. If deliberate noncompliance is not found, then the question becomes: Have others committed the same error within the system? A yes answer here suggests the presence of a systems error.

FAILURE MODES AND EFFECT ANALYSIS FOR IN SITU SIMULATIONS

A **failure modes and effect analysis** (FMEA) is a prospective method to identify system risks. The technique involves assigning scores to the severity, likelihood, and detectability of a potential patient safety issue. Those scores, known as *risk priority numbers,* are then used to prioritize problem-solving efforts. The technique was originally created as a way to brainstorm about what could go wrong with steps in a process. More recently FMEA has been used as a method to analyze events in in situ simulations. Davis, Riley, Gurses, Miller, and Hansen (2008) conducted 10 in situ simulations based on two labor and delivery simulations involving an emergency cesarean section: need for blood product and neonatal resuscitation. Video recordings of the scenarios were reviewed for active and latent failures and were combined with brainstorming to arrive at a list of six active latent and four active failure modes. The identified simulation scenario dealing with a lack of clear roles in an emergency cesarean section, which led to confusion and fragmented care, received the highest risk priority number. In this situation, recognition of the need for better teamwork led to an action plan that included TeamSTEPPS training. This is just one example of the many ways simulation can be used in conjunction with other strategies to improve patient safety.

EXEMPLARS

Two exemplars using two or more of the characteristics presented in this chapter are provided in this section. The first exemplar depicts a standardized patient scenario to develop error disclosure skills, and the second exemplar illustrates a high-fidelity simulation to promote communication skills.

Standardized Patients Exemplar

Elements: Stressor, adverse events, teamwork, improving communication, error disclosure

Site: Indiana University Schools of Nursing and Medicine, Bloomington, Indiana

Target students: First-semester junior nursing students, first-semester/first-year medical students

Preparation: Nursing and medical students jointly attend an onsite seminar on compassionate care, an interactive and emotionally challenging seminar that focused students on patient and family perspectives of care. The seminar is followed by specific training about error disclosure, using the principles from a live training session recorded at the University of Washington (2011). Student teams (one medical student and one or two nursing students) are provided the general scenario and are allowed to meet with one another to discuss approaches before the simulation.

Setup: Standardized patients from the school of medicine are used. Standardized patients are prepared by faculty on the scenario and the level of student (beginning) is chosen. Student teams are provided the following scenario. The teams are to communicate a medication error to a son or daughter of the patient in a private consultation area. All simulations are digitally recorded, and two live evaluators are in the room but away from the table where the communication about the error will occur between the team and the family member.

Scenario: Mr. Smith is an 86-year-old male who is transported to the emergency department from an extended care facility. Mr. Smith is believed to have a urinary tract infection and possibly sepsis because he is somewhat confused. Upon arriving to the emergency department, Mr. Smith is given a penicillin derivative antibiotic intravenously. He is allergic to penicillin, but his armband was lost in transit. Mr. Smith has a respiratory emergency as a result of the penicillin administration, is intubated, and is placed on a ventilator. He is transferred to the intensive care unit. Overnight, Mr. Smith is able to be weaned from the ventilator but is still confused and does not recognize his son/daughter.

Debrief: The initial debrief is with the standardized patient. Standardized patients identify both the desirable and undesirable attributes of the team performance, using "I" statements to explain how they felt about certain statements or posturing. The two evaluators also provide their feedback of the performance with suggestions on improvements. Students share their own evaluation of their performance, which is perhaps the most enlightening part of the debriefing. Digital recordings are reviewed by faculty who then construct a large group debriefing of all medical and nursing students, together in their teams. This debriefing strategy provides the group with a thematic analysis of the communication and behavior patterns observed across scenarios.

Evaluation: Because this experience is a highly emotional experience for beginning level students, teams do not receive a grade; rather, their debriefings serve as an evaluation. The evaluation approach for this scenario creates a nonpunitive approach to managing the difficult topic of error disclosure.

High-Fidelity Human Patient Simulator Exemplar

Elements: Stressor, safety checks, interruptions, handoff, procedural checks, improving communication, TeamSTEPPS

Site: Indiana University Schools of Nursing and Medicine, Bloomington, Indiana

Target students: Junior and senior nursing students, and first- and second-year medical students

Preparation: Students teams are formed between junior nursing students and first-year medical students. These teams are sustained through graduation for nursing students and the second year for medical students. Student teams are introduced by way of a "mini" TeamSTEPPS seminar conducted by faculty at the start of each year. The seminars contain key information regarding how to communicate in teams using the handoff tools, shout outs, and closed loop communication, among other techniques. A beginner-level seminar is held for junior nursing and first-year medical student teams, whereas a more advanced seminar is held for senior nursing and second-year medical student teams. Interactive strategies using case studies with team clickers are used to create the team-building experience. For simulations involving advanced cardiac life support (ACLS) skill sets, the teams are jointly trained and certified in ACLS.

Setup: High-fidelity human patient simulators are used. Students are provided with a brief scenario in advance of the simulation event. Because the key purpose of the simulation is to promote teamwork in order to prevent patient errors, teams are encouraged to meet to prepare as well as to discuss roles during the scenario. All simulations are digitally recorded. A faculty member from both nursing and medicine is present in the debrief room for evaluation.

Scenarios: Scenarios are developed that require and promote communication and teamwork for the appropriate level of the team. The current scenarios are listed in Table 3.1.

Debrief: Debriefing for all scenarios includes an immediate team debrief with both nursing and medicine faculty. The debriefing includes descriptive observations of the desirable and undesirable behaviors for individual communication, team communication, and team "procedural" performance. Digital recordings are reviewed by faculty for the purpose of choosing an exemplar to show in a large group debriefing of all medical and nursing students, again, together in their teams. In this debriefing, teams watch the exemplar video and are then asked what key communication strategies were used that promoted good teamwork and safe patient care. Teams are asked to reflect on their own performance and strategize how they could enhance their performance in subsequent simulations as well as in the clinical setting.

TABLE 3.1

High-Fidelity Human Patient Simulator Scenarios

Year and Level of Students	Scenario
First semester, junior nursing students First semester, first-year medical students	**BLS:** The team is coming to the simulation lab to do a team simulation. They will need to know Basic Life Support (BLS). Students do not get the following information: When the team comes into the simulation lab, they find the environmental support staff person on the floor calling for help. The students need to assess the patient, and when the patient becomes unresponsive, use the automated external defibrillator (AED).
Second semester, junior nursing students Second semester, first-year medical students	**Asthma:** The team will be providing care for a 14-year-old girl who presents to the emergency department with an exacerbation of asthma. The team is told they will need to be able to attend to the exacerbation, including all relevant teaching to the patient and mother based on the assessment and treatment sequencing. The scenario starts with nursing students assessing the patient, then providing a handoff to the medical student.
First semester, senior nursing students First semester, second-year medical students	**ACLS:** The patient presents to the emergency department complaining of chest pain. Students are told that the scenario will require use of their advanced cardiac life support (ACLS) skill set. Teams must manage the scenario, including appropriate disposition of the patient. The scenario starts with nursing students assessing the patient, then providing a handoff to the medical student.
Second semester, senior nursing students Second semester, second-year medical students	**Detective SimMan:** The patient presents to the emergency department with symptomology of one of the following issues: diverticulitis, cholecystitis, bleeding upper gastrointestinal ulcer, pneumonia, or acute myocardial infarction (AMI). Students are told that the scenario will require use of their ACLS skill set. Teams must manage the scenario, including appropriate disposition of the patient. The scenario starts with nursing students assessing the patient, then providing a handoff to the medical student.

Evaluation: Individual communication and team communication are scored using the Indiana University Simulation Integration Rubric, which has been tested successfully for internal consistency and discriminant validity. A third area, procedural performance, which is the ability of the team to manage the patient through the correct sequence of actions for the best patient outcome, is also scored. Procedural performance and team communication elements are both team scores, which is the same score for each team member regardless of individual contribution. The individual communication score is a score unique to each student. The bulk of the scoring is team based. This scoring approach promotes "group think," which is emphasized in teamwork as a desired behavior to get the patient to the right goal. The group is encouraged to be verbal, discussing all possibilities and strategies, along with the rationale for treating the patient.

SUMMARY

Ethical standards require that providers take proactive measures to protect their patients. Drivers in the current socioeconomic climate call on health care providers to create safer systems and build cultures of safety. Simulation offers an active strategy to develop essential safety-focused knowledge, skills, and attitudes in both individuals and teams. Scenarios conducted in either a simulation laboratory or in the clinical setting can help identify active provider errors and latent system weaknesses that are amenable to improvements. Almost any simulation designed to teach the performance of a procedure can be enhanced to teach patient safety by including safety checks, dealing with interruptions, performing in the presence of stressors, preventing known adverse events, or conducting handoffs.

Poor communication poses a particular threat to patient safety. Perhaps one of simulation's greatest strengths is that it provides a venue for teamwork and the opportunity to practice communication and group problem solving. Structuring simulations with the TeamSTEPPS framework can be particularly effective in helping providers develop group think skills and the mindset that patient safety is everyone's responsibility. Combining simulation training with other quality improvement strategies, such as an FMEA, can serve as an excellent way for organizations to proactively protect their patients and workers. Given simulation's dual strengths as a teaching strategy and assessment tool, one can only anticipate that providers in both the academic and service sectors will continue to explore simulation's role in patient safety.

■ Key Concepts

- Ethical behavior requires that providers protect their patients. QSEN has identified 8 prelicensure and 15 graduate safety competencies necessary for practice.
- In the current socioeconomic climate financial drivers, such as the Accountable Care Act, and professional drivers, such as QSEN, call on health care providers to create safer systems and build cultures of safety.
- Cultures of safety characteristics include leadership, just culture, teamwork, evidence-based practices, patient-centeredness, open transparent communication, and learning from mistakes.
- Simulations can specifically be designed to teach preferred responses to high-risk situations such as interruptions, stressors, and handoffs. They can also be designed to improve practice after an adverse event.

- Simulation is a vector for developing interprofessional communication and teamwork, both key components in improving patient safety. Using the TeamSTEPPS framework as part of the simulation design can be particularly effective in helping providers develop the mindset that patient safety is everyone's responsibility.
- Simulation can be used to test system vulnerability and latent failures, especially when done in situ or in conjunction with other quality improvement techniques such as a FMEA.
- Safety simulations can be successfully designed using either standardized patients or a human patient simulator. Standardized patients add value to the debriefing by identifying both the desirable and undesirable attributes of the team performance.

References

Agency for Healthcare Research and Quality (AHRQ). (2013). *Handoffs and signouts.* Retrieved from http://psnet.ahrq.gov/primer.aspx?primerID=9

Agency for Healthcare Research and Quality (AHRQ). (n.d.). *TeamSTEPPS®: National implementation.* Retrieved from http://TeamSTEPPS.ahrq.gov/

American Association of Colleges of Nursing (AACN). (2012). *Graduate-level QSEN competencies: Knowledge, skills and attitudes.* Retrieved from http://www.aacn.nche.edu/faculty/qsen/ competencies.pdf

American Association of Colleges of Nursing (AACN). (2013). *Quality and safety education for nurses.* Retrieved from http://www.aacn.nche.edu/qsen/home

American Nurses Association (ANA). (2001). *Code of ethics for nurses with interpretive statements.* Retrieved from http://www.nursingworld.org/MainMenuCategories/EthicsStandards/CodeofEthicsforNurses/Code-of-Ethics.pdf

Association of periOperative Registered Nurses. (2012). *Patient handoff toolkit.* Retrieved from http://www.aorn.org/Secondary.aspx?id=20849

Barnsteiner, J. (2011). Teaching the culture of safety. *OJIN: The Online Journal of Issues in Nursing, 16*(3), 5.

Barnsteiner, J., Disch, J., Johnson, J., McGuinn, K., Chappell, K., & Swartwout, E. (2013). Diffusing QSEN competencies across schools of nursing: The AACN/RWJF Faculty Development Institutes. *Journal of Professional Nursing, 29*(2), 68–74.

Centers for Medicare & Medicaid Services (CMS). (2013a). *Administration implements new health reform provision to improve care quality, lower costs.* Retrieved from http://www.healthcare.gov/news/factsheets/2011/04/valuebasedpurchasing04292011a.html

Centers for Medicare & Medicaid Services (CMS). (2013b). *Hospital-acquired conditions (HAC) in acute inpatient prospective payment system (IPPS) hospitals.* Retrieved from http://www.cms.gov/Medicare/Medicare-Fee-for-Service-Payment/HospitalAcqCond/downloads/hacfactsheet.pdf

Centers for Medicare & Medicaid Services (CMS). (2013c). *Hospital value-based purchasing: Measure explanations.* Retrieved from http://www.healthcare.gov/news/factsheets/2011/04/valuebasedpurchasing04292011b.html

Centers for Medicare & Medicaid Services (CMS). (n.d.). *Hospital compare: What information can I get about hospitals?* Retrieved from http://www.medicare.gov/HospitalCompare/About/HOSInfo/Hospital-Info.aspx

Cronenwett, L., Sherwood, G., Barnsteiner, J., Disch, J., Johnson, J., Mitchell, P., Sullivan D. T., & Warren, J. (2007). Quality and safety education for nurses. *Nursing Outlook, 55*(3), 122–131.

Davis, S., Riley, W., Gurses, A. P., Miller, K., & Hansen, H. (2008). Failure modes and effects analysis based on in situ simulations: a methodology to improve understanding of risks and failures. *Advances in Patient Safety: New Directions and Alternative Approaches, 3*, 145–160.

Hohenhaus, S., Powell, S., & Hohenhaus, J. T. (2006). Enhancing patient safety during hand-offs: Standardized communication and teamwork using the "SBAR" method. *American Journal of Nursing, 106*, 72A–72B.

Institute of Medicine (IOM). (2000). *To err is human: Building a safer health care system.* National Academy of Sciences. Retrieved from http://www.iom.edu/~/media/Files/Report%20Files/1999/To-Err-is-Human/To%20Err%20is%20Human%201999%20%20report%20brief.pdf

Institute of Medicine (IOM). (2003). *Health professions education: A bridge to quality.* The National Academies Press. Retrieved from http://www.nap.edu/catalog/10681.html

Interprofessional Education Collaborative Expert Panel (IPEC). (2011). *Core competencies for interprofessional collaborative practice: Report of an expert panel.* Retrieved from http://www.aacn.nche.edu/education-resources/ipecreport.pdf

Mitchell, P., Wynia, M., Golden, R., McNelis, B., Okun, S., Webb, C. E.,...Von Kohorn, I. (2012). *Core principles & values of effective team-based health care.* Institute of Medicine. Retrieved from https://www.nationalahec.org/pdfs/VSRT-Team-Based-Care-Principles-Values.pdf

National Patient Safety Foundation (NPSF). (2013). *Events and forums.* Retrieved from http://www.npsf.org/events-forums/patient-safety-awareness-week/

National Quality Forum (NQF). (2010). *Serious reportable events in healthcare 2011.* Retrieved from http://www.qualityforum. org/Publications/2011/12/Serious_Reportable_Events_in_Healthcare_2011.aspx

Patterson, M. D., Blike, G. T., & Nadkarni, V. M. (2008). In situ simulation: Challenges and results. *Advances in patient safety: New directions and alternative approaches, 3.* Retrieved from https://www.ahrq.gov/professionals/quality-patient-safety/patient-safety-resources/resources/advances-in-patient-safety-2/vol3/Advances-Patterson_48.pdf

Patterson, M. D., Geis, G. L., Falcone, R. A., LeMaster, T., & Wears, R. L. (2013). In situ simulation: Detection of safety threats and teamwork training in a high risk emergency department. *BMJ Quality & Safety, 22*(6), 468–477.

Reason, J. (1997). *Managing the risks of organizational accidents.* Hants, England: Ashgate.

Reason, J. (2000). Human error: Models and management. *British Medical Journal, 320*, 768–770.

Roesler, R., Ward, D., & Short, M. (2009). Supporting staff recovery and reintegration after a critical incident resulting in infant death. *Advances in Neonatal Care, 9*(4), 163–171.

Sammer, C. E., Lykens, K., Singh, K. P., Mains, D. A., & Lackan, N. A. (2010). What is patient safety culture? A review of the literature. *Journal of Nursing Scholarship, 42*(2), 156–165.

The Joint Commission. (2013). *National patient safety goals.* Retrieved from http://www.jointcommission.org/standards_information/npsgs.aspx

The Joint Commission. (2012). *Sentinel events.* Retrieved from http://www.jointcommission.org/assets/1/6/CAMH_2012_Update2_24_SE.pdf

University of Washington. (2011). *Video example of error disclosure* [video]. Retrieved from http://collaborate.uw.edu/educators-toolkit/error-disclosure-toolkit/video-example-of-error-disclosure.html

4

Meaningful Debriefing and Other Approaches

Kristina Thomas Dreifuerst, PhD, RN, ACNS-BC, CNE
Sara L. Horton-Deutsch, PhD, CNS, RN
Henry Henao, MSN, RN, ARNP, FNP-BC, CHSE

■ Learning Objectives

1. Summarize how the concept of debriefing is used in simulation and clinical learning environments.
2. Design debriefing opportunities for learners that incorporate the essential components.
3. Compare the different theories of reflection and how they can be incorporated into debriefing.
4. Articulate the relationships between reflection, mindfulness, and debriefing.
5. Use different methods of meaningful debriefing to explore the learner's thinking related to correct as well as incorrect actions in the simulation or clinical environment.

■ Key Terms

- Clinical reasoning
- Debriefing
- Reflection
- Thinking

THE CONCEPT OF DEBRIEFING

The world of health care is ever-changing. Health care professionals face a highly complex environment. There is increasing pressure to be prepared to care for seriously ill patients who have intense needs while using fewer resources. Similarly, interprofessional health care educators are challenged to incorporate new and innovative teaching and learning strategies that are learner centered yet effectively teach students the knowledge and skills they need to practice well. Concurrently, experiential clinical learning environments in health care are changing. Many professional disciplines have increased their use of simulation to both augment and replace traditional clinical practice environments. The goal of every clinical experience, including simulation, is to develop in students tacit and explicit cognitive knowledge as well as the skills and professional attitudes necessary for success. As a result, best practices for teaching and learning in simulation and clinical environments are being advanced.

One area of simulation gaining increasing interest and research focus is the component of **debriefing**. Debriefing is a time of **reflection** that occurs after the clinical or simulation experience in which the instructor or facilitator and the learner revisit the experience to reflect, review what occurred, discuss with other participants, correct errors in practice, and solidify the learning that will be taken forward to subsequent patient encounters (Dreifuerst, 2009; Shinnick, Woo, Horwich, & Steadman, 2011). At a minimum, debriefing includes a discussion of what went right, what went wrong, and what should be done differently. Those, however, are just the beginning steps for meaningful debriefing. The ability to guide reflection and also reveal the thinking behind the actions and decisions gives the clinical instructor as facilitator the opportunity to provide participants with feedback for fostering meaningful learning (Arafeh, Hansen, & Nichols, 2010; Dreifuerst, 2009; Issenberg, McGaghie, Petrusa, Lee Gordon, & Scalese, 2005; Shinnick et al., 2011; Yaeger & Arafeh, 2008).

Although reflection can occur naturally as a reaction to an event, it often manifests in an unstructured way that does not consistently enhance learning, and it may be hindered by emotions related to the overall experience (Fanning & Gaba, 2007). Guided or *facilitated* debriefing by educators provides intentional, systematic educational experiences to support and create a context for meaningful learning (Arafeh et al., 2010). Using a nonjudgmental yet structured method of debriefing, in which the clinical or simulation experience is reviewed by all participants and presented from the student's perspective, allows educators to encourage reflective **thinking** and uncover the intentional and unintentional cognitive processes that inform decision making in learners (Cantrell, 2008; Decker & Dreifuerst, 2012; Dreifuerst, 2009; Issenberg et al., 2005; Shinnick et al., 2011). It also gives a structure for emotional response and release.

The most common goals of debriefing are to recognize and release emotions, reinforce learning objectives, enhance cognition, develop problem-solving skills, promote reflective learning, and bridge what occurred in simulation to the traditional clinical environment (Johnson-Russell & Bailey, 2010). These goals hold true for debriefing simulation as well as for debriefing traditional clinical experiences in which students and educators reflect on what has happened in an effort to link forward the learning that has occurred with the next clinical experience or simulation in which the student will be called upon to reason and make decisions.

Facilitated debriefing is a guided discussion, not a traditional instructional session, which supports the shift from an instructional paradigm to a learning paradigm in experiential learning environments (Candela, 2012). Clinical instructors acting as debriefing facilitators are encouraged to ensure that debriefing does not become a teacher-centered lecture. Rather, the emphasis should be on guiding the reflection on what occurred using open-ended questions or prompts to engage all participants in the discussion. Through this process, the participants in debriefing can uncover the thinking that underpinned their actions during the experience and, together with the clinical instructor or facilitator, correct the misconceptions and recognize the correct reasoning and actions.

Debriefing has been identified as the most important component of simulation for student learning, with evidence of cognitive gains and improved **clinical reasoning** as a direct result, particularly when Socratic-style questioning is used to identify the thinking behind nursing decisions made in complex clinical situations (Dreifuerst, 2012; Shinnick et al., 2011). Through debriefing, the less experienced clinician has the opportunity to analyze taken-for-granted assumptions and compare them to others, including the clinical instructor's expert cognitions, and then develop a new understanding about how to proceed in a future clinical situation.

Fonacier, McNelis, and Ebright (2013) suggest that in this manner, debriefing is an opportunity for the clinical instructor to identify otherwise missing elements of the students' interpretation of what they are seeing, hearing, and thinking about while interacting with their patient, which impact clinical reasoning. This is particularly relevant when the actions during the simulation are correct but the thinking is misguided. Furthermore, if clinical instructors are unaware of students' actual thought processes, they are unable to redirect incorrect cognitive assumptions toward more appropriate and safe clinical judgments or affirm correct ones. Moreover, when routine and consistent debriefing does occur consistently, it becomes an anticipated part of the learning process.

THE ESSENTIALS OF DEBRIEFING

Prebriefing

Immediately preceding the clinical experience or simulation, the clinical instructor or debriefing facilitator should take time for prebriefing. The prebriefing phase is used to establish ground rules and set expectations for the entire experience, including the debriefing, and to present an overview of how participants will be expected to interact. Typically this includes a review of principles of confidentiality that will be expected of everyone involved. During the prebrief, all participants should be oriented to the method of debriefing that will be used and any instruments or tools that might be part of the experience. Objectives of the clinical experience or simulation are presented along with a description of the expectations of the participants including the facilitator-as-guide role (Rudolph, Simon, Rivard, Dufresne, & Raemer, 2007). The clinical instructor should also clearly articulate the consequences of the experience if it is used for high-stakes testing or routine assessment rather than just an experiential learning event.

Location

The debriefing experience should occur in a location that facilitates a robust discussion among participants. Although the location can be highly dependent upon the facilities available, generally the preferred location is removed from the simulator or patient, is private, and allows for comfortable seating. When the debriefing involves a group of people, a seating arrangement that ensures all participants can see and hear one another is important, promoting the open dialogue and respectful conversation that are typical components of debriefing. For this reason, traditional classroom-style seating is not recommended. Using a part of a classroom or simulation center that is used concurrently by others is also not advocated because of the lack of the ability to have uninterrupted, confidential conversations.

Timing

Most debriefing occurs immediately following the simulation or clinical experience. This follows the traditional underpinnings of debriefing taken from the military and the airline industry (Fanning & Gaba, 2007). In both those traditions, the debriefing occurs directly after the experience, when all of the thought processes and decision-making elements are fresh in the minds of the participants and the debriefing facilitator. When it is not possible to debrief immediately, one alternative is to have the participants reflect using written, audio, or video journaling to capture their initial thoughts and incorporate them into formal debriefing with a facilitator at a later time.

Time

Although there are few published data regarding how much time should be used for debriefing and the best ratio of time in simulation to time debriefing, it is clear that investing adequate opportunity for this component of simulation is important. According to Shinnick et al. (2011), the greatest cognitive gains occurred after debriefing simulation rather than during the patient care experience. From these results, they recommend that time to debrief and the quality of debriefing be considered the most important considerations when designing simulation experiences (Shinnick et al., 2011, p. e110). The component of time, then, cannot always be predetermined. Time can be highly dependent on the circumstances of the simulation and the clinical experience as well as the learner's actions, decisions, and judgment. As the debriefing unfolds, and the participants begin to reflect on what occurred and the thinking associated with their actions, the clinical instructor or debriefing facilitator might uncover numerous misunderstandings or poorly understood concepts. Whenever possible, it is important to correct these during debriefing. If time is a limiting factor, a plan for follow up needs to be established within a short time frame to ensure that the mistakes are not incorrectly learned and embedded into the participant's frame of knowledge, assumptions, and feelings that he or she incorrectly takes from the simulation.

Objectives

Most teaching–learning experiences have associated objectives. For simulation pedagogy, these can be related to the clinical experience, the debriefing experience, or both. All participants, including the learners as well as the clinical instructors and debriefing facilitators, should be aware of the objectives for the experience beforehand. These objectives should be reviewed not only in the prebrief but also as part of the debriefing. Objectives are written at appropriate levels for the learners involved in the experience and reflect the intended learning outcomes (Ironside, Jeffries, & Martin, 2009).

Participants and Roles

All participants in the simulation experience should actively participate in the debriefing regardless of the role they assumed for the patient care component. Students who act as observers or in supporting roles can be as involved as those assuming the roles of principal or assisting health care professionals in the scenario. Each participant recounts what occurred from the perspective of the role he or she played in the experience, and all contributions should be considered equally valuable for understanding the thinking and actions in the simulation. Clinical instructors and facilitators can guide the discussion to be highly interactive and inclusive as part of creating a nonjudgmental and nonthreatening debriefing experience and fostering reflection and reflective learning in students (Decker & Dreifuerst, 2012).

Reflection

Theories of Reflection

Transformational learning occurs when adults question their beliefs and actions in the world. Critical reflection is a form of transformational learning in which students are encouraged to examine their beliefs and assumptions and reflect on how these shape and limit their responses and observations in clinical settings as a way to further professional growth and development (Durgahee, 1997; Krmpotic, 2003). Ultimately, transformational learning through reflection is learning that changes behavior, attitudes, and skills into a new way of thinking and acting.

Reflection is an essential component in human learning and development and has been embraced by well-known learning theorists for over a century (Dewey, 1933; Kolb, 1984; Schön, 1983). According to Dewey (1933), reflection leads to increased control by guiding learners to deeper insights and understandings resulting in intentional versus impulsive or routine activity. However, reflection takes time and requires engaging in a thoughtful process, including perplexity, elaboration, hypothesis, comparing hypothesis, and taking action (Dewey, 1933, pp. 106–115).

Similarly, Kolb's (1984) theory of experiential learning focuses on how adults learn from their experiences. His model sets forth four stages of learning from experience:

1. *Concrete experience:* Focusing on practical experiences that result in knowledge
2. *Reflective observation:* Focusing on what the experience means and its association to previous learning
3. *Abstract conceptualization:* Relating reflective observations to what is already known
4. *Active experimentation:* Applying new concepts and theories to practice

According to Kolb (1984), the process is cyclical, and each experience perpetuates more learning. He views reflection as the engine that propels the learning cycle along to further learning, action, and more reflection.

Schön (1983, 1987) was also concerned with how learners use reflection to build professional knowledge and skill. Schön focused on dynamic and adaptive knowledge required in clinical settings. Schön set forth two learning processes that contribute to clinical expertise: reflection-in-action (reflecting while engaged in experience) and reflection-on-action (reflecting after the experience). Dreifuerst (2009) extended this work by identifying reflection-beyond-action (the relation between reflection and anticipation).

Views on reflection and how adults learn have been progressing since the original work by Dewey (1933), where he defined it as active, persistent, and careful consideration of beliefs, supported by knowledge and resulting in conclusive, introspective thoughts. Through reflection, learners gain a detailed view of a situation from the ability to see it from multiple perspectives. This process of rational thinking delays action until the situation is understood, a goal for action is defined, alternative actions are considered, and a plan for implementation is fully developed. This approach includes attention to feelings and beliefs throughout the reflective process and leads to changes in behaviors, skills, and attitudes toward a new way of thinking, thus culminating in transformative learning (Cranton, 2006).

Reflection and Learning

As facilitators of learning, clinical instructors serve as models and mentors for practice by asking reflective questions to help integrate knowledge and experience, which leads to a sense of prominence (Benner, 2010). Often clinical instructors use models and frameworks to help guide learner reflections. These structures need to be flexible and iterative, occurring in a back-and-forth discussion where learners continuously deepen reflective ability, leading to new knowledge and understanding within a given context (Sherwood & Horton-Deutsch, 2012).

Mezirow's (1981) model examines the depth of reflection through a series of processes spanning from consciousness (the way we think about something) to critical consciousness (where we pay attention and analyze our thinking processes). Each level has three sublevels: consciousness includes affective, discriminate, and judgmental reflectivity, and critical consciousness includes conceptual, psychic, and theoretical reflectivity.

Similarly, Freshwater (2008) identified three levels of reflection to guide learners: descriptive, dialogue, and critical. In *descriptive reflection,* clinicians engage in reflection-on-action, whereby practice becomes conscious, is accomplished through journals or reporting thoughts that occurred after an incident to make sense of it, and uses process outcomes to influence future actions. In *dialogic reflection,* practice becomes deliberative through discourse with others to gain feedback on how they are thinking. In *critical reflection,* practice is transformative and is improved as clinicians provide reasoning for actions by engaging in critical conversations about practice with self and others. These structured models can be particularly useful for novice learners. Other reflective models include the reflective cycle of Gibbs (1988) and the learning stages of Boyd and Fales (1993).

John's (2006) model of structured reflection focuses on preparing learners for reflection in a more nonprescriptive way and offers cues to access the depth and breadth for learning through experience. Over time, the cues become internalized and are constantly refined. The cues relate to the four fundamental ways of knowing illuminated by Carper (1978): aesthetic, ethical, empirical, and personal. The cues offer a systematic mode of reflective inquiry. This type of less-structured module is often useful with more advanced learners.

Mindfulness

Mindfulness, defined as paying attention, in the moment, on purpose, and without judgment (Kabat-Zinn, 1990), is a core principle of reflective learning. It allows for expanded awareness by cultivating the courage to observe oneself and inspires flexibility and openness of heart and mind. Reflective practice incorporates this form of self-awareness with other awareness through genuine appreciation and mutual respect demonstrated through listening, attending, and being present with another person. Mindfulness and reflection are both concerned with learning from moment-to-moment experience and aim to realize presence and desirable practice, respectively. These approaches are deliberative and intuitive and support patient-centered care, collaboration, and open communication and foster a culture of safety (Horton-Deutsch, 2012).

Mindful awareness of one's external and internal milieu subsumes the constantly changing and collaborative nature of reflective practice. Although the benefits of such skills might be readily apparent, the means to cultivate this inner capacity are often not incorporated into the educational environment. Paths to bring learners into the present moment include diaphragmatic breathing, brief meditations, or focused activities where everyone practices paying attention and "being with" a routine activity. Educators who create space for, embody, and share mindful practices in the educational environment encourage learners in developing engaged and spirited inquiry of active learning that is responsive to the complex nature of health care (Horton-Deutsch, Drew, & Beck-Coon, 2012).

METHODS OF MEANINGFUL DEBRIEFING

Gather-Analyze-Summarize

The gather-analyze-summarize (GAS) approach has been described as a foundational element that all debriefing models contain (Wang, Kharasch, & Kuruna, 2011). GAS is a simple yet effective three-step process to navigate the stages of debriefing, which can be guided by a facilitator or participant. Upon completion of a simulation experience, the guide will elicit all participants to gather (written or verbally) any relevant data from the clinical experience such as actions, behaviors, conclusions, and patient outcomes related to the care that was delivered. This could be as broad or targeted as the objectives and time frame allow. The facilitator continues to prompt and probe the participants until there is saturation of information.

After all relevant information has been collected, it is then analyzed by the facilitator and participants together in a manner consistent with the learning objectives or in response to issues that emerged during the experience. A video recording of the simulation experience played back during analysis can be potentially useful in this phase because it makes evident the aspects of care the participants might have overlooked or underestimated as well as recognizes strong clinical performance and judgment (Grant, Moss, Epps, & Watts, 2010). To complete the GAS process, the facilitator then summarizes the experience and emphasizes the learning achieved before the debriefing concludes.

Debriefing for Meaningful Learning

Debriefing for Meaningful Learning© (DML) is a systematic method of debriefing designed to lead participants, with the guidance of a facilitator, through a consistently delivered, reflective process that promotes clinical reasoning and judgment skills. Through the use of a worksheet that guides the process of reflection-in-action, reflection-on-action (Schön, 1983), and reflection-beyond-action (Dreifuerst, 2009), the participants experience the development of clinical reasoning and thinking like a nurse (Tanner, 2006) or other health care provider. The facilitator role is vital in the DML method. Facilitators engage participants by using Socratic questioning to elicit their ideas and beliefs, judgments, and decision making. Facilitators help participants challenge taken-for-granted assumptions when the actions are determined to be correct as well as when they are assessed as incorrect in order to unpeel the thinking behind the actions (Dreifuerst, 2012).

DML consists of six elements that were adapted from the E-5 framework for effective teaching (Bybee et al., 1989) into a new E-6 learning framework (Dreifuerst, 2010). The six elements—engage, evaluate, explore, explain, elaborate, and extend—occur iteratively during the debriefing process to challenge thoughts and stimulate interest and inquiry from participants. Although the DML was initially designed for prelicensure nursing students, it has been adapted for use in educating other health professionals (Dreifuerst & Decker, 2012). A critical component of DML is that the debriefing facilitator must be a clinician capable of caring for the patient in the scenario being discussed. This is essential because the facilitator needs to be able to recognize when the actions are correct and incorrect as well as when the thinking is on target or misconstrued. It is a method that adapts to any type of clinical situation or patient care scenario.

Plus-Delta

Plus-delta is a technique designed to involve participants in the process of guided debriefing using a facilitator (Fanning & Gaba, 2007). After a clinical or simulation experience, participants and facilitators gather to reflect on the experience. The facilitator begins by soliciting input from all participants by asking: "What went well?" and "What could have been done differently?" These open-ended questions help to organize behaviors and actions into a two-column table where what went well goes into the plus area and what could have been done differently goes into the delta area.

In the plus column, facilitators and participants list behaviors or actions of individuals or the team that they would consider positive or well done in the simulation experience. These are the positive or plus aspects of the experience. The delta column, represented by the Greek symbol for change (Δ), gives facilitators and participants an opportunity to list behaviors or actions they would like to modify or improve upon in the future. The resulting list serves to guide discussion and gauge consensus from participants (Fanning & Gaba, 2007). By virtue of this technique's simplicity, a participant can be identified as the facilitator, and a clinical teacher is not an essential component of the method. Plus-delta is often used with more experienced participants in simulation or clinical settings such as with practicing clinicians or graduate students. Because it can be used across a wide variety of simulation experiences, this technique has also been adopted by interprofessional teams, particularly when the facilitator represents only one of the health care professions of the members of the team (Dreifuerst & Decker, 2012).

Novice facilitators also often rely on plus-delta as a "rescue" technique when challenged to find a way of initiating postsimulation discussion because of its simplicity and ease of use (Hart, McNeil, Griswold-Theodorson, Bhatia, & Joing, 2012). It is also commonly used when the primary objective of the simulation is to associate decision making with tasks performed. A criticism of this technique is that although it is primarily useful for tasks, it does not consistently explore the deeper understanding of cognitive reasoning that leads to clinical decisions within the simulation experience (Hart et al., 2012). However, if the objective of simulation is to teach a technical skill, plus-delta is an appropriate technique to implement.

Debriefing with Good Judgment

The debriefing with good judgment (DGJ) approach, developed by Rudolph, Simon, Dufresne, and Raemer (2006), is based on the reflective practice work of Schön (1983). A major tenet of DGJ is an emphasis on the facilitator's ability to share critical judgment in a challenging, but psychologically safe, environment that values the clinical expertise of the facilitator.

Three elements comprise the DGJ debriefing approach. The first is a conceptual model that includes frames, actions, and results. The second element is a principle that links curiosity about and respect for the participant, with an assessment (or judgment) of the participant's performance. The third element of DGJ is a communication strategy called advocacy/inquiry. A schema, or cognitive frame, is defined by the knowledge, assumptions, and feelings that participants bring to and subsequently take from the simulation. Frames establish a view, which leads to actions that are then reflected as clinical outcomes (results) in a simulation experience.

The facilitator uses communication skills to enable participants to address feelings they are having about the clinical or simulation experience, reveal their frame, and then, when necessary, guide them to shift or reframe their assumptions. During reframing, the facilitator helps the participants call attention to relevant knowledge that could lead to improved outcomes in future performances. In developing these skills, facilitators are strongly encouraged to analyze their own frames and judgments related to the clinical or simulation experience and consider contrasting their own view with that of the participant in an honest and unambiguous yet provocative manner. This is done using an advocacy–inquiry style of communication.

Advocacy is an assertion or statement based on observations. In this debriefing method, advocacy is paired with a question or inquiry, which is delivered in a manner that reflects genuine curiosity on the part of the facilitator. *Inquiry* aims to reveal and understand a participant's frame. The following is an example of advocacy/inquiry: "I saw that you initiated intravenous therapy but did not use the infusion pump for this medication (advocacy). I'm interested in understanding what led you to this decision (inquiry). Tell me about your thinking in this situation."

The goals of the facilitator using DGJ are to identify a problem, determine a frame through advocacy/inquiry, investigate if other frames related to the problem exist within the group, guide in reframing thinking, and propose an alternative approach to the identified problem.

EE-CHATS

The acronym EE-CHATS stands for emotion, experience counts, communication, higher order thinking, accentuate the positive, time, and structure. Overstreet (2010) identified these seven components that can be used to guide novice and expert facilitators through the process of facilitating debriefing. It does not prescribe an order in which to address each element as they occur iteratively, but the EE-CHATS method provides a comprehensive interdependent approach to debriefing discussions for clinical and simulation experiences.

Facilitators explore a participant's emotions throughout the simulation experience using dialogue and directed questioning. Emotions enhance learning by tying events or experiences to feelings (Schön, 1983). It is important to address emotion early on in the debriefing as this can allow the participant to redirect thinking to learning from what has transpired (Dreifuerst, 2010). During EE-CHATS, expert facilitators share real-life experiences that relate to the clinical or simulation scenario and encourage participants to do so also. Both verbal and nonverbal forms of communication are considered part of this type of debriefing. Journaling can allow for more thoughtful reflection, particularly if it is guided and coached (Petranek, 2000).

Facilitators also need to engage in purposeful listening and less talking when using this method of debriefing. The goal for debriefing using EE-CHATS is for students to develop higher-order thinking as well as the ability to demonstrate extension or transfer of knowledge and apply it to future clinical situations. Emphasizing or accentuating behaviors that form a positive frame to encourage reflection during this vulnerable time is another element of EE-CHATS (Wickers, 2010). Time is an important element in EE-CHATS. The method advocates long periods of time for extensive conversation among participants. The liberal use of silence to elicit thoughtful responses is a function of allowing for sufficient time to pass. Overall, EE-CHATS uses a structure that allows the debriefing to focus and reflect-on-action (Schön, 1983) yet is open enough to allow a tangent conversation related to patient diagnosis or parallel signs and symptoms as well as a discussion to explore the participant's emotional response to a clinical experience or feelings about the use of simulation.

3D Model

The 3D model of debriefing is presented as a framework to facilitate learning from any clinical experience. It consists of three concepts: defusing, discovering, and deepening (Zigmont, Kappus, & Sudikoff, 2011). The 3D model is based on adult learning theories including Kolb's experimental learning cycle (Kolb, 1984), and other outcomes learning models (Zigmont, Kappus & Sudikoff, 2010). This method of debriefing is heavily influenced by the debriefing with good judgment (Rudolph et al., 2007) approach, which was discussed earlier. The 3D model incorporates commonly used debriefing facilitation techniques from health care, aviation, and psychology.

Defusing

After the prebriefing and the clinical or simulation experience, participants gather for a debriefing session and are encouraged to engage in what Kolb (1984) calls defusing. This is a time of reflective observation and giving observations personal meaning. The defusing phase allows participants to verbally express the emotions from their experience and diminish any anxiety or stress. The discussion ensues with a lively dialogue and examination of the actions and decision-making points that occurred during the simulation or clinical experience to reach a consensus on *what* occurred in this phase, which is an important function that will prepare participants for the next phase.

Discovering

Discovering employs reflection to evaluate performance. This phase also allows facilitators to gather insight into the participant's internal process of decision making (mental models). Mental models are identified by engaging in dialogue and determining rationales behind certain behaviors. Once these gaps have been identified, learning can be directed. The advocacy/inquiry approach (Rudolph et al., 2007) was used to identify these mental models.

Deepening

Deepening is the final step in the 3D debriefing method where learning is solidified and becomes internalized knowledge for the participant. Returning to the scenario and attempting to demonstrate successful corrections to the case are considered opportunities to apply new knowledge or understanding in simulation. Through active experimentation, participants achieve their desire to take the new mental model and apply it as soon as possible to replace their previous frame.

These are examples of the most commonly used debriefing methods, however, many more exist. Further research is needed to determine the best practices in debriefing and under what circumstances particular methods work best. There is a need for more research to investigate the relationship between time spent debriefing and meaningful learning and ways to adapt when there are time constraints. As simulation pedagogy evolves, there will also be a continued need for studies that explore how debriefing methods should also evolve.

SUMMARY

Debriefing is an important component of simulation and traditional clinical learning experiences. During debriefing, participants reflect on the experience and recount what occurred to understand actions and behaviors as well as decisions and judgments. A single best method of debriefing in all simulation and clinical environments remains elusive; however, there are several central components that should be included to optimize meaningful learning. Debriefing should include an opportunity for participants to diffuse their emotions, reflect on practice, and receive affirmation for their correct thoughts and actions, as well as points for improvement identified.

Novices particularly can benefit from debriefing that is facilitated by an experienced clinician who uncovers the thinking underpinning their correct as well as incorrect actions to ensure that clinical judgment and reasoning processes make sense. Reflection and the learning it potentiates are key outcomes of debriefing. Clinical instructors and debriefing facilitators can model reflection during meaningful debriefing and coach learners to develop a reflective practice.

Key Concepts

- Debriefing is an important component of simulation and traditional clinical learning.
- Reflection is a central component of meaningful debriefing, and participants may need to learn how to do it.
- The amount of time needed to debrief is highly dependent on what occurred during the simulation or clinical experience and the thinking and judgments that underpin the actions of the participants.
- It is important to take time during debriefing to explore the participant's thinking around correct as well as incorrect actions and to recognize both.

References

Arafeh, J. M. R., Hansen, S. S., & Nichols, A. (2010). Debriefing in simulated-based learning facilitating a reflective discussion. *Continuing Education, 24*(4), 302–309.

Benner, P., Sutphen, M., Leonard, V., & Day, L. (2010). *Educating nurses: A call for radical transformation.* San Francisco, CA: Jossey-Bass.

Boyd, E. M., & Fales, A. W. (1983). Reflective learning key to learning from experience. *Journal of Humanistic Psychology, 23*(2), 99–117.

Bybee, R. W., Buchwald, C. E., Crissman, S., Heil, D. R., Kuebis, P. J., Matsumoto, C., & McInerney, J. D. (1989). *Science and technology education for the elementary years: Frameworks for curriculum and instruction.* Washington, DC: National Center for Improving Science Education.

Candela, L. (2012). From teaching to learning: Theoretical foundations. In D. M. Billings & J. A. Halstead (Eds.), *Teaching in nursing: A guide for faculty* (4th ed., pp. 202–243). St. Louis: Elsevier.

Cantrell, M. A. (2008). The importance of debriefing in clinical simulations. *Clinical Simulation in Nursing, 4*(2), e19–e23.

Carper, B. (1978). Fundamental patterns of knowing in nursing. *Advances in Nursing Science, 1*(1), 13–23.

Cranton, P. (2006). *Understanding and promoting transformative learning: A guide for educators of adults.* San Francisco, CA: Jossey-Bass.

Decker, S. I., & Dreifuerst, K. T. (2012). Integrating guided reflection into simulated learning experiences. In P. R. Jeffries (Ed.), *Simulation in nursing education: From conceptualization to evaluation* (2nd ed., pp. 91–102). New York: National League for Nursing.

Dewey, J. (1933). *How we think: A restatement of reflective thinking to the educative process.* Boston: D.C. Heath. [Originally published in 1910].

Dreifuerst, K. T. (2009). The essentials of debriefing in simulation learning: A concept analysis. *Nursing Education Perspectives, 30*(2), 109–114.

Dreifuerst, K. T. (2010). Debriefing for meaningful learning: Fostering development of clinical reasoning through simulation [doctoral dissertation]. *Indiana University Scholar Works Repository.* Retrieved from http://hdl.handle.net/1805/2459.

Dreifuerst, K. T. (2012). Using debriefing for meaningful learning to foster development of clinical reasoning in simulation. *Journal of Nursing Education, 51*(6), 326–333.

Dreifuerst, K. T., & Decker, S. L. (2012). Debriefing: An essential component for learning in simulation pedagogy. In P. R. Jeffries (Ed.), *Simulation in nursing education: From conceptualization to evaluation* (pp. 105–129). New York: National League for Nursing.

Durgahee, T. (1997). Reflective practice: Nursing ethics through story telling. *Nursing Ethics, 4*(2), 135–146.

Fanning, R. M., & Gaba, D. M. (2007). The role of debriefing in simulation-based learning. *Simulation in Healthcare, 2*(2), 115–125.

Fonacier, T. L., McNelis, A. M., & Ebright, P. (2013, January 2). *Preparing students to think through the complexities of practice in post-clinical conferences.* Retrieved from http://qsen.org/faculty-resources/learning-modules/module-sixteen/

Freshwater, D. (2008). Reflective practice: The state of the art. In D. Freshwater, B. Taylor, & G. Sherwood (Eds.), *International textbook of reflective practice in nursing* (pp. 1–18). Oxford, UK: Blackwell.

Gibbs, G. (1988). Learning by doing: A guide to teaching and learning methods. Further Education Unit, Oxford Polytechnic, Now Oxford Brookes University. Retrieved from http://www2.glos.ac.uk/offload/tli/lets/lathe/issue1/issue1/pdf#oage=5.

Grant, J. S., Moss, J., Epps, C., & Watts, P. (2010). Using video-facilitated feedback to improve student performance following high-fidelity simulation. *Clinical Simulation in Nursing, 6*(5), e177–e184.

Hart, D., McNeil, M. A., Griswold-Theodorson, S., Bhatia, K., & Joing, S. (2012). High fidelity case-based simulation debriefing: Everything you need to know. *Academic Emergency Medicine, 19*(9), E1084–E1084.

Horton-Deutsch, S. (2012). Learning through reflection and reflection on learning: Pedagogies in action. In G. Sherwood & S. Horton-Deutsch (Eds.), *Reflective practice: Transforming education and improving outcomes* (pp. 103–134). Indianapolis: Sigma Theta Tau International.

Horton-Deutsch, S., Drew, B. L., & Beck-Coon, K. (2012). Mindful learners. In G. Sherwood & S. Horton-Deutsch (Eds.), *Reflective practice: Transforming education and improving outcomes* (pp. 79–99). Indianapolis: Sigma Theta Tau International.

Ironside, P. M., Jeffries, P. R., & Martin, A. (2009). Fostering patient safety competencies using multiple-patient simulation experiences. *Nursing Outlook, 57*(6), 332–337.

Issenberg, S. B., McGaghie, W. C., Petrusa, E. R., Lee Gordon, D., & Scalese, R. J. (2005). Features and uses of high-fidelity medical simulations that lead to effective learning: A BEME systematic review. *Medical Teacher, 27*, 10–28.

Johns, C. (2006). *Engaging reflection in practice: A narrative approach.* Oxford, United Kingdom: Blackwell Publishing, Ltd.

Johnson-Russell, J., & Bailey, C. (2010). Facilitated debriefing. In W. M. Nehring & F. R. Lashley (Eds.), *High fidelity patient simulation in nursing education* (pp. 369–386). Sudbury, MA: Jones and Bartlett.

Kabat-Zinn, J. (1990). *Full catastrophe living: Using the wisdom of your body and mind to face stress, pain, and illness.* New York: Delta.

Kolb, D. A. (1984). *Experiential learning: Experience as a source of learning and development.* Englewood Cliffs, NJ: Prentice-Hall.

Krmpotic, J. (2003). Reflective process in the study of illness stories as experienced by three nurse teachers. *Reflective Practice, 4*(1), 19–33.

Mariani, B., Cantrell, M. A., Meakim, C., Prieto, P., & Dreifuerst, K. T. (2013). Structured debriefing and students' clinical judgment abilities in simulation. *Clinical Simulation in Nursing, 9*(5), e147–e155.

Mezirow, J. (1981). Critical theory of adult learning and education. *Adult Education, 3*(1), 3–24.

Overstreet, M. (2010). EE-CHATS: The seven components of nursing debriefing. *Journal of Continuing Education in Nursing, 41*(12), 538–539.

Petranek, C. (2000). Written debriefing: The next vital step in learning with simulations. *Simulation & Gaming, 31*(1), 108–118.

Rudolph, J. W., Simon, R., Dufresne, R. L., & Raemer, D. B. (2006). There's no such thing as "nonjudgmental" debriefing: A theory and method for debriefing with good judgment. *Simulation in Healthcare, 1*(1), 49–55.

Rudolph, J. W., Simon, R., Rivard, P., Dufresne, R. L., & Raemer, D. B. (2007). Debriefing with good judgment: Combining rigorous feedback with genuine inquiry. *Anesthesiology Clinics, 25*(2), 361–376.

Schön, D. A. (1983). *The reflective practitioner: How professionals think in action.* New York: Basic Books.

Schön, D. A. (1987). *Educating the reflective practitioner.* San Francisco, CA: Jossey-Bass.

Sherwood, G., & Horton-Deutsch, S. (2012). *Reflective practice: Transforming education and improving outcomes.* Indianapolis: Sigma Theta Tau International.

Shinnick, M. A., Woo, M., Horwich, T. B., & Steadman, R. (2011). Debriefing: The most important component in simulation? *Clinical Simulation in Nursing, 7*(3), e105–e111.

Tanner, C. (2006). Thinking like a nurse: A research-based model of clinical judgment in nursing. *Journal of Nursing Education, 45*(6), 204–211.

Wang, E. E., Kharasch, M., & Kuruna, D. (2011). Facilitative debriefing techniques for simulation-based learning. *Academic Emergency Medicine, 18*(2), e5–e5.

Wickers, M. P. (2010). Establishing the climate for a successful debriefing. *Clinical Simulation in Nursing, 6*, e83–e86.

Yaeger, K. A., & Arafeh, J. M. R. (2008). Making the move: From traditional neonatal education to simulation-based training. *Journal of Perinatal & Neonatal Nursing, 22*(2), 154–158.

Zigmont, J. J., Kappus, L. J., & Sudikoff, S. N. (2011). The 3D model of debriefing: Defusing, discovering, and deepening. *Seminars in Perinatology, 35*(2), 52–58.

5

Interprofessional Education Using Clinical Simulations

Janice C. Palaganas, PhD, RN, NP, CEN
Mary Elizabeth Mancini, PhD, RN, NE-BC, FAHA, ANEF, FAAN

■ Learning Objectives

1. Discuss how health care simulation can be used to achieve the competencies associated with interprofessional collaborative practice through interprofessional education.
2. Provide practical recommendations to facilitate interprofessional education using health care simulation.

■ Key Terms

- Interdisciplinary learning
- Interprofessional collaborative practice
- Interprofessional education
- Multiprofessional education
- Multidisciplinary simulation
- Simulation-based interprofessional education

Interprofessional collaborative practice is recognized as a necessary element for achieving high-quality, cost-effective, patient-centered care (Aspden, Wolcott, Bootman, & Cronenwett, 2007; IOM, 2010). Interprofessional education (IPE) is increasingly being embraced as an essential mechanism for students in the health professions to achieve the competencies associated with effective interprofessional collaborative practice (Aspden et al., 2007; CCNE, 2009; Howard, 2012; Interprofessional Education Collaborative Expert Panel (IPECEP), 2012; IOM, 2010; NLNAC, 2012).

The concepts associated with interprofessional teamwork and education are not new. The notion of a team approach to health care has been around for decades. In spite of this, these important concepts still have not been fully integrated into all schools of health professions. This reflects not only the challenge of changing the status quo, an apprenticeship model of learning, but also the difficulties of bringing students from various health professional schools together for learning. This chapter will provide a brief overview of the key elements of interprofessional collaborative practice and outline examples of how health care simulation is being leveraged to provide a foundation for IPE in the academic settings as well as opportunities for education in the clinical setting with practicing health care providers.

INTERPROFESSIONAL COLLABORATIVE PRACTICE

Interprofessional collaborative practice has been defined by the World Health Organization (2010) as occurring "[w]hen multiple health workers from different professional backgrounds work together with patients, families, carers [sic], and communities to deliver the highest quality of care."

For more than four decades, the Institute of Medicine (1972, 2003) and others such as the Joint Commission (2008) have made the case that creating a safer, more patient-centered health care system requires members of the health professions to work together in collaborative teams. The challenge has been that although there has been agreement on the goal and the competencies, there has not been clarity on how to achieve them.

In the 2003 report "Health Professions Education: A Bridge to Quality," the Institute of Medicine proposed four core competencies for working in interprofessional teams: provide patient-centered care, utilize informatics, employ evidence-based practice, and apply quality improvement techniques. These competencies were further refined in 2011, when the Interprofessional Education Collaborative (IPEC, 2011) released its "Core Competencies for Interprofessional Collaborative Practice." The IPEC, which includes representatives from the American Association of Colleges of Nursing, American Association of Colleges of Osteopathic Medicine, American Association of College of Pharmacy, American Dental Education Association, Association of American Medical Colleges, and the Association of Schools of Public Health, identified two goals and four interprofessional competency domains, which are illustrated in Figure 5.1.

Under each of the four general domains, the IPEC identified specific competencies that nurses and other health care providers should acquire (Table 5.1). These competencies can and should be used to set specific learning objectives in simulations.

INTERPROFESSIONAL EDUCATION

Interprofessional education occurs "when two or more professions learn with, from and about each other to improve collaboration and the quality of care" (CAIPE, 2005). This can be contrasted to multidisciplinary or **multiprofessional education**, which occurs "when members (or students) of two or more professions learn alongside one another: in other words, parallel rather than interactive learning" (Freeth, Hammick, Reeves, Koppel, & Barr, 2005, p. xv). This distinction between interprofessional and multiprofessional education

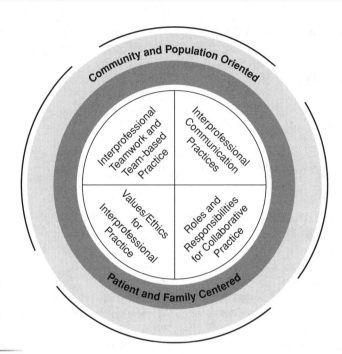

FIGURE 5.1 Interprofessional collaborative practice domains. Although being community and population oriented, the provision of patient- and family-centered care is the goal of interprofessional collaborative practice. The specific competencies associated with interprofessional collaborative practice can be organized into four basic domains: (1) values and ethics for interprofessional practice, (2) roles and responsibilities for collaborative practice, (3) interprofessional communication practices, and (4) interprofessional teamwork and team-based practices. © 2011 American Association of Colleges of Nursing, American Association of Colleges of Osteopathic Medicine, American Association of Colleges of Pharmacy, American Dental Education Association, Association of American Medical Colleges, and Association of Schools of Public Health. As found in Interprofessional Education Collaborative Expert Panel. (2011). *Core competencies for interprofessional collaborative practice: Report of an expert panel.* Washington, DC: Interprofessional Education Collaborative.

is an important one for educators to consider when developing educational activities for learners across the health professions.

Given more than 40 years of attempts toward interprofessional collaborative practice, one might assume that schools for health professionals would have integrated the concepts in meaningful ways into their curricula. Unfortunately, most are still struggling to identify substantive ways to integrate interprofessional education opportunities into their programs. With an accepted granular list of interprofessional collaborative practice competencies, nursing educators are now able to turn their attention to identifying mechanisms to develop these competencies in prelicensure students and postgraduate learners.

TABLE 5.1

Interprofessional Collaborative Practice Competencies

Domain 1: Values/Ethics for Interprofessional Practice

VE1. Place the interests of patients and populations at the center of interprofessional health care delivery.

VE2. Respect the dignity and privacy of patients while maintaining confidentiality in the delivery of team-based care.

VE3. Embrace the cultural diversity and individual differences that characterize patients, populations, and the health care team.

VE4. Respect the unique cultures, values, roles/responsibilities, and expertise of other health professions.

VE5. Work in cooperation with those who receive care, those who provide care, and others who contribute to or support the delivery of prevention and health services.

VE6. Develop a trusting relationship with patients, families, and other team members.

VE7. Demonstrate high standards of ethical conduct and quality of care in one's contributions to team-based care.

VE8. Manage ethical dilemmas specific to interprofessional patient/population-centered care situations.

VE9. Act with honesty and integrity in relationships with patients, families, and other team members.

VE10. Maintain competence in one's own profession appropriate to scope of practice.

Domain 2: Roles/Responsibilities

RR1. Communicate one's roles and responsibilities clearly to patients, families, and other professionals.

RR2. Recognize one's limitations in skills, knowledge, and abilities.

RR3. Engage diverse health care professionals who complement one's own professional expertise, as well as associated resources, to develop strategies to meet specific patient care needs.

RR4. Explain the roles and responsibilities of other care providers and how the team works together to provide care.

RR5. Use the full scope of knowledge, skills, and abilities of available health professionals and health care workers to provide care that is safe, timely, efficient, effective, and equitable.

RR6. Communicate with team members to clarify each member's responsibility in executing components of a treatment plan or public health intervention.

RR7. Forge interdependent relationships with other professions to improve care and advance learning.

RR8. Engage in continuous professional and interprofessional development to enhance team performance.

RR9. Use unique and complementary abilities of all members of the team to optimize patient care.

(continued)

TABLE 5.1

Interprofessional Collaborative Practice Competencies *(Continued)*

Domain 3: Interprofessional Communication

CC1. Choose effective communication tools and techniques, including information systems and communication technologies, to facilitate discussions and interactions that enhance team function.

CC2. Organize and communicate information with patients, families, and health care team members in a form that is understandable, avoiding discipline-specific terminology when possible.

CC3. Express one's knowledge and opinions to team members involved in patient care with confidence, clarity, and respect, working to ensure common understanding of information and treatment and care decisions.

CC4. Listen actively, and encourage ideas and opinions of other team members.

CC5. Give timely, sensitive, instructive feedback to others about their performance on the team, responding respectfully as a team member to feedback from others.

CC6. Use respectful language appropriate for a given difficult situation, crucial conversation, or interprofessional conflict.

CC7. Recognize how one's own uniqueness, including experience level, expertise, culture, power, and hierarchy within the health care team, contributes to effective communication, conflict resolution, and positive interprofessional working relationships.

CC8. Communicate consistently the importance of teamwork in patient-centered and community-focused care.

Domain 4: Teams and Teamwork

TT1. Describe the process of team development and the roles and practices of effective teams.

TT2. Develop consensus on the ethical principles to guide all aspects of patient care and teamwork.

TT3. Engage other health professionals—appropriate to the specific care situation—in shared patient-centered problem-solving.

TT4. Integrate the knowledge and experience of other professions—appropriate to the specific care situation—to inform care decisions, while respecting patient and community values and priorities/ preferences for care.

TT5. Apply leadership practices that support collaborative practice and team effectiveness.

TT6. Engage self and others to constructively manage disagreements about values, roles, goals, and actions that arise among health care professionals and with patients and families.

TT7. Share accountability with other professions, patients, and communities for outcomes relevant to prevention and health care.

TT8. Reflect on individual and team performance for individual, as well as team, performance improvement.

TT9. Use process improvement strategies to increase the effectiveness of interprofessional teamwork and team-based care.

TT10. Use available evidence to inform effective teamwork and team-based practices.

TT11. Perform effectively on teams and in different team roles in a variety of settings.

USING SIMULATION FOR INTERPROFESSIONAL HEALTH CARE EDUCATION

Interdisciplinary learning "involves integrating the perspective of professionals from two or more professions, by organizing the education around a specific discipline, where each discipline examines the basis of their knowledge" (Howkins & Bray, 2008, p. xviii). Simulation, with its full range of methodologies, is an effective approach to providing interprofessional health care education where students can truly learn from, with, and about one another in contextually relevant ways that focus on providing patient-centered care. **Simulation-based** (or simulation-enhanced) **interprofessional education** describes simulations that are created intentionally to focus on interprofessional learning objectives where students from two or more professions learn with, from, and about one another during the simulation. **Multidisciplinary** (or interdisciplinary) **simulations** describe simulations that are created using clinical, diagnosis-centered, or task-focused learning objectives, and students from two or more professions participate in the simulation, learning in parallel but not intentionally from and about one another during the simulation (Palaganas, 2012). This is an important distinction to understand. Many activities that are labeled IPE are actually multidisciplinary simulations with no specific intent to foster the development of the competencies required for effective interprofessional collaborative practice.

Educators in health professions schools are embracing simulation and using immersive simulations as well as standardized patients, screen-based simulation, virtual reality, and serious gaming. However, many educators are struggling with how to use these various simulation methodologies in an effective and efficient manner to facilitate the development of the competencies of interprofessional collaborative practice. Looking at the work of early adopters can provide guidance for those interested in starting or refining a program of simulation-enhanced IPE.

EXAMPLES OF SIMULATION-ENHANCED INTERPROFESSIONAL EDUCATION

In September 2011, the National League for Nursing (NLN) held a think tank on simulation-enhanced IPE (NLN, 2012). The purpose of the think tank was to identify nursing's perspective on the use of simulation-enhanced IPE. The attendees agreed that although consensus had not been reached on a best-practice model for IPE, simulation-based learning experiences were key to acquiring the requisite competencies for collaborative practice. Several examples of various approaches to simulation-enhanced IPE were identified as useful for other schools to consider.

The University of Colorado

The University of Colorado at Denver includes IPE for students in all of their health profession programs. Students from nursing, medicine, pharmacy, physical therapy, and dentistry have mandatory time requirements for interprofessional clinical activities including specifically designed immersive simulations focused on developing interprofessional collaborative competencies (NLN, 2012).

The Center for Education at St. Mary's Medical Center

The Center for Education at St. Mary's Medical Center in Huntington, West Virginia, supports the medical center's nursing, medical imaging, and respiratory care programs. On their common clinical learning day, students from the three programs rotate through an exercise that simulates an interprofessional emergency response team. In advance of their clinical learning day, all students review the roles and functions associated with an emergency response team and come prepared to respond if they are called on as a member of the simulated emergency response team. Not every student is called on every week, so students must remain prepared in case they are called. After the in situ simulation experience occurs, the students debrief as an interprofessional group with their faculty. Although coordination of this activity requires close collaboration among faculty members across the three programs, it provides an exemplar of how IPE can be done in the clinical setting (NLN, 2012).

The University of Kansas

Not every nursing school is situated on the campus of an academic health science center. There are often large distances between schools, causing specific challenges to IPE. Nursing students, medical students and residents, and pharmacy students at the University of Kansas participate in an interprofessional simulation that uses an electronic health record (EHR) as a bridge to learning across campuses. This simulation starts on the medical school campus. Here medical students review a pediatric patient's chart, learn the electronic order entry process, and write electronic orders in an EHR to admit the patient. Forty miles away, pharmacy students access the EHR, verify the medications, and assign each of the medications ordered to products within the formulary. Once the pharmacy students have completed their activities, the nursing students access the EHR and review the case before meeting with medical students and a pediatric resident for a simulation involving the hospitalized pediatric patient. Following completion of the immersive simulation scenario, nursing and medical students and faculty debrief together, helping students understand the unique roles and responsibilities of each discipline (NLN, 2012).

Texas Tech University

Finding the time to develop reliable scenarios and tools for conducting IPE is a challenge. At Texas Tech University Health Sciences Campus, faculty have embraced and adopted a well-established, externally developed training program called TeamSTEPPS® (Team Strategies and Tools to Enhance Performance and Patient Safety) as a mechanism for health profession students to learn with and from one another (Agency for Healthcare Research and Quality [AHRQ], 2008). TeamSTEPPS is an evidence-based interprofessional training system designed by the U.S. Department of Defense and the Agency for Healthcare Research and Quality. The goal of the training is to improve quality, safety, and efficiency of health care through the development of individual as well as group skills and attitudes associated with high-performing teams. Using various simulation techniques, learners focus on achieving four core competencies: team leadership, situational (or mutual performance) monitoring, mutual support, and communication. As the various health profession programs on campus have embraced the development of these competencies in all health professionals, students are expected to use the TeamSTEPPS competencies whenever they participate in any simulation activities as well as in their clinical settings (NLN, 2012).

For educators working with practicing health care practitioners, using TeamSTEPPS materials is an excellent way to provide IPE in the clinical setting. Identifying intact interprofessional teams such as those in the operating room, labor and delivery suite, and emergency department for training will maximize the opportunity for successful training.

Another example of an integrated IPE experience involves the medical and nursing schools at New York University. The purpose of the teaching, technology, teamwork (NYU3T) program (2013) is "to provide NYU medical and nursing students with longitudinal exposure to a diverse patient population and systematic interdisciplinary education in the competencies of team-based care" (NYU, 2013). Focused on creating a physical and virtual environment that fosters IPE and developing a curriculum for interdisciplinary team training, the project uses web-based learning modules, virtual patients, manikin-based interprofessional simulations, and clinical "cross-overs" where students shadow students in other disciplines. Materials from this project, including the curriculum, are available on the NYU website (New York University Langone Medical Center, 2013).

OVERCOMING BARRIERS TO SIMULATION-ENHANCED INTERPROFESSIONAL EDUCATION

Beyond the barriers associated with any simulation (e.g., time, resources, space), participants in the NLN think tank identified a number of factors that limit nurse educators' ability to incorporate simulation-enhanced IPE into nursing courses and curricula (SSH & NLN, 2013). These include:

- Scheduling issues when working with multiple programs
- Unequal number of students in each program, creating a challenge to provide enough IPE opportunities for each student nurse to work with medical students, pharmacy students, and allied health profession students
- Lack of colocated or geographically proximate health professions programs with which to partner
- Lack of recognition by administrations of the impact of IPE on faculty workload
- Faculty and administrative resistance to change
- State-to-state variability on the amount of simulation allowed within a program
- Role confusion both inside and outside the boundaries of the nursing discipline due to the various levels of education allowing different points of entry into practice

The Society for Simulation in Healthcare and the NLN, with support from a grant from the Josiah Macy Jr. Foundation, held an invitational meeting of 22 organizations representing various professional health care disciplines (including nursing, medicine, pharmacy, dental, and allied health), accreditors of academic programs in the health professions, professional societies (including the NLN), regulatory, and patient safety

TABLE 5.2

Challenges to Simulation-Enhanced Interprofessional Education in Health Care

1. *Reasons for Slow Adoption:*
   - Lack of *substantive* and specific accreditation mandates (e.g., exit competency and certification requirements)
   - Insufficient infrastructure and resources (funding, faculty development and incentives, educational materials)
   - Limited support for research (appropriate evaluation instruments, assessment tools, evaluation strategies) that demonstrate impact of simulation-enhanced interprofessional education on actual quality care and patient safety

2. *Logistical Challenges:*
   - Lack of curriculum mapping across discipline-specific educational programs (matching students)
   - Conducting interprofessional education when the discipline ratios are disproportionate
   - Finding space
   - Scheduling time when disciplines have existing schedules
   - Coordinating interprofessional education activities when educational programs are not colocated

3. *Challenges to Current Culture:*
   - Faculty and administrative resistance
   - Traditional compartmentalization, "silos"

experts. The purpose of the program was to identify ways to overcome barriers to effectively and efficiently integrate simulation into IPE in the academic and clinical settings. Although there was great variability in the examples of simulation-enhanced IPE activities reported by the invitees, there was consistency in the gaps, challenges, and opportunities identified across the organizations. Table 5.2 lists the reasons identified for slow adoption of simulation-enhanced IPE in health care, typical logistical challenges to implementing simulation-enhanced IPE, and cultural challenges to be overcome if change is to occur (SSH & NLN, 2013).

A number of strategies have been identified to address the commonly identified challenges associated with running simulation-enhanced IPE. These include:

- *Identify champions within each partner school:* Using simulation as an enabling mechanism for IPE and ultimately enhancing interprofessional collaboration require a champion from each discipline involved. Once identified, a working group can be established to address the issues of matching the level of learners so as to maximize interaction and impact, determining if the IPE will be mandatory or optional, finding time for IPE experiences within the current constraints of individual programs' academic schedule or clinical schedules, and identifying a cadre of individual faculty willing to participate in development and evaluation of the IPE experiences.

- *Clarify the learning objectives for the IPE:* Simulation allows for multiple learning objectives. A key to success is to ensure that all faculty members involved are clear on the objectives for the experience (e.g., Is the focus on learning specific discipline-related content or skills or addressing specific competencies associated with effective interprofessional collaborative practice?).

- *Select the appropriate simulation methodology:* A common simulation method used for IPE is immersive simulations with high-technology manikins. However, this is not the only simulation methodology that can be used for IPE. Scenarios using standardized patients as well as emerging technologies (e.g., virtual simulations, Second Life, and multiplayer gaming) should be considered when trying to overcome barriers related to limited access to a simulation center, distance between campuses or locations, and scheduling challenges. Being creative and open to leveraging the full array of simulation methodologies will open up more options for IPE. For example, if money is limited, consider recruiting retired health care professionals to serve as standardized patients. Before deciding to develop IPE materials internally, consider using established tools and scenarios available through open sources. Excellent materials for use in both health professions programs and in clinical settings can be found on the websites for the Agency for Healthcare Research and Quality (AHRQ) and MedEdPortal.[1]

- *Provide faculty development:* The faculty team's level of knowledge and comfort with the competencies of interprofessional collaborative practice and simulation, as well as their professional values and teaching capabilities, can greatly influence learning outcomes. Although most faculty are comfortable within their discipline, interacting with faculty and students from other disciplines can be challenging. Ensuring there is time for the faculty to get to know one another and articulate their program and individual expectations is important. In addition, simulation as a teaching and learning methodology might be new to some faculty. Training as a team with the equipment that will be used will help minimize unexpected challenges and stresses during the IPE experience.

- *Prepare for interprofessional debriefing:* It is critical that the individuals who will be facilitating the debriefing discuss in advance how they plan to debrief an interprofessional group of learners. It will be important that the faculty or facilitators intentionally reflect on their personal assumptions about roles, values, and beliefs. Providing psychological safety and support during IPE comes with an additional challenge as students and faculty might be uncomfortable with self-disclosure in front of other disciplines. The interaction among the faculty members during the scenario and the debriefing is an opportunity to role model interprofessional respect, communication, and teamwork. As students progress to practicing

---

[1]www.ahrq.gov and https://www.mededportal.org

professionals, they will need to be able to engage in respectful peer-to-peer evaluation and in situ, postevent debriefings. These are skills they will develop during interprofessional debriefings while in their professional training. As such, educators engaged in IPE should embrace the opportunity that debriefing provides.

- *Decide in advance how the impact of IPE will be evaluated:* Because IPE, especially when it involves simulation, is new to many nursing programs, it is important to develop evaluation criteria early in the process. Remember to use validated and reliable evaluation instruments (Hammick, Freeth, Koppel, Reeves, & Barr, 2008; Howkins & Bray, 2008). Attending to this step will help build the body of evidence of what works and why investing time and effort in IPE is worthwhile. Disseminating findings will help overcome objections and provide the data necessary to stimulate change.

RESOURCES FOR SIMULATION-ENHANCED IPE

As programs embrace simulation-enhanced IPE, there are a number of directly related resources available to help faculty develop an IPE program that achieves the desired outcome of enhanced interprofessional collaborative practice:

- The Centre for the Advancement of Interprofessional Education is an international think tank focused on promoting and developing interprofessional education. Their website has an abundant list of resources.
- The Josiah Macy Foundation provides examples of simulation-enhanced IPE activities.
- The MedEdPortal focused on IPE provides easy access to peer-reviewed materials and information related to IPE.
- The NLN Simulation Innovation Resource Center, an online e-learning site for nursing faculty, is a resource for IPE scenarios.
- The Society for Simulation in Healthcare provides examples and networking for educators interested in simulation-enhanced IPE.
- The TeamSTEPPS website provides information on training that is directly related to competencies that fit into every health profession curriculum and at all levels of nursing education.
- The University of Washington Center for Health Science Interprofessional Education, Research and Practice provides a robust repository of IPE resources including free educational presentations and webinars on curriculum design and development.[2]

---

[2]The web URLs for these are, respectively: http://www.caipe.org.uk, www.josiahmacyfoundaiton.org, https://www.mededportal.org/ipe/, www.sirc.nln.org, www.ssih.org, http://teamstepps.ahrq.gov, http://collaborate.uw.edu/resources-and-publications/ipe-resources.html.

■ Key Concepts

- Health care simulation has been demonstrated to be an effective tool to achieve the competencies associated with interprofessional collaborative practice through interprofessional education.
- The creation of simulation activities specifically targeting the IPE competencies associated with interprofessional collaborative practice will provide a foundation for effective interprofessional education.
- Engaging in effective simulation-enhanced interprofessional education requires faculty to establish directed learning objectives, select the appropriate simulation method, and prepare for the IPE experience.

References

Agency for Healthcare Research and Quality. (2008). *TeamSTEPPS: Team strategies & tools to enhance performance & patient safety instructor guide.* Washington DC: AHRQ Publications.

Aspden, P., Wolcott, J. A., Bootman, J., & Cronenwett, L. R. (Eds.). (2007). *Preventing medication errors.* Washington, DC: National Academies Press. Retrieved from http://www.nap.edu/catalog.php?record_id=11623

Center for the Advancement of Interprofessional Education (CAIPE). (2005). Defining IPE. Retrieved from http://www.caipe.org.uk/about-us/defining-ipe

Commission on Collegiate Nursing Education (CCNE). (2009). *Standards for accreditation of baccalaureate and graduate degree nursing programs.* Washington, DC: Author.

Djukic, M., Fulmer, T., Adams, J. G., Lee, S., & Triola, M. M. (2012). NYU3T: Teaching, technology, teamwork: A model for interprofessional education scalability and sustainability. *Nursing Clinic of North America, 47*(3), 333–346.

Freeth, D., Hammick, M., Reeves, S., Koppel, I., & Barr, H. (2005). *Effective interprofessional education: Development, delivery & evaluation.* Oxford, UK: Blackwell.

Hammick, M., Freeth, D., Koppel, I., Reeves, S., & Barr, H. (2008). A best evidence systematic review of interprofessional education. *Medical Teacher, 29*(8), 735–751.

Howard, V. M. (2012). President's message: Interprofessional Education and Healthcare Simulation Symposium. *Clinical Simulation in Nursing, 8*(3), e77.

Howkins, E., & Bray, J. (2008). *Preparing for interprofessional teaching.* Oxon, UK: Radcliffe Publishing.

Institute of Medicine (IOM). (1972). *Educating for the health team.* Washington, DC: National Academy of Sciences.

Institute of Medicine (IOM). (2003). *Health professions education: A bridge to quality.* Washington, DC: The National Academies of Science.

Institute of Medicine (IOM). (2010). *The future of nursing: Leading change, advancing health.* Washington, DC: National Academies Press. Retrieved from http://www.iom.edu/Reports/ 2010/The-Future-of-Nursing-Leading-Change-Advancing-Health.aspx

Interprofessional Education Collaborative Expert Panel (IPECEP). (2011). *Core competencies for interprofessional collaborative practice: Report of an expert panel.* Washington, DC: Author.

Joint Commission. (2008). *Health care at the crossroads: Strategies for improving the medical liability system and preventing patient injury.* Retrieved from www.jointcommission.org/assets/1/18/Medical_Liability.pdf

National League for Nursing Accrediting Commission. (NLNAC). (2012). *NLNAC accreditation manual.* Atlanta, GA:

Author. Retrieved from http://www.nlnac.org/manuals/NLNACManual2008.pdf

National League for Nursing (NLN). (2012). *A nursing perspective on simulation and interprofessional education (IPE): A report from the National League for Nursing's think tank on using simulation as an enabling strategy for IPE.* Retrieved from http://www.nln.org/facultyprograms/facultyresources/pdf/nursing_perspective_sim_education.pdf

New York University Langone Medical Center (NYULMC). (2013). *NYU3T: Teaching, technology, teamwork.* Retrieved from http://dei.med.nyu.edu/research/nyu3t

Palaganas, J. (2012). *Exploring healthcare simulation as a platform for interprofes-sional education* (Doctoral dissertation). Retrieved from ProQuest Dissertations and Theses database, http://gradworks.umi.com/35/47/3547895.html

Society for Simulation in Healthcare & National League for Nursing (SSH & NLN). (2013). *A report from the Inter-professional Education and Healthcare Simulation Symposium.* Retrieved from http://ssih.org/uploads/static_pages/ipe-final_compressed.pdf

World Health Organization (WHO). (2010). *Framework for action on interprofes-sional education and collaborative practice.* Geneva: Author. Retrieved from http://whqlibdoc.who.int/hq/2010/WHO_HRH_HPN_10.3_eng.pdf

6

Serious Gaming Using Simulations

Eric B. Bauman, PhD, RN
Penny Ralston-Berg, MS

■ Learning Objectives

1. Compare the potential types of learners in the intended nursing and clinical education audience.
2. Debate the need for engagement in nursing and clinical education.
3. Define just-in-time learning.
4. Describe how just-in-time learning contributes to clinical education.
5. Summarize how the traditional pedagogy of experiential learning and problem solving impacts clinical education.
6. Summarize how the contemporary pedagogy of created spaces, socially situated cognition, and design experience impacts clinical education.
7. Outline the similarities, differences, and crossover of games and simulations.
8. Recognize strategies for successful integration of games.
9. Identify the key questions to ask when integrating games into the curricula.
10. Explain the perspectives from which technology in the curriculum must be evaluated.

■ Key Terms

- Created environment or space
- Designed experience
- Digital immigrant
- Digital native
- Just-in-time learning

This chapter provides an introduction to game-based learning for nursing and clinical education. We will frame our discussion with an emphasis on audience, engagement, and the concept of targeted just-in-time learning. The chapter also includes a review of traditional and contemporary pedagogies that support game-based learning and covers several other topics integral to the successful integration of serious games into nursing and other health sciences curricula. To end the chapter, we will address how games can expand traditional learning spaces, the notion of games and curricular fit, and evaluation.

AUDIENCE

Successfully creating or selecting a game for inclusion into a new or existing lesson or curriculum starts with an examination of your intended audience. Today's traditional students possess a level of media savvy that often exceeds that of their instructors and faculty (Bauman, 2010). Furthermore, making assumptions about media literacy based on common assumptions and stereotypes is fraught with error and erroneous information.

Close to 99 percent of U.S. teens report that they play videogames of some sort (Ito, 2009). However, the Entertainment Software Association (2011) reports that the average age of sampled game players is 37 and that a greater proportion of game players are women over the age of 18 than there are boys under the age of 17. These demographics do not support many of the stereotypes associated with videogame players. Although it is true that teenage boys continue to play videogames, the overall audience and appetite for videogames are much more diverse and broad.

Prensky (2001) coined the terms *digital native* and *digital immigrant*. Although these terms are now well over 10 years old, they continue to illustrate an important challenge. Almost all of our students are **digital natives**, those who grew up immersed in digital technology, who may have spent more time playing videogames than they did reading by the time they began college (Prensky, 2003). The digital native is able to leverage digital technology intuitively. "*Digital natives* are fluent in the language of the digital environment. They possess an innate sense of media literacy" (Bauman, 2012, pp. 79–80, emphasis in original).

Many nursing leaders and faculty are digital immigrants. **Digital immigrants** generally represent those of us who were born prior to the digital media explosion and have had to adapt to an increasingly inclusive digital environment. Although adapting to digital environments is possible, the digital immigrant faces the same challenges that any nonnative speaker encounters when immersed into a new sociocultural environment. Immigrants are often biased by their previous nonnative experiences. They carry the artifacts of the old world with them and must learn to negotiate in a modern and rapidly advancing technocracy. The reality for many digital immigrants is that they will rarely achieve native levels of digital literacy (Bauman, 2012; Prensky, 2001).

The challenge for leadership and faculty occurs when the needs and expectations of the modern-day student are juxtaposed with the traditional learning models and curricula that many faculty are comfortable with. Failing to meet student expectations as they relate to access and delivery of the curriculum will simply push the best and brightest students to those campuses and institutions that are best suited to meet their needs (Bauman, 2012).

ENGAGEMENT

Engagement is an often-debated concept in education. Some teachers resent the notion of the teacher as entertainer. Others insist that education, particularly clinical education, should not be fun, and that clinical education is serious business. Both of these perspectives are misguided. Engaging learning opportunities can be fun and nothing is lost by creating learning experiences that are enjoyable. To the contrary, leveraging technology, including games, to create active learning experiences increases learner engagement (Gee, 2003).

If we accept that contemporary learners expect to leverage technology to achieve academic and later clinical mastery, then we must explore and integrate digital pedagogy, including game-based learning, into the clinical curricula. We have already embraced the digital environment for many aspects of nursing education. Literature searches to support best practices and clinical preparedness have moved from the library stacks to the laptop and even mobile devices. Is it such a stretch to accept that didactic preparation and even some forms of simulation are moving away from the face-to-face learning medium and into the digital game-based medium? "Interactivity and engagement are hallmarks of games and online environments; they are also known to lead to deeper learning" (Oblinger, 2004, p. 15).

JUST-IN-TIME LEARNING

Just-in-time learning supports advancement through learning exercises and experiences. In other words, just-in-time learning allows a student to acquire knowledge to support continuous learning in a situated and contextually relevant manner. Just-in-time learning facilitates a solution to a challenge in real time, rather than sometime in the future. Good videogames seed the game environment with pearls to support first proficiency and later mastery. In this way, needed and relevant information need not be recalled from some distant lecture with little if any contextual meaning, but rather information becomes available to learners and is reinforced as they need it to progress through a problem (Gee, 2003). Videogames often leverage this type of design to increase player engagement and support player success (Bauman, 2012; Squire, 2006). Simulations accomplish this through real-time feedback, decision making, opportunity for self-correction, and mastery through practice (Aldrich, 2009a).

Just-in-time learning mirrors actual clinical practice. In actual practice, nurses and other clinicians work to solve ill-structured problems. They do not have all of the needed information about any given patient prior to actually encountering the patient. In actual clinical settings, known patient information in the form of a shift or handoff report is not always available. Yet traditional problem-based learning presents students with an "if/then" style of learning that is detached from actual practice. Nursing students often prepare for clinical encounters 12 to 24 hours before they actually take care of patients. The information they glean in preparation is often irrelevant by the time they actually care for their patient. Modern videogame design supports a model of information availability that more accurately models actual clinical practice.

In game design, information is presented through immersion in the environment, authentic patient interaction, and situational feedback. Games implore students to leverage their environment to mobilize information rather than recall memorized facts (Oblinger, 2004). Games and simulations also encourage independent thought and decision making based on the experience rather than following a predescribed decision path (Aldrich, 2009a).

PEDAGOGY

Traditional Pedagogy Supporting Game-Based Learning

Experiential Learning: Kolb, Benner, and Schön

Experiential learning models are often used to frame theoretical discussions that support clinical education as well as simulation and game-based learning. In addition to providing the theoretical framework for these discussions, they also provide the groundwork for the introduction of more contemporary theories specifically explicated for learning that takes place with or is facilitated by videogames. As is the case with all theories, founding authors have no control, nor can they really foresee, how their theories will be used to support theoretical foundations.

Kolb's (1984) experiential learning cycle includes four elements moving in a clockwise fashion. Each element relates to another so the cycle remains continuous. The elements of Kolb's learning cycle are experience, reflection, conceptualization, and experimentation. The *experience* element of Kolb's model relates to information or knowledge acquired through firsthand or practical experience of the learner. *Reflection* refers to a process that is unique to the learner. It is the learner's interpretation of his or her experience. *Conceptualization* refers to the analytical abilities and integration of ideas and applications of existing concepts associated with learners' experience and reflection. Finally, *experimentation* occurs when the learner applies decision making and problem-solving skills to implement new concepts into his or her current practice. Experimentation gives rise for the potential to create a new experience, beginning the cycle again (Bauman, 2007; Kolb, 1984; Merriam & Caffarella, 1999). Kolb's experimental learning model represents an important foundation in adult learning theory because it fits well with the concept of lifelong learning. From the perspective of game-based learning, it is important because it implicates the student in his or her own learning process. In other words, learners are not seen as passive subjects to be informed by teachers; instead, students are responsible for knowledge creation.

Benner (1984) argued that nurses enter the profession as novices and that over time they progress to expert-level clinicians. The move from novice to expert occurs as nurses gain relevant experience upon which to draw. The distinction between novices and experts is ultimately made by the quality of decisions a nurse is capable of making while thinking in action. Experts are able to make decisions by drawing not only from content acquired in the classroom or through some other form of didactic transfer of knowledge, but also through past practice experience. In traditional nursing education, students or prenovices and those just entering the profession simply do not have clinical experience from which they can draw upon to solve complex clinical challenges.

As students and later novices acquire more clinical experience, they begin to recognize patient presentation, diagnostic, and practice patterns specific to their area of expertise. Pattern recognition skills represent a hallmark component differentiating the clinical ability among novices and experts. Principles deployed in simulation and game-based learning that situates meaningful experiences bolster and augment actual clinical encounters. Experts come to recognize patterns that often lead them to conclusions much more quickly and more accurately than novices. This can explain why experts may not perform as well as students (novices) on standardized tests or practical exams based on check-off lists, but often clinically outperform novices (Bauman, 2007; Bauman & Games, 2011; Benner, 1984; Gee, 2003; Murray et al., 2002).

Schön's (1983) discussion of effective professional practice also represents an experiential theoretical perspective. Schön discusses the role of thinking or reflection-in-action, but also emphasizes the importance of thinking or reflection-on-action. In Schön's theory, the professional engages in an internal dialogue with a problematic situation or experience. This internal conversation or back-talk, a form of self-generated feedback, helps guide and inform decision making. The distinction to be noted for clinical education is that the student or prenovice may have no ability or reference point to accurately reflect-in or think-in-action. Students who are just beginning nurses' training do not yet have a vetted context for reflection and must rely on their teachers to provide guided reflection until they have more experience situated within the context of the profession (Bauman, 2010, 2012; Bauman & Games, 2011; Games & Bauman, 2011).

Problem Solving: Barrows and Jonassen

Barrows's (1986) taxonomy of problem-based learning methods identifies four objectives important to clinical education: structuring knowledge, reasoning, self-directed learning, and motivation. These objectives facilitate successful future performance in a clinical setting and are best met by "the use of problems in the instructional sequence" (p. 481). He suggests that desired outcomes, cost, and feasibility can impact the selection of a problem-based learning method. Methods range from traditional lectures to cases to simulations with varying degrees of student responsibility for their own learning. For example, a more traditional case-based lecture is a less expensive option and requires little additional preparation or production of resource materials. However, a problem-based simulation with a high degree of learner control requires advanced planning, instructional design, and more time and effort of content experts, plus more information vetting, instructor facilitation, and assessment methods. Barrows adds that evaluation is critical to the problem-based learning process. Without evaluation, students will not be properly motivated to participate, and instructors might not be able to determine whether the learning objectives were met.

Also related to problem-based learning, Jonassen's (1997) instructional design models distinguish between well-structured and ill-structured problem solving. He contends well-structured problems "are constrained problems with convergent solutions that engage the application of a limited number of rules and principles within well-defined parameters" (p. 65). Such problems in clinical practice tend to point students down a prescribed path toward a "correct" answer based on the constraints. Jonassen defines ill-structured problems as having "multiple solutions, solution paths, fewer parameters which are less manipulable, and contain uncertainty about which concepts, rules, and principles are necessary for the solution or how they are organized and which solution is best" (p. 65). Ill-structured problems are more appropriate in preparing students for clinical practice in that they encourage decision making based on presented variables and situations. Without a predetermined path, students receive a more life-like experience.

Contemporary Pedagogy Supporting Game-Based Learning

Created Environments or Spaces

Created environments or spaces are engineered, built, or programmed to accurately replicate a perceived or existing space. These spaces aim to produce sufficient authenticity and fidelity to allow for the suspension of disbelief. They can be fixed in the case of manikin or standardized patient simulation laboratories resembling elaborate theatrical sets or can exist within a virtual reality or game-based environment (Bauman, 2007, 2010, 2012).

Created spaces should support curriculum objectives and narratives. However, when designing these spaces, educators must understand that there are drawbacks in providing too much fidelity. This may be distracting to learners who are just beginning to explore the virtual world and game-based learning environments. For example, compare a very engaging theatrical production that has attendees on the edge of their seats with a terrible multimillion dollar movie steeped with special effects. The goal of your environment is to support the production or narrative. Although we want students to engage in the game, to leave no stone unturned, we also want some value in doing so. When students engage in the game-based environment, the interactivity and fidelity of the environment should map back to the lesson plan and the curriculum.

Created spaces, particularly digital or game-based spaces, offer educational designers and teachers the ability to provide practice environments that are otherwise unavailable. Availability refers to clinical venues as well as the variables of time and location. Created spaces provide consistency among students and the experiences that are expected of them in school. For example, a game-based environment can provide labor and delivery experiences for every nursing student, whether or not he or she has the opportunity to attend a "live" delivery. Further, a game-based created labor and delivery environment can be used to support other kinds opportunities that support clinical experiences, including manikin-based labor and delivery experiences.

As clinical venues become more and more sparse, we often turn to simulation-based technology to fill essential gaps in clinical training and preparedness. However, the cost of operating physical simulation laboratories is expensive and time consuming. We need students to come to their simulation labs as prepared as possible. Yet we struggle to find time to run students through several simulation experiences per semester. Clinical competency and later mastery require multiple repetitions. This sort of repetition simply cannot and should not occur on actual patients, and supervised simulation laboratory time is often not available to orient students for optimal success. Digital game-based environments and mobile applications provide students with access to situated and engaging learning opportunities without regard to time and location.

Socially Situated Cognition

Nursing and other forms of clinical education are not simply about students moving through a curriculum and meeting benchmarks that attempt to demonstrate competence or proficiency. Nor is the educational process limited to what an individual student is thinking. Rather education, particularly educational processes that prepare students for professional or clinical practice, is situated within a material, social, and cultural world. In other words, the process of learning to become a nurse and actually practicing as one are situated within a contextually specific environment with a host of values and expectations (Bauman, 2007; Bauman & Games, 2011; Games & Bauman 2011; Gee, 2003).

Game-based environments have the ability to immerse students into *created environments* that provide a context for the roles that students hope to assume professionally. The roles that students play in virtual or game-based environments provide a situated context of nursing practice that allow students to complete activities and to interact with others in ways that authentically foreshadow and model future practice. In the traditional supervised clinical experience, the student can only be a student. He or she is identified as a student by the nature of who that student is at that given moment in time.

Immersion into a game-based world requires players to "try on" different identities that exist within a virtual community (Bartle, 2004; Bruckman, 2004; Games & Bauman, 2011; Gee, 2003). Virtual communities can be designed to model communities of practice. Within the confines of the game narrative, players are not biased in terms of role assignment. This is to say that a student playing the role of the charge nurse or triage nurse is in fact a nurse within the confines and context of his or her immersion in the game-based environment. This sort of immersion and role assignment provides students with facets of acculturation into the profession of nursing that are simply not available in actual supervised clinical experiences.

The negotiation of who the student is now and what role he or she is playing during game play is something Gee (2003) calls the projective identity. The projective identity is the learners' reflection on assumptions and implications associated with the reconciliation of their game and real-world identities. Students' real-world identities are initially fairly rigid; they are preconceived and biased. Identities assigned in the context of a game environment are immediately assignable and malleable. From an academic context, game-based identity can represent learners' future identity (Bauman & Games, 2011; Games & Bauman, 2011).

As previously discussed, pattern recognition as a component of thinking and reflecting-in-action is a key component of experiential learning theory and is also an essential facet of socially situated cognition. We teach nurses and other clinicians to recognize patterns to develop their diagnoses. Until students gain experience identifying patterns and have the opportunity to compare these patterns to unfolding narratives, they are not able to make sense of real-time clinical events occurring in front of them. The progression from novice to expert is not simply a measure of time-in-state, but rather a function of meaningful and deliberate practice within the context of nursing. Lived and situated experience need not be confined to the real world taking place in classrooms and supervised clinical venues, but valuable experiences that support pattern recognition can and should be acquired in both game-based and real-world environments, which leads to quality decision making on the path from novice to expert (Bauman, 2010; Bauman & Games, 2011; Games & Bauman, 2011).

Designed Experience

According to Squire's (2006) theory of **designed experience**, "participants learn through a grammar of *doing* and *being*" (p. 19, emphasis in original). Designed experiences guide learners not only through new domains of knowledge but also introduce them to new context-dependent skills in situated environments that support an authentic narrative. This is accomplished by presenting learners with targeted problem-solving opportunities that provide consequential feedback and allow learners to test the limits of their new capabilities and the boundaries of the roles they are performing (DeVane & Bauman, 2012).

Another key element of designed experiences is that students see learning as the embodiment of performance. Students are encouraged to move beyond skill and drill-style task-oriented exercises. This is a departure from viewing technology, including games and simulation, as a simple mechanism for knowledge transfer. Games are not simply "teaching machines" (Skinner, 1960), but rather have the potential to encourage complex thinking and facilitate behavioral change. Players or learners co-create knowledge and experience that propels them through educational processes. From this context, a student nurse not only learns how to start an intravenous line or give a medication, but also experiences the rewards or consequences of doing so within a carefully thought-out narrative in a created space based on participation structures that encourage learning through context-rich performance (Bauman, 2007; DeVane & Bauman, 2012; Games & Bauman, 2011).

The notion of learning as performance is consistent with nursing education and practice. Nursing and many other clinical disciplines are performance based. The process of becoming a nurse moves beyond knowledge transfer. One cannot learn to become a nurse simply by reading textbooks. The process of becoming a nurse is more than the sum of its parts; it is cognitive, behavioral, and social. This process takes place through performance. Instructors and mentors constantly evaluate learner performance as a measure for clinical readiness and entry into the profession. Seeing learning as performance might help future nursing faculty and leaders frame technology, including digital games, as an integral part of the nursing curriculum.

Ecology of Culturally Competent Design

Bauman (2010) and Bauman and Games (2011) developed the ecology of culturally competent design to provide a framework to evaluate and design videogames in the context of practice professions, including nursing and other forms of clinical education. The ecology of culturally competent design focuses on four elements: activities, context, narrative, and character.

Activities

Activities refers to what a learner or student will do in a game or virtual environment. The most powerful activities are authentically situated with attention to environmental fidelity and account for social and behavioral facets of practice, culture, and diversity. Activities should be based on expert knowledge of the communities and individuals represented within game-based environments (Bauman, 2010; Bauman & Games, 2011; Games & Bauman, 2011).

Context

Context refers to the way a learner is able to interact with the game environment. In the most meaningful and engaging games, context is fluid and malleable. It is defined and redefined by the interaction that exists between learners and their environment, as well as others inhabiting the environment (Bauman, 2010; Bauman & Games, 2011; Games & Bauman, 2011). For example, the way students interact with the digital environment as well as with one another in a videogame will drive other elements of game play. If a player fails to wash his or her hands before beginning a procedure, a situated consequence may occur later during game play. However, this consequence and practice error might be mitigated if another student who is also engaged in the same videogame points out this error and reminds the first student to wash his or her hands prior to starting the procedure.

Narrative

Narratives should be an intentional and integrated part of the game environment. Game narratives should situate identity and engage learners to the extent that experiences in a game provide important patterns that can be recalled during actual clinical performance. Game narratives can provide memories with a collection of patterns that help students recognize and make sense of real-world experiences in the same way that traditional manikin-based simulation can provide important clinical experiences to drive effective real-world practice (Bauman, 2010; Bruner, 1991; Games & Bauman, 2011; Gee, 1991, 2003).

Character

The element of character at sophisticated levels of game play should represent students' in-game identities as the projective identity (Gee, 2003). Recall from our earlier discussion that the projective identity is a negotiation of a player's in-game existence with the player's actual real-world identity. Games and Bauman (2011) concur, positing:

> Identity necessarily and purposely drives in-world interaction and experience. The virtual world provides cues to encourage reflection on the role of character and identity during the process of professional acculturation associated with the clinical affinity group that the student hopes to join. (p. 195)

GAMES, SIMULATIONS, AND THEIR APPLICATIONS

Definitions of Games and Simulations

Abt (1987) defines a game as "an activity among two or more independent decision makers seeking to achieve their objectives in some limiting context" (pp. 6–7). He adds that although some may think of games as adversarial, in which players attempt to "win" over opponents, some games are cooperative and require players to work together to overcome a common challenge. Cruickshank and Telfer (1980) define games as "contests in which both players and opponents operate under rules to gain a specified objective" (p. 75). In terms of games for learning, Schwartzman (1997) characterizes games as having structure or rules, a purpose or goal, an identified desirable outcome, and rewards for successful play. A more modern definition from Alrich (2009b) describes games as "fun, engaging activities usually used purely for entertainment, but they may also allow people to gain exposure to a particular set of tools, motions, or ideas" (p. 1).

Cruickshank (1968) defines simulations as "creation of realistic experiences to be played out by participants in order to provide them with life-like problem-solving experiences related to their present or future work" (pp. 190–191). Aldrich (2009b) describes simulations as using "rigorously structured scenarios carefully designed to develop specific competencies that can be directly transferred into the real world" (p. 1). Aldrich contends simulations are a good fit for nonlinear, dynamic content in which learners perform analysis, decision making, and implementation within a changing environment.

Crossover between Games and Simulations

Aldrich's (2009b) HIVE (highly interactive virtual environment) model illustrates distinctions and connections among games, simulations, and virtual worlds. All take place in some sort of virtual environment or world. He also points out other similarities in that successful implementation of each requires support structures to ensure ease of use and adequate preparation; tools that build community either inside or as a separate function outside the activity; and action from the players, meaning they are attempting or doing something within the environment (Aldrich, 2009b). Aldrich notes there are also distinct differences between games and simulations. Although both games and simulations focus on achieving goals and include the use of rules, feedback based on performance, and specific tools to function within the environment, games tend to be more fun and engaging when compared with simulations. The more complicated the game, the stricter the rules become, which in turn requires more high-order strategy and competency from the player. Scenario-based simulations are more rigorous and focus on building specific competencies to be transferred to real-life practice (Aldrich, 2009b).

Combinations of Games and Simulations

It is important to note that virtual worlds do not have any inherent purpose other than to provide an environment in which to be. Content, activities, games, or simulations must be added to virtual worlds to give them purpose—learners need a reason to be there (Ralston-Berg & Lara, 2012). In terms of instruction, games provide an opportunity for learning to take place within a virtual environment.

There are several concepts and game design elements that can be used to promote purpose, engagement, and intrinsic value within digital environments. Many schools are now exploring how to best use digital virtual worlds or environments for nursing education. Virtual worlds host a synchronous digital environment. The environment is a persistent network of people (students), represented as avatars or player characters, facilitated by networked computers (Bell, 2008). It is important to understand that there is a distinction between game environments and virtual worlds. Not all virtual worlds are game environments. They become game environments when they attend to the elements previously discussed in the contemporary theory section of this chapter. The ability of players to engage in some sort of activity is key to any game experience.

Metagaming

Metagaming refers to the use of out-of-game resources or strategy to effect in-game success (Carter, Gibbs, & Harrop, 2012). In teaching and learning paradigms, we might consider this cheating. But in game-based learning, it is often rewarded. Moving through multiple levels of a game requires achievement. As players demonstrate proficiency, they are allowed to "level-up" or advance through the game narrative. We know that clinical practice is distributive. What we really want students to learn is how to make informed decisions that will drive desired outcomes. When it comes to patient care and patient safety, we do not want them to guess. From this perspective, perhaps we should be teaching our students how to metagame complex problems.

Minigames

Minigames are games that exist within games or virtual environments. They often provide brief in-world encounters to engage players in a process, provide just-in-time information, or orient them in a specific environment or needs skill required to negotiate the environment. For example, in the game "Grand Theft Auto," several of the orientation tasks really focus on teaching the player how to negotiate the virtual environment. For example, your first mission in the narrative is walking to a location in the virtual world. Along the way you are presented with a bicycle to ride and later a car to drive. These skills are needed to interact within the "Grand Theft Auto" environment and engage in deeper game play. Similarly, imagine a game in a hospital environment. To begin with nursing playing, the player might be asked to transport patients from the emergency department to various departments and wards in the hospital. Later, players might be asked to engage in tasks that orient them to various types of equipment found in the hospital, perhaps airway devices and a defibrillator. These exercises really only serve to orient the players to the virtual environment. The real mission assignments ask the players to respond on different types of rapid response teams such as the intravenous team, behavioral emergency team, and later, as skills are developed through various levels of play, the code blue resuscitation team.

Gamification

Gamification has been described as "the use of game-design elements in non-games contexts" (Deterding, Dixon, Khalid, & Nacke, 2011, p. 9). Gamification aims to encourage targeted behaviors and provide incentives for completion of tasks that might be undesirable or boring. The term and concept of gamification continues to be controversial. We routinely ask our students to do uncomfortable and perhaps undesirable and even boring things to prepare them for clinical practice. Not everything about the practice of nursing is or will be fun. That said, if we could use gamification to initially engage challenging topics we might be able to bring emphasis to important content that might otherwise be ignored. The key with gamified homework is to promote the intrinsic value of mastery, rather than the extrinsic nature of most coursework. Students are extrinsically motivated to complete tasks because they are graded. They are intrinsically motivated when successfully completing a project represents value to self.

EXPANDING THE LEARNING SPACE

Tearing Down the Ivory Towers

Digital games expand the learning space. They provide a level of situated interactivity not found in traditional didactic learning. Games are interactive in a way that textbooks and e-readers are not. Digital games can be deployed through online learning platforms or as standalone applications. E-learning platforms provide a distributed model of educational delivery that moves beyond the confines of the traditional classroom. In general, online courses have made important technological breakthroughs, allowing teachers and educational designers to add video, forums, quizzes, and homework assignments. However, for all of their convenience and flexibility, e-learning platforms do not provide the same sort of social interaction and acculturation that occurs during face-to-face activities. That is to say, in well-developed courses, the content delivered through e-learning platforms remains valid but occurs through different processes. This can be challenging in disciplines like nursing that are inherently social and require a high degree of social interaction and modeling of processes to promote professional acculturation.

Today's videogames are designed to be interactive and increasingly socially interactive. Commercial massively multiplayer online games (MMOGs) are literally played by millions of people at the same time. They provide synchronous real-time interaction with a digital environment that is coinhabited by many other players. Games like "World of Warcraft" and "Starcraft II" represent two of the more popular MMOGs being played around the world. These games focus on missions to be completed by groups of players. The game is inherently social and interactive. These activities occur in real time without the confines of time or physical space. Players are rewarded for completing both individual in-game tasks, but also face challenges that cannot be completed without multiplayer cooperation and interaction (Gaydos & Bauman, 2012).

Videogames and digital applications are capable tools that should be explored and used to introduce nursing students and those seeking continuing education opportunities to new task-related and collaborative processes that promote team training. Interprofessional education and team training have been identified as a deficiency in clinical education that negatively impacts patient care. Leape (2009) argues that nurses, physicians, and others must work together to redesign flawed processes to prevent harm to patients. Leape et al. (2012) also argue that dysfunctional and disrespectful workplaces, particularly large academic hospitals, are a threat to professional development, career longevity, and patient safety.

Need for Role Clarity and Collegiality

Some of the challenges associated with complex workplaces arise from a lack of role clarity. Novice clinicians are just learning their own roles and likely have even less understanding of the roles of other types of clinicians whom they must work with. Simply transitioning from student to novice clinician, whether the novice is a new medical resident or new graduate nurse, is challenging. Existing videogames and digital learning environments that focus on teamwork can be deployed in prelicensure settings and during orientation so new graduates can familiarize themselves with not only their roles and responsibilities, but also the roles and responsibilities of other types of clinicians. The challenge for educators is to bridge the gap where nursing students go to class with other nursing students and medical students go to class with other medical students.

Professional boundaries do not get explored until after graduation, in the workplace, where poor etiquette can be deadly for patients. Game environments break down the walls between the classrooms and expand the learning space in ways that can foster collaboration and acculturation under the watchful eyes of an interprofessional faculty team. These multidiscipline or interprofessional learning experiences are often not possible in traditional clinical or health sciences learning models. Yet in a game-based learning environment, students can assume multiple roles within their chosen discipline as well as those roles found in health care representing other disciplines. In this way, the nursing student might play the role of the attending physician and the medical student might play the role of the triage or charge nurse. This sort of collaborative play has the ability to foster role clarity and future collegiality.

Mobile Applications: Designing with Mobile Delivery in Mind

Ownership of tablets, e-book readers, smartphones, and other devices continues to increase. As of January 2012, it is estimated that 29 percent of Americans own at least one digital reading device (Rainie, 2012). As of February 2012, 46 percent of adults in the United States owned smartphones. Within that group, college graduates aged 18 to 35 years old showed ownership of 60 percent or more of these devices (Smith, 2012).

Distributive game-based and virtual environments are now commonplace in the entertainment world. More and more often, social games, social media, and multimedia entertainment venues are being made available on mobile devices. Just a few years ago, the term mobile device used to refer to laptops. Now the term more often refers to tablet computers and smartphones. Many colleges and universities make lectures available by streaming video or portable download. Massive open online courses are beginning to emerge as legitimate coursework and can often be accessed on mobile or smart devices. As learning opportunities become more mobile, they become more accessible. But games possess something the streaming lecture does not—interactivity and distributed social interaction.

Consider a mobile game or application that begins as a didactic trainer to prepare students for a manikin-based simulation experience. For example, there are numerous game-style mobile applications that focus on cardiac resuscitation. Students can download and play these applications in preparation for their simulation laboratory experience. If the application is well thought out, it might become a long-lasting cognitive aid to support supervised clinical experiences and even independent clinical practice. As long as this sort of game is well vetted and clinically relevant, teachers, faculty, and leadership should accept it just as we have historically accepted the numerous pocket guides that forever weighed down our white coats. Moreover, these types of games and applications provide just-in-time learning and information to facilitate problem solving and best practices.

The Synergistic Approach to Integrating Games and Simulations

In the current digital environment, knowledge is no longer privileged. The scholar or professor no longer controls access to discipline-specific information. Rather, the job of the professor is to facilitate learning by vetting information and crafting its inclusion into the curriculum so that it provides authentic, situated, transformative learning experiences. A quality learning experience often requires the synergy of a professor, or content expert, working in collaboration with a team of specialized experts such as game designers, instructional designers, multimedia specialists, or programmers (Aleckson & Ralston-Berg, 2011).

The professor or content expert who works with game designers familiar with educational games is more likely to provide overarching game narratives and interactive environments that incorporate microgames and simulations to encourage learner success. However, nursing and other clinical faculty should be careful to remember that they must provide more than content expertise to the game designers. They must also provide the rules, problems, and cues for reflection within the targeted clinical culture (in this case nursing). The players or learners will create an emergent experience based on their intentions, feelings, and activity within the game environment. Immersing students in a game that is carefully crafted to mimic nursing tasks and nursing performance builds situated and experiential knowledge, allowing players to experiment in an authentic-feeling space (DeVane & Bauman, 2012).

Considerations for Alternate Delivery Formats: Time, Budget, Staffing Needs, and Resources

Effective, efficient, and appealing instruction can be delivered through many technology methods (Ralston-Berg & Lara, 2012). The key when considering alternate delivery formats is to weigh the cost, effort, and resources required to create or maintain the instruction against its ability to meet desired learning outcomes. Questions to be considered include:

- What is the initial startup cost in terms of technology, design, development, and delivery?
- How much preparation is required to ready learners for participation?
- Are resources needed throughout the delivery of the instruction?
- Are facilitators or faculty able to manage and maintain the instruction?

- Are there ongoing subscription, server, or other maintenance costs?
- Is ongoing technical support for learners necessary?

With all the questions related to cost and resources, it is important that learning objectives remain the top priority. Aleckson and Ralston-Berg (2011) describe low-fidelity solutions, which are inexpensive and easily implemented, in contrast to high-fidelity solutions, which are more expensive to develop and require orientation as well as ongoing support for users. On this continuum of complexity, higher-order learning objectives require more complex solutions and therefore increased costs, while lower-level objectives require more simple solutions (Aleckson & Ralston-Berg, 2011). It is important to ask the following questions in this regard:

- Does the complexity of the technology match the complexity of the learning objectives?
- Are we spending too much time and resources on a simple learning outcome?
- Could the learning objective be met just as effectively by other methods?

EVALUATING FOR FIT WITHIN THE CURRICULUM

Ralston-Berg and Lara (2012) contend that to accomplish a good fit between technology and curriculum, the instruction must be effective, efficient, and appealing; technology without good fit becomes a distraction to learning. The instruction must provide necessary support and practice for learners to succeed, align all activities with desired learning outcomes, and engage the learner. Learning objectives must be clear, whether faculty are selecting existing games to integrate into the curriculum or are working with educational and game designers to design an original game. The following cues can be used when embarking on the process of integrating games into clinical curricula:

- Clarifying learning objectives and outcomes
- Matching activities to objectives
- Alignment of objectives, activities, and assessments

Aldrich (2009a) proposed that some types of learning objectives are more appropriate for specific technologies. For example, he suggests virtual worlds can be used to convey emotion, proximity, and community at a distance. He also suggests that games and simulations can increase engagement when integrated with other course activities; meet the same objectives as in-person lab experiences; or present difficult materials in an alternate format. Ralston-Berg and Lara (2012) argue that "learning objectives should align throughout the activities in an instructional unit" (p. 138) and not be limited to the game or simulation. When an instructional unit is designed, the team must weave the objectives through all parts of the unit.

EVALUATING OUTCOME

Games must be carefully selected when they are integrated into curricula to ensure they map back to the lesson objectives and meet students' learning needs. To this end, best practices in curriculum and instruction dictate that curriculum changes, including the introduction of new technology, must be evaluated from several perspectives. This is an important consideration for faculty-content experts as well as stakeholders and administrators who are in a position to support evaluation as part of the design and development process.

It should be noted that digital games are very good at collecting data. Commercial games continuously evaluate players in terms of proficiency and mastery. In general, one cannot move through a game narrative or finish a game without achieving predetermined benchmarks. Furthermore, learning is an inherent part of game play. You cannot be a good basketball player without learning the rules and skills of the game. In any type of game, players are evaluated based on performance. Evaluation is built into game play, and the nature and design of digital games allow for sophisticated collection of data based on learner performance.

Student Achievement

Perhaps most important in terms of academic success is the variable of student achievement. Although graduate nursing education focuses on professional development and research, undergraduate nursing education at most schools is fundamentally about preparation for entry into practice. To this end, it is important to understand which facets of your curriculum are driving student achievement and how. Games should not be introduced to students merely because they are cool. Educational games should address a curriculum gap or objective. At the very least, games should provide situated supplemental opportunities that are seen to have intrinsic value for learners.

Instructor Performance

As discussed earlier, games allow participants to co-create knowledge. From this perspective, even if an instructor is not an active player character within an assigned game, the instructor should understand that students and their peers will, and should, evaluate them based on the game-based learning and technology integrated into their courses. Using videogames as filler is not appropriate. Teachers should be well versed in the games they deploy in their courses. Any games or technology used should be relevant, hold instructional value, and promote learning objectives.

Evaluating Courses and Curricula in the Context of Game-Based Learning

Those instructors who are comfortable using manikin-based technology in their courses understand that developing new simulation scenarios and even implementing existing scenarios are iterative processes. This is also true for the deployment of games into curricula. The type of game and where and how it is introduced are all variables for consideration. Remember, course and curriculum objectives should come first. Everything else, including the integration of games, should follow. In other words, you must determine how simulation or game-based learning can help you meet your curriculum objectives.

SUMMARY

We support the acceptance and inclusion of both games and simulation into nursing curricula. This chapter reviewed the traditional and contemporary pedagogies that support integration of game-based learning into nursing curricula and introduced readers to contemporary elements of game design. The use of mobile and smart technology as a mechanism to expand traditional learning spaces was also discussed. The importance of good fit was emphasized as it relates to the integration of game-based technologies into nursing and other clinical curricula. Further, we emphasize that games should be used to *support* nursing education, not *replace* it. Leveraging technology, including manikin-based simulation and game-based learning, often requires a hybrid approach that uses game technology to address gaps and challenges in curriculum content and delivery. Technology integration requires a team of specialized experts to work with the faculty content expert. Finally, we emphasize the need to evaluate games from multiple perspectives using an iterative process when choosing and integrating games into the curriculum.

■ Key Concepts

- The media savvy of today's students often exceeds that of their instructors and faculty.
- Just-in-time learning is a process by which students acquire knowledge through solving challenges in real time.
- Just-in-time learning supports advancement through situated and contextually relevant learning exercises and experiences.
- Traditional pedagogy suggests ill-structured problems with multiple solutions, and paths encourage firsthand or practical experience, reflection, and decision making in students, moving them from novice to expert clinicians.
- Nursing and other clinical students learn through performance within material, social, and cultural worlds where learning is cognitive, behavioral, and social.
- Although both games and simulations focus on achieving goals and include the use of rules, feedback based on performance, and specific tools to function within the environment, games tend to be more fun and engaging when compared with simulations.
- To successfully integrate games into the curriculum, consider collaboration with a team of design and media experts, the desired delivery mode of the game, the opportunities for roles and teamwork within the game, and the alignment of the game to existing learning objectives.
- Budget, available resources, timeline, and support required for faculty and users must be considered when integrating games into the curricula.
- Evaluators should consider student achievement, instructor performance, and how well game-based learning helps meet curriculum objectives.

References

Abt, C. C. (1987). *Serious games.* Lanham, MD: University Press of America.

Aldrich, C. (2009a). *Learning online with games, simulations, and virtual worlds: Strategies for online instruction.* San Francisco: Jossey-Bass.

Aldrich, C. (2009b). Virtual worlds, simulations, and games for education: A unifying view. *Innovate, 5*(5).

Aleckson, J., & Ralston-Berg, P. (2011). *MindMeld: Micro-collaboration between e-learning designers and instructor experts.* Madison, WI: Atwood.

Barrows, H. S. (1986). A taxonomy of problem-based learning methods. *Medical Education, 20*(6), 481–486.

Bartle, R. (2004). *Designing Virtual Worlds.* Indianapolis, IN. New Riders Games.

Bauman, E. (2007). *High fidelity simulation in healthcare.* Ph.D. dissertation, University of Wisconsin–Madison. Dissertations & Theses CIC Institutions database. (Publication no. AAT 3294196; ProQuest document ID: 1453230861).

Bauman, E. (2010). Virtual reality and game-based clinical education. In K. B. Gaberson & M. H. Oermann (Eds.), *Clinical teaching strategies in nursing education* (3rd ed., pp. 182–212). New York: Springer.

Bauman, E. B. (2012). *Game-based teaching and simulation in nursing & healthcare.* New York: Springer.

Bauman, E. B., & Games, I. A. (2011). Contemporary theory for immersive worlds: Addressing engagement, culture, and diversity. In A. Cheney & R. Sanders (Eds.), *Teaching and learning in 3D immersive worlds: Pedagogical models and constructivist approaches* (pp. 248–270). Hershey, PA: Information Science Reference, IGI Global.

Bell, M. (2008). Toward a definition of virtual worlds. *Journal of Virtual Worlds Research, 1*(1), 1–5.

Benner, P. (1984). *From novice to expert: Excellence and power in clinical nursing practice.* Menlo Park, CA: Addison-Wesley.

Bruckman, A. (2004). Co-evolution of technological design and pedagogy in an online learning community. In Barab, S. Kling, R. & Gray, J. (Eds.) *Designing for virtual communities in the service of learning.* Cambridge: Cambridge University Press.

Bruner, J. (1991) The narrative construction of reality. *Critical Inquiry, 18,* 1–20.

Carter, M., Gibbs, M., & Harrop, M. (2012). Metagames, paragames and orthogames: A new vocabulary. FDG '12 Proceedings of the International Conference on the Foundations of Digital Games, May 29–June 1, Raleigh, NC.

Cruickshank, D. R. (1968). Simulation. *Theory into Practice, 7*(5), 190–193.

Cruickshank, D. R., & Telfer, R. (1980). Classroom games and simulations. *Theory into Practice, 19*(1), 75–80.

Deterding, S., Dixon, D., Khalid, R., & Nacke, L. (2011). From game design elements to gamefulness: defining gamification. In *Proceedings of the 15th International Academic MindTrek Conference: Envisioning Future Media Environments* (pp. 9–15). ACM.

DeVane, B., & Bauman, E. B. (2012). Virtual learning spaces: Using new and emerging game-based learning theories for nursing clinical skills development. In E. B. Bauman (Ed.), *Game-based teaching and simulation in nursing & healthcare* (pp. 47–73). New York: Springer.

Entertainment Software Association. (2011). Sales, demographic and usage data: Essential facts about the computer and video game industry. Retrieved from http://www.theesa.com/facts/pdfs/ESA_EF_2011.pdf

Games, I., & Bauman, E. (2011). Virtual worlds: An environment for cultural sensitivity education in the health sciences. *International Journal of Web Based Communities, 7*(2), 189–205.

Gaydos, M., & Bauman, E. B. (2012). Assessing and evaluating learning effectiveness: Games, Sims and Starcraft 2. In E. Bauman (Ed.), *Games and simulation for nursing education* (pp. 179–203). New York: Springer.

Gee, J. P. (1991). Memory and myth: a perspective on narrative. In A. McCabe & C. Peterson (Eds.), *Developing narrative structure* (pp. 1–26). Mahwah, NJ: Erlbaum.

Gee, J. P. (2003). *What videogames have to teach us about learning and literacy.* New York: Palgrave-McMillan.

Ito, M. (2009). *Hanging out, messing around, and geeking out: Kids living and learning with new media.* Boston: MIT University Press.

Jonassen, D. H. (1997). Instructional design models for well-structured and III-structured problem-solving learning outcomes. *Educational Technology Research and Development, 45*(1), 65–94.

Kolb, D. (1984). *Experiential learning: Experience as the source of learning and development.* Upper Saddle River, NJ: Prentice-Hall.

Leape, L. L. (2009). Errors in medicine. *Clinica Chimica Acta, 404*(1), 2–5.

Leape, L. L., Shore, M. F., Deinstag, J. L., Mayer, R. J., Edgman-Levitan, S., Meyer, G. S., & Healy, G. B. (2012). Perspective: A culture of respect, part 1: The nature and causes of disrespectful behavior by physicians. *Academic Medicine, 87,* 845–852.

Merriam, S. B., & Caffarella, R. S. (1999). *Learning in adulthood: A compressive guide* (2nd ed.). San Francisco: Jossey-Bass.

Murray, D., Boulet, J., Ziv, A., Woodhouse, J., Kras, J., & McAllister, J. (2002). An acute care skills evaluation for graduating medical students: A pilot study using clinical simulation. *Medical Education, 36*(9), 833–841.

Oblinger, D. G. (2004). The next generation of educational engagement. *Journal of Interactive Media in Education, 8,* 1–18.

Prensky, M. (2001). Digital natives, digital immigrants. *On the Horizon, 9*(5), 1–6.

Prensky, M. (2003). *Digital game based learning. Exploring the digital generation.* Washington, DC: Educational Technology, U.S. Department of Education.

Rainie, L. (2012). Tablet and e-book reader ownership nearly double over the holiday gift-giving period. Pew Internet and American Life Project. Retrieved from http://libraries.pewinternet.org/2012/01/23/tablet-and-e-book-reader-ownership-nearly-double-over-the-holiday-gift-giving-period/

Ralston-Berg, P., & Lara, M. (2012). Fitting virtual reality and game-based learning into an existing curriculum. In E. Bauman (Ed.), *Games and simulation for nursing education* (pp. 127–145). New York: Springer.

Schön, D. A. (1983). *The reflective practitioner: How professionals think in action.* New York: Basic Books.

Schwartzman, R. (1997). Gaming serves as a model for improving learning. *Education, 118*(1), 9–17.

Skinner, B. F. (1960). Teaching machines. *The Review of Economics and Statistics, 42*(3 Pt 2), 189–191.

Smith, A. (2012). Nearly half of American adults are smartphone owners. Pew Internet and American Life Project. Retrieved from http://www.pewinternet.org/Reports/2012/Smartphone-Update-2012.aspx

Squire, K. (2006). From content to context: Videogames as designed experience. *Educational Researcher, 35*(8), 19–29.

7

Second Life and Other Virtual Emerging Simulations

Sarah Knapfel, RN, BSN, CCRN
Gina Moore, PharmD, MBA
Diane J. Skiba, PhD, FAAN, FACMI

■ Learning Objectives

1. Define the concept of a virtual world.
2. Identify uses of virtual worlds in health care.
3. Analyze the benefits and challenges of using virtual worlds in education.

■ Key Term

- Avatar
- Second Life
- Virtual world

Since the early days of electronic bulletin board systems, **virtual worlds** have played a part in our lives. Early examples included text-based role-playing communities. With the advent of the World Wide Web and increased bandwidth, virtual worlds have evolved. Today, imagine connecting through the Internet to an immersive online environment that mimics the real world. Imagine being able to walk, talk, and interact with the environment and feeling as if you were "right there" within the environment. These environments can be virtual hospitals, clinics, or even a bioterrorism event. All of this is possible in the virtual world. The concept of virtual worlds (VWs) is not new to higher education or health care.

What is confusing about this field are the many acronyms used to describe the virtual world, such as MUDs (multiuser dungeons/dimensions/domains), MUVEs (multiuser immersive environments), HIVEs (highly interactive virtual environments), and CVEs (collaborative virtual environments). Some of these environments are used within a gaming environment such as "World of Warcraft," which is a massive multiplayer online role-playing game. There are even virtual reality therapies in which patients are given goggles to wear that immerse them in different worlds from their current physical space.

Definitions

Although the different terms share some common features, there was a need to further clarify what constituted a virtual world. In higher education, Educause's (2006) "7 Things You Should Know About Virtual Worlds" initially crafted a simpler definition where a "virtual world is an online environment whose 'residents' are **avatars**. They are immersive, animated, 3D environments that operate over the Internet, giving access to anyone in the world." One important feature highlighted by Bell (2008) was the concept of persistence, meaning the virtual environment remained consistent after the user exited. Bell offered a definition of a virtual world as "a synchronous, persistent network of people, represented as avatars, facilitated by networked computers." Schroeder (2008) expanded this definition by stating that "virtual worlds are persistent virtual environments in which people experience others as being there with them—and where they can interact with them." In addition to "being there," VWs also encompass "online social spaces...virtual environments that people experience as ongoing over time and that have large populations which they experience together with others as a world for social interaction." The dialogue surrounding the definition was an important step when the business, education, and research communities began their use of VWs.

Although educational institutions had experiences using various VWs since the 1990s, most were experiments tied to funding. In 2003, the **Second Life**® (http://secondlife.com/) platform was introduced and described as a place for companies to advertise and market their products. In 2005, Forbes' "Knowledge@Wharton" series began dialogue about the potential of virtual commerce. Because VWs such as Second Life created a virtual marketplace, it was just a matter of time before virtual economies would expand. The only question is by how much? It was certainly seen as an area to watch closely. In 2007, DFC Intelligence (2007) predicted that massive multiuser game players would generate $13 billion in revenue within the next five years. Skiba (2007) noted in her initial review of Second Life that several major companies, such as IBM, Coca-Cola, and Audi were early adopters and part of the ever-growing landscape of real estate in Second Life. It was not until the release of platforms such as Second Life, which offered educational discounts, that the VW growth was catalyzed in the higher education market.

PLATFORM FOR EDUCATION DELIVERY

As the world continues to transition from the era of Web 1.0 to Web 2.0, higher education shifted as well, moving from flat, web-based education and interfaces to interactive and dynamic ones (Johnson, Vorderstrasse, & Shaw, 2009). This shift opened the door for changes in how health care professionals could be taught. As educators moved their teaching platforms and adapted pedagogy toward the technology and culture of the information age, there was a shift in educational strategies (Wang & Braman, 2009), including VW environments.

In higher education, there were many examples of schools and universities experimenting with Second Life and other virtual platforms as a means to augment online education and as a mechanism to advertise their campuses. One early example was a continuing education course offered by Harvard's Law School in 2006. The course, CyberOne: Law in the Court of Public Opinion, contained course video, lectures, and interactive experiences for participants in a courtroom that mimics one at the Harvard Law School, which was offered by the Law School and the Harvard Extension School jointly. (To learn more about this groundbreaking course, visit the website on the Berkman Center for Internet & Society at http://cyber.law.harvard.edu/node/4809.)

Another early adopter was Dartmouth College with their Media Lab. The Department of Homeland Security provided funding to create a multiuser immersive environment to train first responders to emergency responses. This has evolved over time to be part of their Virtual Terrorism Response Academy and provides a game-like training in the areas of chemical, biological, radiological, nuclear, and explosive threats. (To learn more, go to http://iml.dartmouth.edu/education/pcpt/vtra/ops-plus/2.0/.)

Another long-standing example is work at the University of Illinois at Chicago School of Public Health. Since 2006, they have been designing and researching the use of "[v]irtual environments of a scale dispensing and vaccination center along with a large convention center and hospital for primary, surge and alternate care simulations" (Hsu et al., 2013).

Three early adopters in nursing were John Miller's company, MUVErs (Medical Simulation in the Virtual World of Second Life), which developed Second Life simulations for use at Tacoma Community College, University of Kansas School of Nursing, in their informatics and operating room nurses specialties and the University of Wisconsin–Oshkosh's College of Nursing bachelor of nursing online program. Skiba (2009) described the groundbreaking work of these three nursing programs and their use of Second Life to create interactive immersive simulations of real-world nursing examples. For example, Miller created emergency department simulations for associate degree students. The University of Kansas used Second Life to foster student engagement in their online educational program in informatics. Students presented posters of their coursework, interacted with avatars in a long-term care facility as they designed database management systems for patient falls, and had interprofessional teams do home assessments of patients. The University of Wisconsin–Oshkosh created a community that was used by students for their public health courses. Students participated in classes, went to their local public health department to do class assignments, and participated in disaster training exercises. They could inspect restaurants and manage the Women, Infants, and Children (WIC) program.

Early adopters also wanted to use VWs to advertise their colleges and showcase their campuses. Case Western Reserve University and Duke University, both early adopters, created replicas of their campus in Second Life. Students could meet with admission counselors and join with other students to take virtual tours of the campus. Although some colleges and universities had virtual campuses that replicated their campus, others took more liberties and created what Young (2010) called "fantasy" versions of traditional campuses.

Several colleges adopted VWs as a means to create a familiar environment for faculty who were not familiar with teaching online. Some colleges thought that by creating a virtual classroom with all the necessary features, faculty would feel more comfortable (Young, 2010). Some faculty embraced the concept and created virtual offices with virtual office hours to interact with both current and potential students. Some faculty believed VWs would augment the distance learning opportunities offered by their campuses. What a better way to interact with distance students than to meet them virtually on campus in the student union or perhaps take a stroll through the campus and talk about their experiences in online courses? Several faculty thought the use of a VW could add a new dimension to their online lectures. So instead of doing voice-over PowerPoint presentations, the faculty stand at a podium in a virtual auditorium and present the lecture to virtual student avatars sitting in the audience.

One such example of the evolving delivery of higher education using VWs was Duke University's (n.d.) School of Nursing. Using the Second Life platform, students attend lectures in a building that has been created to look similar to the real Duke University campus in Durham, North Carolina. Students enter the building where they will find a classroom for lectures, seats for students to sit in, an instructor podium, and a board for accessing discussions and PowerPoint presentations. The environment created in Second Life allows students and faculty to interact beyond the traditional discussion board by using an avatar to create lifelike situations and allow students to feel an increased sense of place and presence. Beyond class discussion and lectures, students are also able to take part in workshops, synchronously engage as a group to do work, attend office hours, and go on virtual field trips. The lifelike representation of a university engages the student and enables facilitation of activity learning from a distance. This method of education also enables the possibility for collaborations among additional institutions.

Although there was a lot of activity in VWs such as Second Life, the business and projections for virtual commerce did not materialize. Companies built sites on Second Life but the virtual dollars did not follow. Several companies that offered VW platforms also went out of business, such as Google's Lively, and this caused much angst in the business world. What happens if the platform goes bankrupt? The simple answer is all your virtual real estate and investments will be gone in a flash.

Academia also became disenchanted with VWs. Universities built grand campuses with tours but few people came. There were several reasons for the loss of interest in platforms like Second Life. First, the pricing structure was changing, eliminating the discounts for educational institutions (Ramaswami, 2011). Second, there were many technical issues that faculty and students encountered. For example, the use of voice was always tenuous and many were frustrated. If one had to text instead of chat, why not use other Web 2.0 tools such as text messaging, blogging, online discussion groups, social networking sites, and other interactive technologies that are part of the daily lives of many faculty and students (Baker, Wentz, & Woods, 2009)?

There were also issues with obtaining broadband access and updated computers with good graphic interface cards. There were also the technical skills needed to create and maintain Second Life properties. These could be cost prohibitive if colleges did not have technical support trained to program. Third, faculty and even some students also noted that Second Life had a steep learning curve. People did not like to look like fools walking into walls, and interacting in the environment was often less than optimal (Young, 2010). Perhaps one of the most compelling reasons was aptly noted by Reneta Lansiquot (Ramaswami, 2011): "Part of what went wrong is that a lot of people tried to replicate a real classroom in Second Life(®), instead of asking, What can I do that I cannot do in real life?"

But despite the hype and diminishing numbers of academic environments building in Second Life, there is still a commitment to use of VWs. As noted by Young (2010), "educators appear more interested than ever in the idea of teaching in video-game like realms." He noted that several new special interest groups, especially Educause's virtual environment group, were increasing in numbers. In addition, new platforms, especially those connected to the open source movement such as OpenSim and Duke's Open Cobalt, were introduced in the hopes of allowing more collaborative efforts in development. There were also other platforms, like Blue Mars and Unity, being offered as alternatives.

According to Ramaswami (2011), "Virtual worlds might find their sweet spot in medical and therapeutics applications." Health care professional faculty were able to answer the question, What can I do in VWs that I cannot do in real life? VWs can be used to teach health care students and the current workforce, but they can also be applied to patients and consumers. For patients and consumers, there is also the benefit of the use of VWs for therapeutic interventions. This is particularly true as more and more health care education becomes dependent on simulation training. It is important for health care professionals to investigate these options for their distant students and as other alternatives to standardized patients and physically located high-fidelity simulations labs. VWs provide these interactive simulated opportunities for students, providers, patients, and consumers. Here are some recent examples.

Simulation Training for Health Care Providers

Simulations in all forms are increasingly accepted and implemented in health care education because of their ability to focus on a student's experience to solve problems, perform skills, and make decisions in a safe and nonthreatening environment (Rogers, 2011). Using methods such as VWs facilitates a way to prepare health care professionals to engage in simulations at a distance and by decreasing the cost of expensive standardized patients while increasing the number of accessible physical labs offering high-fidelity manikins.

VWs are most often used for the purposes of training health care professionals. This environment for simulation can create real-life scenarios with virtual patients in which an individual can be trained on a particular set of skills. Simulation training can address an array of different competencies and anatomical regions including training for palpitation for subsurface breast tumors and esophageal intubation (Mantovani, Castelnuovo, Gaggioli, & Riva, 2003). "Heart Murmur Sim" in Second Life is an example of using VWs to improve assessment and identification skills of health care providers. The simulation creates an environment for cardiac auscultation training by allowing students to tour a clinic while testing their knowledge on different types of heart sounds and murmurs (Boulos, Hetherington, & Wheeler, 2007).

Cook (2012) designed and evaluated a VW simulation for family nurse practitioner students and also created a primary care pediatric simulation for use by family nurse practitioner students in Second Life. These care-based interactive virtual experiences were supplemental to students' traditional clinical practice experience. The cases were developed using constructivist learning theory and experiential learning principles.

Schools of pharmacy are also developing VWs to educate pharmacists. The University of North Carolina School of Pharmacy uses Second Life to practice presentations for the North Carolina Association of Pharmacists, and students can participate in virtual orientation in a neonatal intensive care unit before going to their real-life clinical rotation. Monash Univeristy's pharmacy school also uses virtual practice environments to prepare their pharmacists (www.monash.edu.au/pharm/innovative-learning/spaces/virtual-environments/). Keele University's School of Pharmacy has created the Keele

Active Virtual Environment (www.keele.ac.uk/pharmacy/vp/kave/kave_video/), which is a three-dimensional immersive environment to care for avatars representing a variety of clinical patients.

The University of Southern California's Institute of Creative Technologies created virtual patients for use by students in their School of Social Work. These virtual patients are built as realistic lifelike avatars. The project uses speech recognition and natural language processes to interact in realistic nonmilitary and military scenarios to educate clinicians in areas such as provider–clinician interactions, interviewing, and diagnoses. (To learn more about the cast of virtual patients, go to: http://ict.usc.edu/prototypes/virtual-patient/.)

Seefeldt et al. (2012) used Second Life to allow pharmacy, nursing, physical therapy, occupational therapy, and physician assistant students to interact around a mock patient case. This pilot study examined the feasibility of using Second Life as a means to foster interprofessional education (IPE). The pilot was undertaken as many IPE programs find it difficult to overcome barriers of time, space, and location. Students found Second Life useful for participating in IPE discussions, but there were some technical difficulties in using the platform, which included issues with the voice component and the students' lack of necessary skills in using the Second Life platform.

Emergency Response Training

The use of VWs to simulate emergency training is one of the most widely used and long-lasting application in health care. This environment allows professionals to learn how to respond when faced with limited supplies, and it simulates the demands and stress of stabilizing multiple casualties. This route of training creates a real-life approach without the time, risk, and cost constraints of typical disaster trainings. As noted by Hsu et al. (2013), "the immersive and participatory nature of virtual reality training offers a unique realistic quality that is not generally present in classroom-based or web-based training, yet retains considerable cost advantages over large-scale real-life exercises and other modalities." This is particularly true for computer-based immersive environments available via broadband access.

As mentioned previously, Dartmouth has extensive experience developing VW scenarios for the Department of Homeland Security. Another example is the Division of Health Sciences' Institute of Rural Health Play2Train Bioterrorism Training developed at Idaho State University (www.isu.edu/irh/projects/). Other examples include the Johns Hopkins Office of Critical Event Preparedness and Response and the University of Florida (https://www.burncentertraining.com/about/). Farra, Miller, Timm, and Schafer (2013) discovered that when VWs were used as a learning strategy for nursing students to practice disaster response, there was a strong positive effect on retention beyond postknowledge.

Mental Health Training

The use of simulation through VWs promotes awareness and can be used as a support tool for psychological teaching and understanding. Yellowlees and Cook (2006) steered a project that involved constructing the simulation of auditory and visual hallucinations of patients with schizophrenia to use as an education tool on hallucinations. Using the

Second Life platform, users felt they gained an enhanced understanding of the experience of hallucinations. The University of Flinders in Australia uses Second Life to train interdisciplinary students to learn about mental health and general medicine (www.flinders.edu.au/nursing/research/mental-health/virtual-teaching-resources. cfm). The University of Colorado's College of Nursing also uses Second Life to allow psychiatric advanced practice nurses to practice different therapies with faculty serving as avatars for a variety of mental health issues. At the University of Akron, Kidd, Morgan, and Savery (2012) designed and implemented a simulation in which nursing students conducted a mental state assessment in virtual homes of patients.

Developing avatars for simulation in a VW also proves beneficial in the creation of personal interactions between provider and patient to help improve the basic interview skills of students. This setting allows a student and a virtual patient to meet and interact in what would be considered a typical health care setting. The student can proceed with a conventional history and physical interview while the simulated patient answers with preprogrammed responses, allowing the student provider to make a diagnosis and plan of care similar to the real-life workflow. VWs are seen to be useful not only to support the achievement of technical skills, but also to augment a complex set of skills including the personal aspects of care (Mantovani et al., 2003).

Educational Resource for Patients and Providers

VWs have become progressively popular for private companies and health care agencies. Several different health-related activities are found to be facilitated within the environments of VWs. Similar to the way that VWs are used for online education, websites offer information on numerous health-related issues that redirect users to associated websites and real-life information such as events on specific topics (e.g., the American Cancer Society has a presence in Second Life). The marketing and promotion of health care services is utilized in VWs by endorsing new or future health services, organizations, fundraising efforts, and real-life health care initiatives (Beard, Wilson, Morra, & Keelan, 2009).

The Centers for Disease Control and Prevention (CDC), an early adopter of virtual worlds, is an example of a health care agency creating numerous mechanisms to interact with consumers. The CDC has designed a broad array of social networking tools that include Facebook, Twitter, Second Life, e-cards, and text message as part of its health campaign. The CDC aims to use this platform to research and evaluate the potential for engaging audiences in actively modeling health behaviors and lifestyle choices while providing videos, links to health information, and an environment for visitors to engage in health-related activities (CDC, n.d.).

The VW platforms can also be used to facilitate the conduction of research. This area can take on many facets ranging from recruiting participants for studies within the virtual arena to a stage for testing new information delivery technologies (Boulos et al., 2007).

VWs can not only benefit providers and their skills, but also empower the individual patient as a source for information and interaction. Varying virtual platforms create a setting for patients to have individualized interaction for reference or support with health care professionals or fellow patients.

Another early adopter was the disability community. Virtual Ability (2012), formed by three friends, had a vision to remove barriers so they could fully participate in the physical community. They called it a sanctuary that ultimately evolved into Virtual Ability Island. Working with Second Life, they created Virtual Ability Island where there are mentors to help orient new users to the many features of Second Life. There are classrooms and other resources to help all members of their community learn how to navigate the virtual world. Virtual Ability Island has an employment orientation and support center within Second Life that was designed to address the needs of people with diverse disabilities. Support can also be delivered to specific populations.

Within the Virtual Ability community, there are several projects that support the various communities. One such community is Cape Able, which supports the hearing-impaired community. Another large community has a particular emphasis on veterans and those with traumatic brain injuries, which helps them find resources that will increase their potential for employment. HealthInfo Island, originally started by the Alliance Library System, is now part of the Virtual Ability Community that provides information about physical, emotional, and mental health. One-way immersion platforms provide support, as is seen on HealthInfo Island in Second Life. Users have the ability to seek answers to their health-related questions by interacting with real-life health librarians and medical experts. The purpose of this island is to supply patients with an avenue to seek information related to health care and to promote awareness on health-related topics (Beard et al., 2009).

Patients' anticipation and anxiety over health procedures can cause unwanted stress. Research suggests that the "priming" of patients using a VW experience may improve clinical outcomes by creating an opportunity for patients to have a greater understanding of the health care system and its procedures prior to setting foot into the hospital or clinic (Beard et al., 2009). Experiencing the interaction or procedure virtually first can increase the patient's familiarity, which in turn will improve his or her confidence and sense of control in regards to his or her health.

As can be seen, the use of VWs in the health care arena is alive and prospering. There are distinct advantages to using VWs in the preparation of new health care professionals, the current health care workforce, as well as patients and consumers. Using VWs allows people to interact in immersive health care scenarios. Health care professionals have not merely augmented online learning or replicated what is done in a classroom, but they have used it to simulate patient experiences in realistic immersive environments without fear of harming patients. Health care is highly dependent on the use of standardized patients and simulations to allow students to practice in safe environments. The use of VWs allows for one more alternative to provide simulated experiences that may prove to be less costly and more accessible to students on campus or those at a distance.

As an alternative method for simulations, it is important to understand the benefits and challenges associated with the development and implementation of VWs. Here is a summary of the benefits and challenges.

Benefits

- *User-centered approach.* Experiences can be tailored to individual learning and performance styles due to the vastly flexible and programmable environment of VWs (Hsu et al., 2013; Mantovani et al., 2003).

- *Increase self-confidence.* Using an avatar within a VW can provide a layer of anonymity and a level of comfort for operators, which will enable them to speak up to ask questions or provide comments as well as to test procedures or emergency response plans without fear or harm (Baker et al., 2009; Hsu et al., 2013).

- *Improve clinical judgment.* Receiving education and training in a VW platform allows users the opportunity to practice newly learned behaviors or skills in real-life situations without the drawback of making mistakes in real life (Johnson et al., 2009).

- *Relatively low cost.* VW interaction and training can remove the travel or other expenses that health care training necessitates. This can include the cost of classroom time or the use of paid actors for trainings such as the classic clinic examination (Beard et al., 2009).

- *Accessibility.* VWs such as Second Life can be accessed by anyone with a Windows or Macintosh computer and a broadband Internet connection (Yellowlees & Cook, 2006). The platform also transcends time, space, and location (Hsu et al., 2013).

- *Flexible, around the clock meeting place.* An online VW is available 24/7 and creates the anytime anywhere benefit of providing education to students who are distance learners. It also improves access to places that would be otherwise difficult to reach (Hansen, 2008). The ability for students to work at their own pace and to participate in scenarios more frequently are also benefits.

- *Realistic scenarios in three-dimensional setting.* The virtual environment makes scenarios come to life and offers a more realistic approach. This lifelike approach also fosters interactive and active learning by having student avatars participate in the scenarios. Simulated environments provide the realism.

- *From an educational standpoint, VWs build upon constructivist theories of learning and allow for experiential teaching strategies* (Cook, 2012).

Challenges

- *Usability.* A VW can represent a challenge for users during their initial interactions in these platforms. Student and faculty orientations are a must. The complexity and uniqueness of the technology creates a need for orientation for users with limited previous skill (Hsu et al., 2013; Mantovani et al., 2003).

- *Initial development can be costly to provide the realism needed* (Hsu et al., 2013).

- *Lack of collaboration.* Proper time must be spent developing the experiences or activities within the VW in order for users to reach the full potential of the intended experience. Additional external services such as blogs or wikis may also be required to support the interaction of avatars within the VW platform (Warburton, 2009).

- *Technical limitations.* Technological bandwidth and hardware requirements must be met in order to properly utilize VWs to their full potential. Latency and program glitches can cause problems and delays (Baker et al., 2009; Hsu et al., 2013).
- *Limited research to demonstrate effectiveness* (Hsu et al., 2013).

As with many educational technologies, the use of VWs is still in its infancy. Although there are some excellent studies examining the effectiveness of these techniques, there is still a gap in our knowledge about the efficiency, effectiveness, and costs compared with other simulated experiences, such as high-fidelity simulation manikins and standardized patients. For health care professional educators, it does provide a realistic and feasible alternative method to provide simulations, especially IPE experiences that transcend time, space, and geographic barriers.

■ Key Concepts

- ■ There are various terms used to describe the virtual world. Important concepts that underlie the definition of virtual world include: immersive, three-dimensional online environment, persistence, social interactions, and avatars as representations of humans.
- ■ In health care, virtual worlds have been used for both formal and informal educational opportunities for health care professionals and for consumers to seek health care information and to engage with others as a form of social support interactions among health care communities, such as the disabled or those suffering from posttraumatic stress disorder.
- ■ There is a lack of substantive research studies that provide evidence on the impact of virtual worlds on educational or health care outcomes.
- ■ The benefits noted include the provision of real-life scenarios that can occur across time and geographic boundaries with the potential of being more cost-effective than physical centers and the use of standardized patients.
- ■ The challenges to using virtual worlds are upfront design costs, technical support, and lack of technical skills and comfort in using virtual world technologies.

References

Baker, S. C., Wentz, R. K., & Woods, M. M. (2009). Using virtual worlds in education: Second Life® as an educational tool. *Teaching of Psychology, 36*(1), 59–64.

Beard, L., Wilson, K., Morra, D., & Keelan, J. (2009). A survey of health-related activities on Second Life. *Journal of Medical Internet Research, 11*(2), e17.

Bell, M. (2008). Toward a definition of "virtual worlds." *Journal of Virtual Worlds Research, 1* (1). Retrieved from http://journals.tdl.org/jvwr/index.php/jvwr/article/view/283

Boulos, M. N. K., Hetherington, L., & Wheeler, S. (2007). Second Life: An overview of the potential of 3-D virtual worlds in medical and health education. *Health Information & Libraries Journal, 24*(4), 233–245.

Centers for Disease Control (CDC). (n.d.). Retrieved from www.ache.org/pubs/hap_companion/thielst/Centers%20for%20Disease%20Control.pdf

Cook, M. J. (2012). Design and initial evaluation of a virtual pediatric primary care clinic in Second Life(®). *Journal of the*

American Academy of Nurse Practitioner, 24(9), 521–527.

DFC Intelligence. (2007, May 30). Digital distribution key to online game market growth. Retrieved from www.dfcint.com/wp/?p=14

Duke University. (n.d.). Innovative Nursing Education Technologies. Second Life. Retrieved from http://inet-nurse.org/?p=457

Educause Learning Initiative. (2006, June). 7 things you should know about virtual worlds. Retrieved from www.educause.edu/library/resources/7-things-you-should-know-about-virtual-worlds

Farra, S., Miller, E., Timm, N., & Schafer, J. (2013). Improved training for disasters: Using 3-D virtual reality simulation. *Western Journal of Nursing Research, 35*(5), 655–671.

Forbes. (2005, October 21). Knowledge@Wharton. Hey buddy, can you spare a Linden dollar? Retrieved from www.forbes.com/2005/10/20/onlinegaming-worldofwarcraft-gaming-cx_1021wharton.html

Hansen, M. M. (2008). Versatile, immersive, creative and dynamic virtual 3-D health-care learning environments: A review of the literature. *Journal of Medical Internet Research, 10*(3), e26.

Hsu, E., Li, Y., Bayram, J., Levinson, D., Yang, S., & Monahan, C. (2013). State of virtual reality based disaster preparedness and response training. *PLOS Currents, 5.* Retrieved from http://currents.plos.org/disasters/article/state-of-virtual-reality-vr-based-disaster-preparedness-and-response-training/

Johnson, C. M., Vorderstrasse, A. A., & Shaw, R. (2009). Virtual worlds in health care higher education. *Journal of Virtual Worlds Research, 2*(2). Retrieved from http://journals.tdl.org/jvwr/index.php/jvwr/article/view/699

Kidd, L. I., Morgan, K. I., & Savery, J. R. (2012). Development of a mental health nursing simulation: Challenges and solutions. *Journal of Interactive Online Learning, 11*(2), 80–89.

Mantovani, F., Castelnuovo, G., Gaggioli, A., & Riva, G. (2003). Virtual reality training for health-care professionals. *Cyber Psychology & Behavior, 6*(4), 389–395.

Ramaswami, R. (2011, September). Is there a second life for virtual worlds? *Campus Technology.* Retrieved from http://campustechnology.com/articles/2011/09/01/is-there-a-second-life-for-virtual-worlds.aspx

Rogers, L. (2011). Developing simulations in multi-user virtual environments to enhance healthcare education. *British Journal of Educational Technology, 42*(4), 608–615.

Schroeder, R. (2008, June). Defining virtual worlds and virtual environments. *Journal of Virtual Worlds Research, 1*(1). Retrieved from http://journals.tdl.org/jvwr/index.php/jvwr/article/view/294

Seefeldt, T., Mort, J., Brockevelt, B., Giger, J., Jorde, B., Lawler, M., Nilson, W., & Svien, L. (2012). A pilot study of interprofessional case discussions for health professions students using the virtual world Second Life. *Currents in Pharmacy Teaching and Learning, 4*(4), 224–231.

Skiba, D. (2007). Nursing education 2.0: Second Life. *Nursing Education Perspectives, 28*(3), 156–157.

Skiba, D. (2009). Nursing education 2.0: A second look at Second Life. *Nursing Education Perspectives, 30*(2), 129–131.

Virtual Ability Inc. (2012). A support environment. Retrieved from www.virtualability.org/

Wang, Y., & Braman, J. (2009). Extending the classroom through Second Life. *Journal of Information Systems Education, 20*(2), 235.

Warburton, S. (2009). Second Life in higher education: Assessing the potential for and the barriers to deploying virtual worlds in learning and teaching. *British Journal of Educational Technology, 40*(3), 414–426.

Yellowlees, P., & Cook, J. (2006). Education about hallucinations using an internet virtual reality system: A qualitative survey. *Academic Psychiatry, 30*(6), 534–539.

Young, J. (2010, February 14). After frustrations in Second Life, colleges look to new virtual worlds. *Chronicle of Higher Education.* Retrieved from http://chronicle.com/article/After-Frustrations-in-Second/64137/

8

Evaluating Teacher Effectiveness When Using Simulations

Cynthia E. Reese, PhD, RN, CNE

◼ Learning Objectives

1. Define effective teaching in simulation.
2. Discuss the role of the teacher in various educational settings.
3. Describe learning theories and evidence informing effective teaching.
4. Consider use of evidence-based teaching strategies when planning and implementing simulations.
5. Identify reliable and valid instrument to evaluate teacher effectiveness in simulation.

◼ Key Terms

- Effective teaching
- Learner-centered teaching
- Scaffolding
- Zone of proximal development

Clinical simulation is an innovative teaching and learning strategy that supports the efforts of educators to prepare students for practice (Bearnson & Wilker, 2005; Bradley, 2006; Hotchkiss, Biddle, & Fallacaro, 2002; Jeffries, 2005; Nehring, Lashley, & Ellis, 2002). Despite the positive implications and increased use of clinical simulations in nursing education, there is little evidence to support overall best practices and no evidence to inform effective teaching in simulated learning environments. As a result, a survey instrument has been developed to serve as a tool for assessment, evaluation, and feedback in the ongoing professional development of nurse educators who use clinical simulations in the teaching learning process.

To address this lack of evidence to describe and measure effective teaching specific to clinical simulation settings, the evidence-based literature associated with effective teaching in the higher-education classroom and nursing clinical education was reviewed. Important components from the literature related to both classroom and clinical teaching were synthesized with learning theory and the National League for Nursing's Jeffries Simulation Framework (NLN/JSF) to define and develop a way to describe and measure effective teaching specifically in simulation contexts. In conjunction with the instrument development, effective teaching behaviors and their importance as perceived by prelicensure nursing students were identified. This chapter defines effective teaching and presents a reliable and valid instrument useful for measuring effective teaching behaviors in simulations.

DEFINITION OF EFFECTIVE TEACHING

Effective teaching in clinical simulations has a powerful impact on student experiences and outcomes of a simulation exercise (Bremner, Auddell, Bennett, & VanGeest, 2006; Nehring et al., 2002). The role of teacher and effective teaching strategies are informed by the **learner-centered**, sociocultural, and constructivist learning theories underpinning the NLN/JSF model. The role of the teacher changes significantly with learner-centered and constructivist teaching as the focus shifts from teacher to learner control of the educational environment. The teacher is viewed as a facilitator of learning who structures learning experiences to allow students to construct knowledge for themselves, in contrast to a lecture-driven, content delivery mode of instruction. Additionally, the educational objectives of the simulation direct the teaching strategies necessary for a successful simulation. For example, a simulation developed for teaching purposes requires the instructor to perform in a more supportive and facilitative role; however, if the simulation is used to evaluate students, the appropriate role is more of an observer (Jeffries, 2007; Jeffries & Rizzolo, 2006).

Effective teaching strategies in simulation have not been identified. However, a definition of effective teaching in simulation has been developed based on the current literature. Effective teaching in clinical simulation is defined as the degree to which the teaching strategies and behavioral characteristics of the instructor promote student achievement of the learning outcomes specified in the simulation experience. It is hypothesized that through the identification and subsequent use of effective teaching strategies, the quality of simulations will improve, which will ultimately improve the abilities of nursing graduates to function safely in the workplace.

LEARNING THEORY AND TEACHING IN SIMULATION

Given the need to develop empirical support for the use of clinical simulation in nursing, a simulation model (Jeffries, 2005) has been developed to guide the design, implementation, and evaluation of simulations. The NLN/JSF model provides a framework grounded in a synthesis of learner-centered, sociocultural, and constructivist learning theories. Chickering and Gamson's (1987) best practices in undergraduate education provided a framework for the development of the educational practices component of the model. The following discussion describes the theoretical underpinnings of effective teaching and the NLN/JSF model.

SOCIAL-CULTURAL LEARNING THEORY

Social constructivism, the educational theory supporting the simulation model, was developed by Vygotsky (1978) and originated from Marxist theory. Vygotsky rejected the reductionist psychology of his day, arguing that to understand an individual, one must first understand the context in which the individual exists (Lattuca, 2002). Learning, in social constructivist terms, is "the development of connections with and appropriation from the socio-cultural context in which we all exist" (Bonk & Cunningham, 1998, p. 33). Palincsar (1998) described learning and understanding as "inherently social; and cultural activities and tools (ranging from symbol systems to artifacts to language) are regarded as integral to conceptual development." As such, the examination of the educational context and setting is essential to understand and facilitate student thinking and learning.

Social constructivist teaching emphasizes active learning methods embedded within an environment in which the role of educator is that of a facilitator or guide. Discussions and interactions among learners as well as between the educator and learners help to transform the learning context into a learner-centered environment. Through these interactions, the educator can model his or her reasoning processes, which serve as a scaffold for the development of student knowledge (Lattuca, 2006). **Scaffolding** is a temporary framework developed by the educator that supports the development of the learner and is gradually withdrawn as the learner develops understanding (Dunphy & Dunphy, 2003; Sanders & Welk, 2005). Scaffolding supports the student initially, and the support is gradually withdrawn as the student actively constructs understanding in a way that makes meaning for him or her (Sudzina, 1997).

A central tenet of sociocultural learning theory is the concept of the **zone of proximal development** (ZPD). Vygotsky (1978) defined the ZPD as "the distance between the actual developmental level as determined by independent problem solving and the level of potential development as determined through problem solving under adult guidance or in collaboration with more capable peers" (p. 85). Thus, productive interactions between peers and educators become a critical element to learn and develop higher-order thinking and problem-solving abilities. Additionally, it is hypothesized that interactions between the learner and a more capable peer become more important than those between educator and learner and should be encouraged (Palincsar, 1998).

Strategies to scaffold student learning, known as *assisted performance* and based on the application of the ZPD, have been created to apply sociocultural learning theory in medical and nursing education (Dunphy & Dunphy, 2003; Sanders & Welk, 2005). Five strategies to assist student performance have been identified as modeling, feedback, instructing, questioning, and cognitive structuring. As the student progresses in knowledge and ability, the scaffolding supports are slowly removed and the student begins to internalize information and perform without assistance. The responsibility for learning shifts during this time from the teacher to the learner, and it is hypothesized that teaching occurs when assistance is offered at certain points in the student's ZPD where assistance is required (Dunphy & Dunphy, 2003; Vygotsky, 1978).

In addition to assisting individual student performance, learning activities reflecting the complexity of real-world problems allow students to make meaning and develop a deeper understanding of realistic situations. Sociocultural learning theory implies that learning occurs best within realistic environments, which is one of the primary advantages of simulations over didactic learning contexts. Thus, the basic tenets of social constructivism fit well with simulation as a teaching and learning strategy, through the simulation model, and the role of educator in clinical simulation.

LEARNER-CENTERED APPROACHES

Weimer (2002) described teaching in a learner-centered environment as a context in which teachers "position themselves alongside the learner and keep the attention, focus, and spotlight aimed at and on the learning process" (p. 76). The learner-centered role of the teacher is generally defined as a facilitator, coach, or guide. Further, Weimer (2002) proposed five key areas for educators to examine to facilitate changes in practice to move toward a learner-centered environment:

1. The balance of power must shift from the teacher to the learner. The focus of the classroom must be on learners.

2. The function of content must be taken into consideration as rote memorization of information leads to "surface learning" as opposed to "deep learning." Deep learning involves relating previous knowledge and what has been learned from different courses to new knowledge. The knowledge is internally analyzed and integrated by the learners into a coherent whole.

3. The role of the teacher. The teaching role is one of a facilitator of learning rather than a transmitter of knowledge seen in traditional teaching.

4. Responsibility for learning. Students bear much of the responsibility for their own learning, as the focus is clearly on the learner. This may pose a challenge to students initially as traditionally educators take responsibility for organizing content and information for students to "learn." Increasing student responsibility for learning may encourage students to develop as independent, autonomous learners.

5. Evaluation purpose and process. Traditional classroom assessments are driven by grades using assessment and evaluation tools developed by the educator. The learner-centered classroom supports the use of evaluation activities which support learning, and provide opportunities to develop self and peer-assessment skills (pp. 8–17).

The use of learner-centered principles in the design, implementation, and evaluation of clinical simulation may improve student outcomes as outlined by the NLN/JSF. The empowerment of students in a learner-centered environment encourages the growth of students into confident, self-motivated learners.

CONSTRUCTIVISM

Constructivism as a theory of learning has developed past its philosophic roots and has garnered support from the fields of neurobiology and cognitive science (Fosnot, 2005, p. 276). A consensus among educational researchers has developed with agreement that knowledge is actively constructed rather than transmitted to the learner. Von Glasersfeld (1996) described two basic aspects of the constructivist model: (1) learning is a constructive activity that the students themselves must carry out, and (2) the task of the educator is not to dispense knowledge but to provide students with opportunities and incentives to build it up. However, what continues to remain challenging for educators are the implications for the application of constructivist theory to education, specifically the implications of constructivism in regard to teaching strategies.

Capra (2002) developed a new biologic model that informs constructivism. Cells and cellular networks are described as complex, nonlinear, open systems; "whole cellular networks" that are living and evolving systems needing a continual flow of matter and energy from the environment to stay alive. An integral facet of this model hypothesizes that when a flow of energy to the system increases, the overall system develops instability, resulting in the development of a "bifurcation point." The *bifurcation* is the location that produces new structures that developed as a direct result of interaction with the environment. As such, an individual's connection with the environment produces changes in the neural structure, which has direct implications for the construction of knowledge based on prior understandings and challenges posed to the learner from the environment (Fosnot, 2005, p. 278).

As support for the value of constructivism continues to develop, challenges remain regarding the practical application of the theory in the educational setting. Constructivism is a theory of learning and not a theory of teaching. However, based on an understanding of constructivism, an educator is able to develop applicable teaching strategies. In a global sense, Fosnot (2005) described the role of the teacher in the constructivist tradition as a facilitator, provocateur, and questioner focusing discussions around "big ideas" and efficient strategies aligned with learning. Richardson (2003) outlined the following characteristics of constructivist pedagogy:

1. Attention to the individual and respect for students' background and developing understandings and beliefs about elements of the domain.

2. Facilitation of group dialogue that explores an element of the domain with the purpose of leading to the creation and shared understanding of a topic.

3. Planned and often unplanned introduction of formal domain knowledge into the conversation through direct instruction, reference to text, exploration of a website, or some other means.

4. Provision of opportunities for students to determine, challenge, change, or add to existing beliefs and understandings through engagement in tasks that are structured for this purpose.

5. Development of students' awareness of their own understandings and learning processes.

Although the characteristics of constructivist teaching have been explicated by Richardson (2003), behaviors corresponding to those characteristics have not been developed. However, these global characteristics of constructivist pedagogy may be relevant to the identification of effective teaching behaviors within clinical simulation. For example, specific behaviors relating to the facilitation of group dialogue during the debriefing period following simulation have been suggested, such as structuring the discussion using preset questions, seating the group in a circle, maintaining eye contact, focusing on the positive aspects of the simulation, and using a nonjudgmental communication style. Thus, the lack of development of specific theory-based teaching behaviors is problematic for the design, implementation, and evaluation of clinical simulations.

A synthesis of the theories and principles underpinning the NLN/JSF model—sociocultural learning theory (Vygotsky, 1978), the principles of learner-centered teaching (Weimer, 2002), constructivist characteristics of teaching (Fosnot, 2005; Richardson, 2003), and Chickering and Gamson's (1987) best practices—provides a set of principles to guide educators working with simulation as a teaching-learning strategy. However, from a practical standpoint, using guiding principles that are not explicit, defined, or measureable is of limited usefulness to front-line educators. There is a pressing need to identify effective teaching behaviors in simulation to enhance, coach, and evaluate teaching within this context.

ROLE OF THE TEACHER AND BEST PRACTICE IN SIMULATIONS

The role of the teacher and effective teaching strategies in simulation have not been clearly defined. However, evidence-based literature exists that describes effective teaching and effective teaching behaviors in traditional classroom and clinical contexts within higher education. This empirical literature was reviewed because simulations have characteristics that are both similar and dissimilar to classroom and clinical teaching. Simulation uses active, experiential learning that is a major component of clinical education (Bremner et al., 2006; Larew, Lessans, Spunt, Foster, & Covington, 2007; McCausland, Curran, & Cataldi, 2004). Additionally, simulations are conducted in a controlled setting, which has similarities with classroom teaching. Theory learned in the classroom can be actively applied and synthesized in the simulation laboratory. Thus, a clinical simulation has similarities to both clinical and classroom teaching. Because simulation is essentially a hybrid of the two and there are no data to define effective teaching specifically in simulation, the literature from both areas has been used to identify best practices that may integrate with simulations.

Several commonalities have been identified in the literature related to best practice in classroom and clinical teaching that can be applied to simulations. The effective teacher in the classroom is dedicated, enthusiastic, knowledgeable, professionally competent, and supportive and communicates well. The difficulty of the material and examination and grading practices are all at a level appropriate for students. In the clinical context, effective teachers are professionally competent and knowledgeable with strong teaching ability. Effective teachers have an ability to develop interpersonal relationships with students and provide constructive feedback to students.

As a result of a synthesis of the learning theories described previously and the clinical and classroom teaching literature, the following best teaching practices in simulation were developed:

1. *Facilitator–learner centered.* The role of the teacher is to provide the structure for and to assist or coach student learning. The focus is squarely on the learner in an environment conducive to learning. Instruction is designed to allow students to control and be responsible for their learning (Vygotsky, 1978; Weimer, 2002).

2. *Feedback and debriefing.* Feedback is the constructive and nonjudgmental appraisal of performance. It can be formative or summative. The type and amount of feedback is assessed (Bienstock et al., 2007; Mogan & Knox, 1987).

3. *Teaching ability*. An ability to design, implement, and evaluate simulations effectively. Specifies a knowledge base and comfort level with simulation technology (Jeffries, 2007).

4. *Modeling*. Modeling is the process of offering behavior for imitation. Modeled activities can be transformed into images and verbal symbols that guide subsequent performance. Faculty or more advanced peers may serve as a model (Dunphy & Dunphy, 2003).

5. *Interpersonal relationships*. This includes faculty to student, student to student, and group interactions or communication. These interactions are based on mutual respect, fairness, and confidentiality (Copeland & Hewson, 2000; Mogan & Knox, 1987).

6. *Expectations*. The level of complexity of the simulation is appropriate for optimal student learning to occur. Generally it is based on the level of the students and assessment of students' ZPD (Sanders & Welk, 2005; Vygotsky, 1978).

7. *Organization*. Organization is based on whether the simulation experience (simulation plus debriefing) flowed smoothly and the simulation design, implementation, and evaluation were orderly, functional, and well structured into a coherent whole.

8. *Enthusiasm*. The instructor is dynamic and energetic and demonstrates excitement and interest toward the subject (Marsh, 1987).

9. *Cuing*. Verbal, nonverbal, or written information or data are provided to the learners to spur their thinking in order to make meaning of the situation (Alfaro-LaFevre, 2004; Larew et al., 2007; Pesut & Herman, 1999).

10. *Questioning*. Questioning calls for an active linguistic and cognitive response, and it provokes creations by the learner (Dunphy & Dunphy, 2003). There are two kinds of questions: those that assess and those that assist. Appropriate questioning allows the educator to know how much assistance is needed to optimize learning (Sanders & Welk, 2005).

DEVELOPMENT OF THE STUDENT'S PERCEPTION OF EFFECTIVE TEACHING IN CLINICAL SIMULATION SCALE

The Student's Perception of Effective Teaching in Clinical Simulation (SPETCS) scale is a 33-item survey instrument developed as an evidenced-based tool to identify and measure effective teaching behaviors specific to simulation (Reese, 2009). The instrument is scored on a five-point Likert scale with two response scales: extent and importance. The extent scale measures students' perception of the extent the instructor used a particular teaching strategy during the simulation, and the importance scale measures perception of the importance of each teaching strategy toward meeting the simulation learning outcomes. Items were written based on the best practices identified in the classroom and clinical teaching literature and related learning theories described previously.

Items for the instrument were reviewed for content validity by seven nationally recognized simulation experts, with a solid content validity index of 0.91. A convenience

TABLE 8.1

Sample Items from the Student's Perception of Effective Teaching in Clinical Simulation Scale

Learner Support	Real-World Application
Cues were used in the simulation to help me progress through the experience.	Participation in this simulation was a valuable learning activity.
The instructor served as a role model during the simulation.	The simulation was realistic.
The instructor encouraged helpful collaboration among participants during debriefing.	The simulation experience allows me to model a professional role in a realistic manner.

Reese, C. (2009). *Effective teaching in simulation: Development of the student perception of effective teaching in simulation scale.* (Doctoral dissertation). Retrieved from https://scholarworks.iupui.edu/bitstream/handle/1805/1901/Rev_Diss_4_4.pdf?sequence=1

sample of undergraduate nursing students ($n = 121$) who participated in high-fidelity simulation with two master teachers in simulation was used for psychometric analysis. The SPETCS was found to be very reliable, with a Cronbach's alpha of 0.95 for the extent scale and 0.96 for the importance scale.

To further examine the validity of the SPETCS, the results were compared with two well-known instruments: the Student's Evaluation of Educational Quality (Marsh, 1987) used in the classroom and the Nursing Clinical Teacher Effectiveness Inventory (Mogan & Knox, 1987) used in the clinical setting. The SPETCS demonstrated evidence of criterion-related validity as all of the correlations were significant ($p < .05$) between the scores of the three instruments.

An exploratory factor analysis with varimax rotation was calculated on the importance scale to determine the major constructs the students identified as important to meeting the learning outcomes of the simulation. Two factors, learner support and real-world application, accounted for 71 percent of the variance. See Table 8.1 for examples of several SPETCS items from each factor.

The SPETCS is an easy-to-administer survey and ideally should be completed by students immediately following a simulation experience. The extent response scale provides feedback to faculty related to students' perception of the extent of effective teaching strategies used in the simulation. The mean score for each item on the scale can be calculated. Areas of strength and areas for improvement can be easily identified, with items with the higher mean indicating an area of strength and those with lower means an area for improvement. Additionally, the mean of the total of scores on the extent scale can be used to determine an overall score of teaching effectiveness, and the results can be trended over time. The importance response scale results, both individual items and total mean score, are useful to determine which teaching strategies students see as central to attainment of simulation outcomes.

TABLE 8.2

Constructs Underlying Factors of Effective Teaching

Factor	Construct
Learner support	Feedback
	Debriefing
	Teaching ability
	Modeling[a]
	Interpersonal relationships
	Enthusiasm
	Cuing
	Questioning
Real-world application	Expectations
	Organization
	Modeling[a]

[a]Modeling is related to both factors.

IMPLEMENTATION OF THE SPETCS

The results from development and testing of the SPETCS provide evidence informing effective teaching practices in simulations. Two major factors, learner support and real-world application, represent global constructs identified in this process. Learner support fits with the learner-centered and constructivist learning theories and clearly relates to what occurred during the simulation experience such as teacher enthusiasm, feedback, cues, and questioning. All of these teaching behaviors were found to facilitate learning during simulation. The second construct, real-world application, relates to the expectation of the learner that participation in simulation has a positive impact on the ability to perform in a clinical setting with actual patients. The simulation fidelity, development of critical-thinking abilities, and learning objectives have been met as components of the real-world application. See Table 8.2 for the components of effective teaching for each major factor.

IMPLICATIONS FOR EDUCATORS IMPLEMENTING SIMULATIONS

Nurse educators have been charged to develop and use evidence-based educational practices to prepare graduates to be able to function in the complex health care environment. The SPETCS has been created to define and evaluate teaching strategies specifically in simulations. A set of teaching strategies and behaviors that learners perceive to be most important to the attainment of the student learning outcomes has been identified. It is suggested that these strategies be taken into consideration when a simulation is planned. The most important teaching strategy is useful feedback from the teacher. In a well-designed simulation, feedback is generally provided during debriefing immediately following the simulation. However, feedback may be given at any time during the simulation depending on the purpose of the simulation.

Debriefing has been found to be important to learners' development of clinical reasoning abilities. Learners should be encouraged to share and discuss the thinking that guided their decisions made during simulation. Careful consideration needs to be given to the debriefing component of the simulation, and adequate time needs to be allotted to support the high-quality learning that occurs during debriefing.

The capability to translate learning from simulation into an improved ability to care for actual patients in the clinical setting is another salient component of simulation. The evidence supports that the creation of simulations that are realistic and allow learners to model psychomotor, cognitive, and affective behaviors needed in the clinical area are necessary components of well-designed simulations. The fidelity of the simulation may be enhanced through the use of moderate to high-fidelity human patient simulators in a realistic setting. The use of realistic props, moulage, and clinical uniforms worn by learners and educators can also support fidelity of the simulation.

SUMMARY

As simulations continue to become more prominent in schools of nursing, it is important for educators to plan and implement quality, evidence-based simulations to maximize the achievement of student learning outcomes. One major component of a quality simulation is the role of the teacher. Learning theory and the literature from classroom and clinical education in conjunction with data from the development of the SPETCS provide evidence informing the role of the teacher.

The role of teacher is based on several elements. The primary element is related to the learner-support factor from the SPETCS. These factors include the objectives of the simulation, the level of the learner, and the degree of scaffolding for learners generally through cues embedded in the simulation. Additionally, the role of teacher changes in an evaluative simulation to that of an evaluator rather than a facilitator of learning.

A secondary element is related to the real-world application factor from the SPETCS. The setting of the simulation dictates the objectives and planning. The simulation needs to be structured based on whether the learners are in a prelicensure (undergraduate) program, a graduate level educational program, or in the practice setting for new graduate orientation or to ensure the competency of new practitioners.

The role of the teacher, as well as the evidence supporting effective teaching strategies and behaviors in simulation, needs to be taken into careful consideration by educators planning and implementing simulations in a variety of settings. Because the use of simulation in nursing education and practice continues to evolve, the development of quality, evidence-based simulations becomes more important to preparing students for practice.

Key Concepts

- Effective teaching in clinical simulations has a powerful impact on student experiences and outcomes of a simulation exercise.
- Effective teaching in clinical simulation is defined as the degree to which the teaching strategies and behavioral characteristics of the instructor promote student achievement of the learning outcomes specified in the simulation experience.
- Literature from clinical and classroom teaching in higher education was reviewed and synthesized with NLN/JSF to develop a definition and measure of effective teaching in simulation.
- The SPETCS is a 33-item survey to measure effective teaching behaviors and the importance of these behaviors to student participants.
- The purpose of the SPETCS is to serve as a tool for assessment, evaluation, and feedback in the ongoing professional development of nurse educators who use clinical simulations in the teaching learning process.
- Two major areas of effective teaching have been identified and supported empirically: real-world application and learner support.

References

Alfaro-LeFevre, R. (2004). *Critical thinking and clinical judgment.* St. Louis, MO: Saunders.

Bearnson, C., & Wilker, K. (2005). Human patient simulators: A new face in baccalaureate nursing education at Brigham Young University. *Journal of Nursing Education, 44*(9), 421–425.

Bienstock, J. L., Katz, N. T., Cox, S. M., Hueppchen, N., Erickson, S., & Pushcheck, E. E. (2007). To the point: Medical education reviews-providing feedback. *American Journal of Obstetrics & Gynecology, 196*(6), 508–513.

Bonk, C. J., & Cunningham, D. J. (1998). *Searching for learner-centered, constructivist, and sociocultural components of collaborative education learning tools in electronic collaborators.* Mahwah, NJ: Erlbaum.

Bradley, P. (2006). The history of simulation in medical education and possible future directions. *Medical Education, 40,* 254–262.

Bremner, M. N., Auddell, K., Bennett, D. N., & VanGeest, J. B. (2006). The use of human patient simulators: best practices with novice nursing students. *Nurse Educator, 31*(4), 170–174.

Capra, F. (2002). *The hidden connections: integrating the biological, cognitive, and social dimensions of life into a science of sustainability.* New York: Doubleday.

Chickering, A. W., & Gamson, Z. F. (1987). Seven principles of good practice in undergraduate education. *AAHE Bulletin, 39*(7), 5–10.

Copeland, H. L., & Hewson, M. G. (2000). Developing and testing an instrument to measure the effectiveness of clinical teaching at an academic medical center. *Academic Medicine, 75*(2), 161–166.

Dunphy, B. C., & Dunphy, S. L. (2003). Assisted performance and the zone of proximal development: a potential framework for providing surgical education. *Australian Journal of Educational and Developmental Psychology, 3,* 48–58.

Fosnot, C. T. (2005). *Constructivism: theory, perspectives, and practice.* New York: Teachers College Press.

Hotchkiss, M., Biddle, C., & Fallacaro, M. (2002). Assessing the authenticity of the human simulation experience in anesthesiology. *AANA Journal, 70*(6), 470–473.

Jeffries, P. (2005). A framework for designing, implementing, and evaluating simulations used as teaching strategies in nursing. *Nursing Education Perspectives, 26*(2), 96–103.

Jeffries, P. R. (Ed.). (2007). *Simulation in nursing education from conceptualization to evaluation.* New York: National League for Nursing.

Jeffries, P. R., & Rizzolo, M. A. (2006). *Designing and implementing models for the innovative use of simulation to teach nursing care of ill adults and children: a national, multi-site, multi-method study.* New York: National League for Nursing.

Larew, C., Lessans, S., Spunt, D., Foster, D., & Covington, B. G. (2007). Innovations in clinical simulation: Application of Benner's theory in an interactive patient care simulation. *Nursing Education Perspectives, 27*(1), 16–21.

Lattuca, L. R. (2002). Learning interdisciplinarity: Sociocultural perspectives on academic work. *Journal of Higher Education, 73*(6), 711–739.

Marsh, H. W. (1987). Students' evaluations of university teaching: Research findings, methodological issues, and directions for future research. *International Journal of Educational Research, 11*(3), 253–388.

McCausland, L., Curran, C., & Cataldi, P. (2004). Use of a human simulator for undergraduate nurse education. *International Journal of Nursing Education Scholarship, 1*(1), article 23.

Mogan, J., & Knox, J. E. (1987). Characteristics of "best" and "worst" clinical teachers as perceived by university nursing faculty and students. *Journal of Advanced Nursing, 12,* 331–337.

Nehring, W., Lashley, F., & Ellis, W. (2002). Critical incident nursing management using human patient simulators. *Nursing Education Perspectives, 23*(3), 128–132.

Palincsar, A. S. (1998). Social constructivist perspectives on teaching and learning. *Annual Reviews of Psychology, 49,* 347–375.

Pesut, D., & Herman, J. (1999). *Clinical reasoning: The art and science of critical and creative thinking.* Albany, NY: Delmar.

Reese, C. (2009). *Effective teaching in simulation: Development of the student perception of effective teaching in simulation scale.* (Doctoral dissertation). Retrieved from https://scholarworks.iupui.edu/bitstream/handle/1805/1901/Rev_Diss_4_4.pdf?sequence=1

Richardson, V. (2003). Constructivist pedagogy. *Teachers College Record, 105*(9), 1623–1640.

Sanders, D., & Welk, D. S. (2005). Strategies to scaffold student learning: Applying Vygotsky's zone of proximal development. *Nurse Educator, 30*(5), 203–207.

Sudzina, M. R. (1997). Case study as a constructivist pedagogy for teaching educational psychology. *Educational Psychology Review, 9*(2), 199–260.

Von Glasersfeld, E. (1996). Introduction: Aspects of constructivism. In C. T. Fosnot (Ed.), *Constructivism: Theory, perspectives, and practice* (Chapter 1). New York: Teachers College Press.

Vygotsky, L. S. (1978). *Mind in society: The development of higher psychological processes.* Cambridge, MA: Harvard University Press.

Weimer, M. (2002). *Learner-centered teaching five key changes to practice.* San Francisco: Jossey-Bass.

9

Developing and Using Simulation for High-Stakes Assessment

Mary Anne Rizzolo, EdD, RN, FAAN, ANEF

Learning Objectives

1. Describe the current process used in schools of nursing to determine if students are competent to progress to the next level in the curriculum.
2. Propose a set of guidelines for developing and using high-fidelity simulations in place of some summative evaluation currently used by faculty in the clinical practice environment that includes the following:
   - Deciding if and when to use simulation for assessment
   - Assembling a simulation-based evaluation team
   - Identifying where simulation-based evaluation will be used in the curriculum
   - Describing the steps in the scenario design and development process
   - Preparing the testing environment
   - Preparing learners for a high-fidelity simulation-based evaluation
3. Plan the evaluation phase for simulation-based assessment including selecting evaluation tools, determining their reliability and validity for your population of students, and choosing and training evaluators.
4. Discuss the challenges associated with implementing high-fidelity simulation-based evaluation.

The recommendations contained in this chapter were derived from the "National League for Nursing Project to Explore the Use of Simulation for High Stakes Assessment," which was conducted from 2010 to 2013. Pamela Jeffries, PhD, RN, FAAN, ANEF, led the team that developed the simulations, Marilyn Oermann, PhD, RN, FAAN, ANEF, and Suzan Kardong-Edgren, PhD, RN, ANEF, CHSE, developed the evaluation plan and designed training for the evaluation team. Manuscripts describing the processes and outcomes of the project are in development.

■ Key Terms

- ■ Formative evaluation
- ■ High-fidelity simulations
- ■ High-stakes assessment
- ■ Summative evaluation

Nurse educators diligently strive to prepare their students to be safe, competent practitioners in an increasingly complex health care environment. However, evaluating students to determine if they are ready to progress to the next level in their curriculum or to certify that they are ready to take the National Council Licensure Examination (NCLEX®) at the end of their program is not an easy task. Traditional programs typically use a combination of multiple choice teacher-made tests and standardized tests purchased from vendors, along with an evaluation of student performance in the clinical setting to determine whether a student advances to the next level. Although well-constructed multiple choice exams offer an objective tool to measure a student's knowledge base, using today's clinical environment is a questionable venue to provide a fair assessment of a student's ability to apply his or her nursing knowledge in a patient care situation. Oermann, Yarbrough, Saewart, Ard, and Charasika (2009) noted that clinical evaluation is "rife with problems," including issues of inconsistency and subjectivity.

In the National League for Nursing's (2012) living document titled "The Fair Testing Imperative in Nursing Education," recommendations for faculty included a statement that "multiple sources of evidence are fundamental to evaluate basic nursing competence. This is especially true when high-stakes decisions are based on the assessment." In recommendations for deans, directors, and chairs of nursing programs, this same document urged them to "[p]rovide appropriate resources for faculty and staff to develop knowledge and skills in using multiple approaches to assessing student learning and nursing competence."

Some types of simulation have been used in the health care professions for several years. Objective simulated clinical exams (OSCEs), which are short and skills based (NLN Simulation Innovation Resource Center, n.d.), have been used in medicine, dentistry, nursing, and other health professions. Holmboe, Rizzolo, Sachdeva, Rosenberg, and Ziv (2011) summarized the use of simulation-based assessment in the health professions, citing examples such as the National Board of Medical Examiners, which has been using OSCEs for Step 2 of the U.S. Medical Licensing Exam (Papadakis, 2004), and successful completion of the Fundamentals of Laparoscopic Surgery course, required by the American Board of Surgery (n.d.), for initial certification in surgery.

In nursing, OSCEs are being used in several countries throughout the world (Walsh, Bailey, & Koren, 2009) and there appears to be growing interest in their use (Mårtensson & Löfmark, 2013; McWilliam & Botwinski, 2010; Selim, Ramadan, el-Gueneidy, & Gaafer, 2012; Smith, Muldoon, & Biesty, 2012). In Quebec, they are part of the RN licensing exam and OSCEs are used throughout Canada to assess skills of graduates of foreign nursing schools. Drexel University is one of the few, and perhaps the only, known prelicensure program in the United States that requires students to pass a high-fidelity simulated encounter with a standardized patient focused on communication skills, obtaining a health history, completing a focused physical assessment, and providing appropriate patient teaching in order to graduate from their program (Wilson et al., 2006).

This chapter will focus exclusively on a set of guidelines for developing and using **high-fidelity simulations** for summative **high-stakes assessment**. Essentially, it addresses using simulation in place of some of the evaluation currently done by faculty in the clinical practice environment. Before reading further, reflect on how fair and effective the existing evaluation process is at your school.

- Have all faculty and adjunct faculty been educated on how to assess the clinical competencies of their students?
- Does every faculty member evaluate their students in the same way?
- Have there been deliberative conversations among faculty to clarify the behaviors and expectations of student practice at the end of each course and at the end of the program?
- Do you know of faculty who never fail a student, even though you have seen evidence of poor practice by that student?
- When your school submits a list of students who have completed your program and are eligible to take the NCLEX exam, are you confident about the competencies of all the students on that list?

THE DECISION TO USE SIMULATION FOR ASSESSMENT

Anyone who has developed a simulation can attest to how time consuming it is. When the simulation is being designed to determine student progression, it requires an even greater investment in time and resources, so the decision to use a high-fidelity simulation for student assessment should not be made lightly. Use simulation for those competencies that cannot be assessed well by other forms of evaluation. In general, that means a simulation that requires learners to "put it all together." Currently, clinical evaluation is used to measure those types of holistic competencies. The advantage of using simulation is that in a simulated clinical encounter, the environment can be deliberately designed and controlled to provide learner assessment that is unencumbered by interruptions and unexpected events. It also delivers an equivalent event to all students and has the potential for a more objective evaluation, because standardized tools and multiple trained raters can be used. But not everyone is convinced that simulation should be used for assessment, as evidenced in a roundtable discussion at the International Nursing Association for Clinical Simulation and Learning conference in 2009 (Kardong-Edgren, Hanberg, Keenan, Ackerman, & Chambers, 2011). Be sure that faculty are on board before undertaking the long process of developing a valid and reliable simulation-based assessment.

THE PROCESS FOR DEVELOPING SIMULATION-BASED EVALUATION

The Simulation-Based Evaluation Team

Once faculty have made the decision to use simulation-based assessment (SBE), the first step is to assemble a team consisting of experts in simulation development, faculty representatives, evaluation experts, and simulation technicians who can provide technical support in the testing environment. When simulation is being used at the end of a program, include practice partners on the team. Berkow, Virkstis, Stewart, and Conway (2008) revealed a wide gap in agreement between academic and practice leaders on competencies of new graduates, so the input of your practice partners will be invaluable. It is recommended that simulation developers at other schools be included on the team so they can participate in piloting the simulations.

Where in the Curriculum Will Simulation-Based Evaluation Be Used?

The first decision for the team is to select the points in the curriculum when the SBE will take place. A required course with a clinical component that occurs early in the curriculum can be a good place to begin, because the level of clinical judgment expected of students is at a basic level at this point. Many schools already require students to validate their skills in the skills lab and use checklists to indicate that the critical elements of each skill have been demonstrated. Adding a high-fidelity simulation that requires students to demonstrate the appropriate level of clinical judgment would acclimate students to a high-stakes testing process early in their curriculum. Bensfield, Olech, and Horsley (2012) found several disadvantages in initiating a simulation-based assessment late in their curriculum. The most concerning was that some students with high grade point averages had significant deficiencies in some essential competencies. When assessment begins early, there is more time available for remediation, successful completion of the program, and a smoother transition into the workforce.

The Scenario Design and Development Process

The next decision is what outcomes or competencies will be evaluated. The simulation experts on the team need to help faculty envision the behaviors that students must exhibit to prove competency; expect that it will take several meetings for that to occur.

The next choice is whether to create the simulations in house or buy them from a vendor and adapt them to meet your needs. The advantage of purchasing is that those simulations have already undergone a pilot process for content validity, so the development phase can be shortened. Whether to use a standardized or simulated patient or a manikin will be dictated by the outcomes and competencies that are being assessed.

Whether you purchase or create your own, expect to go through many iterations and revisions before everyone is satisfied. It is essential to get consensus from faculty that the final simulations reflect the performance that is expected of learners at that evaluation point in the curriculum. Getting that consensus may not be an easy task, particularly if faculty have not engaged in this type of conversation before. Agreeing to a list of competencies that appear in a written document does not necessarily translate into agreeing that the simulations you purchased or designed can assess those competencies.

Design Pointers

Begin the scenario by providing a prerecorded report on the patient by the nurse going off duty. This can save facilitator time and reduce unintentional cueing by the person giving the report. In the scenario progression outline, anticipate common student actions and provide specific script guidelines for facilitators (if the student asks X, you respond with Y). At the end of the scenario, some type of debriefing is needed to determine whether students used good clinical judgment to guide their interventions. A verbal report is one approach that can be used, and it provides facilitators with an opportunity to ask the student for clarification if needed. There should be guidelines for this as well, because questions can also cue the student to a correct response.

Creating Multiple Forms

To protect the security of your scenarios, you will want to create several versions of each one. A set of medical or surgical scenarios can start out with the same diagnosis or surgical procedure, but then each could develop a different complication requiring nursing intervention. Changing the names, sex, and other minor details can provide numerous additional variations. However, during the pilot phase, be sure to confirm with other simulation experts, preferably those at other schools, that all versions are equivalent and parallel in nature and measure the same competencies.

Piloting

Apply your networking skills to identify simulation experts and faculty at other schools who are interested in SBE, particularly those who are ready to undertake a similar journey of student assessment. Use listservs and discussion boards and make contacts at simulation events. Propose creating a multisite project, and be sure to publish your results!

Begin the pilot phase by having simulation experts review written versions of the scenarios to identify areas that need clarification and revision, then find students to run the scenario. Using students at other schools to run through the simulations will protect the security of your simulations, and the simulation facilitators at another school can provide a more objective review of the scenarios. Video record all student performances so they can be reviewed at convenient times. Video recording can also be used later to train facilitators and raters. Expect that this pilot phase will take a long time to complete. Scenarios often need to be run repeatedly with different groups of students to refine them, to ensure that the time allowed for students to complete simulation activities is fair, and to ensure that versions are parallel.

THE TESTING ENVIRONMENT

While the simulations are being piloted and refined, take time to consider how you will prepare the testing environment. It should be a fairly quiet area with minimal noise and distractions. The setup of the room should be as similar as possible for every SBE session. The simulation template will provide a list of all needed supplies, any moulage required, and resources such as textbooks that should be available to students. Taking pictures of the room can provide additional guidance to those who will set it up for testing and to ensure that props are consistently in the same place for all simulations. Bringing facilitators together for training on how to set up and run the scenarios can help to minimize variability in the testing environment.

Advantages and Guidelines for Video Recording

If your school has not used video to record student performances, an important step is getting signed consent from those being videotaped. Most schools have students sign a broad consent form at the beginning of their program that covers using video for both **formative** and **summative evaluation**. Using video to record student performance for SBE has several advantages. Final student performances can be viewed by several trained evaluators at a time that is convenient for each of them. However, video equipment is expensive, and significant preplanning is required to determine the best placement of cameras and microphones. Generally three camera views are required to provide good coverage of the simulation area. Students and facilitators also need orientation and instructions related to the equipment. Although this increases the amount of time needed to set up the testing environment, having the recordings has many advantages for ensuring a fair student assessment and it provides rich data for quality assurance and research.

PREPARING STUDENTS FOR HIGH-STAKES ASSESSMENT

Although preparing the testing environment is important, preparing the student for SBE is, of course, even more important. Students should have multiple experiences with simulation as a teaching and learning strategy before it is used for assessment. There needs to be a clear distinction between when simulation is being used to learn and when it is being used for evaluation. Clear instructions should be provided in advance related to how long the simulation will run and any other information the student needs to know to be successful.

There is much work needed in this aspect of SBE, but some is already under way. Willhaus (2013) conducted research on student anxiety during simulation. Cordeau (2012) explored two research questions: (1) What is the specific social psychological problem in high-stakes, clinical simulation? (2) What is the social psychological process used to cope with the problem? This type of scholarly work will eventually provide the evidence needed to prepare students for this new approach to evaluation.

EVALUATION OF STUDENT PERFORMANCE

Evaluation Tools

Developing evaluation tools is complex and requires expertise. It is suggested that you seek a tool that provides a holistic approach to evaluation rather than a long checklist of items. There are several existing tools that can be used. Adamson, Kardong-Edgren, and Willhaus (2013) provided an extensive list of instruments. The evaluation experts on your SBE team are essential for selecting a valid and reliable tool that best meets your needs and determining how it should be piloted to confirm its reliability and validity for your students. They will also be invaluable in developing the plan to select and train raters.

Selecting Evaluators

It is very hard for anyone who has taught a student to move into the role of evaluator and be fully objective in that role (Chambers, 1998; Oermann et al., 2009; Stroud, Herold, Tomlinson, & Cavalcanti, 2011). The team should establish some criteria for the selection of raters. They should have experience with simulation and be familiar with the competencies expected of students at whatever point in the curriculum you are using SBE. Some faculty are better suited than others to the task of evaluation. Ideally, faculty from outside your school can be recruited to participate.

Training Evaluators

Raters will need training to understand the tool that has been selected. Have authors and evaluators come together to discuss the meaning of each competency item on the tool and then come to a consensus on the evidence required for scoring student performance on each item. Several training sessions may be required to help evaluators distinguish between competent and incompetent behaviors. Multiple training sessions and refreshers will also need to occur to ensure test–retest and interrater reliability. Finally, a decision needs to be made on the final score that students need to achieve to "pass."

CHALLENGES AND THE LONG ROAD AHEAD

Many of the challenges associated with implementing SBE, such as time commitment and security, have already been addressed, but there are innumerable research questions that must be asked and answered. Here are but a few:

- What outcomes must be measured to determine whether SBE is a superior method of assessment?
- How do the results of simulation-based assessments compare with traditional faculty clinical evaluations of those same students?
- How much experience should students have with simulation as a teaching or learning tool before it is used for assessment purposes?
- How many variations of a simulation are enough?
- How much does it cost to do this process correctly?
- What is the impact of SBE on retention, graduation rates, and success on the NCLEX?
- Are there specific qualities associated with faculty who are comfortable and consistent in the evaluator role?

- What are the best methods to use to train raters?
- Are there differences in scores when student performance is viewed live vs. viewed in a prerecorded video?

But perhaps the most important question of all is: What is the reliability and validity of what we are doing now?

The process that is outlined in this chapter is a huge undertaking. Can steps be omitted? Can the process be streamlined? We will not know the answers to those questions until we collect the evidence that will document what is essential. If this is too onerous a task for schools to undertake, perhaps it can be delegated to organizations or vendors. The answers will only come as research provides the data to help us make those decisions.

Wolf et al. (2011) wrote about the process they used at their school to combine formative and summative evaluations, accompanied by remediation, over the course of their curriculum and the benefits they perceived. Read that article, then reflect again on the questions that were posed at the beginning of this chapter to help you and your faculty decide on the next steps that your school should take in the student evaluation process.

■ Key Concepts

- Multiple sources of evidence are fundamental to evaluate basic nursing competence.
- Faculty need resources and training to develop the necessary knowledge and skills for using multiple approaches to assess student learning.
- Today's clinical environment is a questionable venue to use to provide a fair assessment of students' ability to apply their nursing knowledge and skills in a patient care situation.
- A high-fidelity simulated clinical encounter has the potential for a more objective student evaluation because it provides an environment that can be deliberately designed and controlled, is unencumbered by interruptions and unexpected events, and delivers an equivalent event to all students, and student performance can be evaluated using standardized tools and multiple trained raters.
- The process for developing and implementing simulation-based evaluation requires a commitment by faculty, the expertise of an entire team of individuals, and an extensive amount of time.
- Research questions must be formulated and answered to provide the data needed to guide all of the aspects of simulation-based evaluation.

References

Adamson, K., Kardong-Edgren, S., & Willhaus, J. (2013). An updated review of published simulation evaluation instruments. *Clinical Simulation in Nursing, 9*(9), e393–e405.

American Board of Surgery. (n.d.) ABS to require ACLS, ATLS and FLS for general surgery certification. Retrieved from http://home.absurgery.org/default.jsp?news_newreqs

Bensfield, L., Olech, M., & Horsley, T. (2012). Simulation for high-stakes evaluation in nursing. *Nurse Educator, 37*(2), 71–74.

Berkow, S., Virkstis, K., Stewart, J., & Conway, L. (2008). Assessing new graduate nurse performance. *Journal of Nursing Administration, 38*(11), 468–474.

Chambers, M. A. (1998). Some issues in the assessment of clinical practice: A review of the literature. *Journal of Clinical Nursing, 7*, 201–208.

Cordeau, M. A. (2012). Linking the transition: A substantive theory of high-stakes clinical simulation. *Advances in Nursing Science, 35*(3), E90–E102.

Holmboe, E., Rizzolo, M. A., Sachdeva, A. K., Rosenberg, M., & Ziv, A. (2011). Simulation-based assessment and the regulation of healthcare professionals. *Simulation in Healthcare, 6*(7 Suppl), 558–562.

Kardong-Edgren, S., Hanberg, A., Keenan, C., Ackerman, A., & Chambers, K. (2011). A discussion of high-stakes testing: An extension of a 2009 INACSL conference roundtable. *Clinical Simulation in Nursing, 7*(1), e19–e24.

Mårtensson, G., & Löfmark, A. (2013). Implementation and student evaluation of clinical final examination in nursing education. *Nurse Education Today,* pii: S0260-6917(13)00004-X.

McWilliam, P., & Botwinski, C. (2010). Developing a successful nursing objective structured clinical examination. *Journal of Nursing Education, 49*(1), 37–41.

National League for Nursing. (2012). The Fair Testing Imperative in Nursing Education. Retrieved from www.nln.org/aboutnln/livingdocuments/pdf/nlnvision_4.pdf

National League for Nursing Simulation Innovation Resource Center. (n.d.). SIRC glossary. Retrieved from http://sirc.nln.org/mod/glossary/view.php?id=183

Oermann, M. H., Yarbrough, S. S., Saewert, K. J., Ard, N., & Charasika, M. (2009). Clinical evaluation and grading practices in schools of nursing: National survey findings. Part II. *Nursing Education Perspectives, 30*(6), 352–357.

Papadakis, M. (2004). The step 2 clinical skills examination. *New England Journal of Medicine, 350*(17), 1703–1705.

Selim, A. A., Ramadan, F. H., el-Gueneidy, M. M., & Gaafer, M. M. (2012). Using objective structured clinical examination (OSCE) in undergraduate psychiatric nursing education: Is it reliable and valid? *Nurse Education Today, 32*(3), 283–288.

Smith, V., Muldoon, K., & Biesty, L. (2012). The objective structured clinical examination (OSCE) as a strategy for assessing clinical competence in midwifery education in Ireland: A critical review. *Nurse Education in Practice, 12*(5), 242–247.

Stroud L., Herold, J., Tomlinson, G., & Cavalcanti, R. B. (2011). Who you know or what you know? Effect of examiner familiarity with residents on OSCE scores. *Academic Medicine, 86*(10 Suppl), s8–s11.

Walsh, M., Bailey P. H., & Koren, I. (2009). Objective structured clinical evaluation of clinical competence: An integrative review. *Journal of Advanced Nursing, 65*(8), 1584–1595.

Willhaus, J. (2013). *Measures of physiological and psychological stress in novice health professions students during a simulated patient emergency.* (Unpublished doctoral dissertation). Washington State University, Spokane.

Wilson, L., Gordon, M. G., Cornelius, F., Glasgow, M. E. S., Suplee, P. D., Vasso, M., Dreher, H. M., Gardner, M., Rockstraw, L., Donnelly, G., Falkebstein, K., & Waite, R. (2006). The standardized patient experience in undergraduate nursing education. Proceedings of the International Council of Nurses. In H-A ParkH-A et al. (Eds.), *Consumer-centered computer-supported care for healthy people* (p. 830). Amsterdam: IOS Press.

Wolf, L., Dion, K., Lamoureaux, E., Kenny, C., Curnin, M., Hogan, M. A., Roche, J., & Cunningham, H. (2011). Using simulated clinical scenarios to evaluate student performance. *Nurse Educator, 36*(3), 128–134.

10

Unfolding Simulation Cases:
Purpose and Process

Mary L. Cato, EdD, RN
Jeanne Cleary, BSN, MAN, RN
Cynthia E. Reese, PhD, RN, CNE
Teri K. Boese, MSN, BSN, RN

■ Learning Objectives

1. Define an unfolding case.
2. Discuss the purpose of an unfolding case.
3. Discuss learning theories that support unfolding cases in nursing education.
4. List elements involved when planning an unfolding case study.
5. Explain implications for use of unfolding cases in nursing education.

■ Key Terms

- Simulation
- Unfolding case

DEFINITION OF AN UNFOLDING CASE

The use of **unfolding cases** is not new to nursing education but has progressed over time to integration into multiple teaching environments. In recent years, unfolding cases have been advanced and revised for various learning environments including the classroom, simulation, lab, and clinical setting. During an unfolding case presentation, learners can experience the clinical situation as it progresses over time where they are exposed to the full context and complexity of the changing story and disease progression (Glendon & Ulrich, 2001).

An unfolding **simulation** case evolves over time in a manner that is unpredictable to the learner and has elements and new situations that develop and are revealed with each encounter. It incorporates the power of storytelling with the experiential nature of simulation scenarios. Students develop problem-solving skills, critical-thinking skills, and increased clinical decision-making skills to address the complex health care needs of a patient and the support system or families of the patient. Unfolding simulation cases can follow the progression of a patient from a basic health assessment through a chronic condition or an acute situation to meet the learning objectives. An unfolding case can take clinical situations and experiences that the student might face and put them into a realistic learning experience that will then evolve over time. Unfolding cases can be simple or complex. An example of a simple respiratory case might be focused respiratory assessment. An example of a complex case might be a patient with respiratory distress who requires multiple interventions. Another example is taking students through an experience of congestive heart failure; the learners could explore the patient's experience as well as how symptoms and treatments might change through an exacerbation of the disease. With unfolding cases, students can be exposed to low-incidence, high-risk situations as well as commonly encountered situations. These cases can be designed to incorporate best practice, and they can utilize the Quality and Safety Education for Nurses (QSEN) principles. Unfolding cases can be developed to immerse participants in experiences or situations they will have a high likelihood of encountering in the first months of practice.

Traditional case studies are problem-oriented descriptions of events or situations that require students to analyze a problem and offer solutions. Case studies and unfolding simulation cases are both based on a patient story. The difference between a case study and an unfolding case is that typically a standard case study focuses on a single issue or problem. Many times a case study is done in a single presentation or uses a single event with a narrower focus than an unfolding case. Generally, a lot of information about the patient or client is provided to the learner. A case study is often an instructive example that is faculty driven, not student driven. Traditional case studies present all the scenario data at once and students develop a single response based on the given information. In contrast, unfolding case studies present data in stages, so that students read, process, and respond to information from one stage before receiving access to additional information from the next stage (Glendon & Ulrich, 2001).

PURPOSE OF UNFOLDING SIMULATION

Using unfolding cases, students are challenged to reflect in order to learn and understand as they engage in purposeful and intentional encounters with patients throughout their lifespan. As an example, the unfolding case may use the same patient and family with changing situations and dynamics. The National League for Nursing's (NLN) "Advancing Care Excellence for Seniors (ACES): Unfolding Cases"[1] demonstrates how patient stories can progress through time. These stories increase the realism and learner understanding of each individual as a patient or client rather than knowing them only as a medical diagnosis. The focus of the ACES cases is care of the older adult. Expected outcomes include:

- Recognition of atypical presentations in older adults
- Identification of geriatric syndromes
- Use of emerging evidence

---

[1]http://www.nln.org/facultyprograms/facultyresources/aces/unfolding_cases.htm

- Best practices to develop and implement plans of care
- Making appropriate judgments regarding the risks and benefits of care decisions
- Collaborating with an interprofessional team

Another example of unfolding cases is Jean Giddens's (2007) "The Neighborhood," where health care is represented in a simulated environment that includes homes, community agencies such as schools and senior centers, outpatient offices and clinics, and hospitals. Members of "The Neighborhood" include families as well as health care professionals in a number or roles such as hospital staff nurse, nurse manager, advanced practice nurse, school nurse, and community agency nurse. Learners are presented with situations involving patients, family members, and health care professionals. A community newspaper features health-related articles that correlate with events taking place within "The Neighborhood."

The evolving nature of an unfolding case lends itself to examining continuity of care experiences and can provide opportunities that can easily change the dynamics of a patient, the family, or a situation. The flexible methodology provides faculty the ability to incorporate each portion of an unfolding case into a course or a curriculum in a manner that fits the desired outcome. Dynamics between the patient, family, health care situation, and the interprofessional team can be incorporated in a manner that will facilitate the desired outcome of the unfolding case.

THEORETICAL BASIS FOR UNFOLDING CASES

Learning theory supports the use of simulation in general and unfolding cases in particular in nursing education. In a simulated clinical environment, students are able to practice caring for patients and families in a realistic way in a context that resembles reality. By providing students with an unfolding case, faculty can simulate the patient's ongoing story, as "learners experience the uncertainty and unpredictability of an actual, evolving clinical case" (Karani, Leipzig, Callahan, & Thomas, 2004, p. 1192).

In "How People Learn," Bransford, Brown, and Cocking (2000) summarized the findings of multiple research studies on cognition and learning. They emphasize that a learner's preexisting knowledge is foundational in adult education, and that learners continue to build on what they know as they enter new situations. In simulation, students can build on what they know from their didactic courses and skills lab training and incorporate that knowledge as they provide care to a patient. An unfolding case carries the idea of building on previous knowledge one step further, as students bring what they know about a patient in one situation to another situation along a trajectory.

Constructivist learning theory has often been cited to support the use of simulation in nursing education. Using real-world settings and case-based learning incorporates the basic principles of constructivism, along with thoughtful reflection, collaboration among learners, use of prior knowledge, and active learning (Jonnasen, 1994). A constructivist learning environment relies less on the provision of didactic content through lectures and focuses instead on concept-based activities and helping students become independent learners (Brandon & All, 2010). When using unfolding cases, students are truly able to build upon what they know and what they have learned with others as they continue to engage in a patient story. Because the patient data are presented in stages, the ongoing patient narrative carries learners from the known to the unknown and back again as they engage with the patient at varying points in time. Depending on the patient and the unfolding case, participants can gain skills in thinking, doing, and reflecting on patient care, all of which will be valuable in the "real world" of nursing.

PROCESS OF DEVELOPING UNFOLDING SIMULATIONS

There are several factors to consider when planning to develop an unfolding case study for use in simulation. First, the curricular objective(s) to be met should be identified. Unfolding cases can be developed to meet a need that has been recognized in a course or program. The case can focus on a particular patient population, a health issue or disruption, or a specific topic such as interprofessional communication. Some unfolding cases have been developed to address the care of the older adult and others focus on the needs of veterans. Still others address gaps in content related to safety or sentinel events that have occurred. So, begin with the end in mind. Understand the purpose and intended outcomes of the unfolding case, and develop the objectives for the overall unfolding case and the objectives for the intended participants.

Once the desired competencies, guidelines, and standards are identified, objectives should be developed that address the appropriate domains of learning. Objectives related to the cognitive, affective, and psychomotor domains of learning can be included as they relate to the overall purpose and desired learning outcomes of the unfolding case.

The unfolding case must be written with a good understanding of who will be participating in the simulation. The complexity and details of the case will vary depending on the knowledge, skills, and abilities the students bring to the simulation. It is important to have high expectations for the students; at the same time the complexity of the unfolding case must not be so difficult that the students cannot meet the objectives.

Determine the period of time over which the case will be run. Participants may see all of the parts of the unfolding case over a period of several hours, weeks, or semesters. If a case is developed that participants will engage in over a longer period of time, the changing abilities of the participant must be taken into account as the case is developed.

Effective simulations can be located in a basic classroom setting or a sophisticated simulation center; as the unfolding case is developed, it is important to consider the environment and the resources available for implementation. The capabilities of the available manikins or standardized patients need to be taken into account. For instance, if the patient dies during the scenario, it is an important cue to not see a rise and fall of the patient's chest; a standardized patient could not be expected to hold his or her breath for an extended period of time, so a manikin that is capable of having chest movement with breathing and cessation of movement when death occurs would be the best patient option. Or, if a roadside accident is part of the unfolding case, consider how this will be staged: Is there a safe place to simulate the scene?

To develop an unfolding case, consider what the story arc will be. Start with setting the stage by introducing the student to the everyday life of the patient (or family or community). One way of doing this is to provide a monologue from the point of view of the patient. The patient can provide the context or back story for the unfolding case.

Using a first-person monologue allows the participant to understand more about the patient; it can also include the patient's responses to his or her objective data (personal demographics, health history) and response to this health challenge. (For examples of monologues, see the NLN's Faculty Programs & Resources development website on the ACES Unfolding Cases, as cited earlier.)

Once the stage is set, determine how the case will unfold. What is the event(s) that triggers students to intervene in the care of the patient? An unfolding case, written so that it reveals new information at several points, may develop in a variety of ways. The complexity of the patient's illness may change as he or she is seen at multiple points in time or in a variety of settings such as a clinic, school, home, or hospital. A case might also unfold by a patient being seen only in the hospital, but on multiple shifts or days as his or her disease trajectory or health issue changes. Hospital admissions and discharges are important points of nursing care to include in unfolding cases.

As the case unfolds, there will be obstacles or conflicts along the way that require the students to think critically and make choices. Just as in the actual patient setting, sometimes there are data that might not be important at the time or there could be missing data. Consider leaving out information that is important to the care of the patient. The student would need to identify what information is missing and formulate a way to gather that information. Students will react to the unfolding simulation in ways that you expect and also in ways you do not expect. Anticipate reactions and interventions as much as possible in order to be ready for the appropriate patient reaction.

The NLN Simulation Design Template[2] can be used to organize the specifics of the unfolding case study that is being developed for simulation. The template prompts the developer to consider a number of simulation design elements that are useful for the successful implementation of a simulation experience. If the patient is in an acute care setting, a chart can be developed with a complete history and physical, reports, and assessments from all departments involved in the care of the patient; this could be a paper chart or an electronic medical record.

Evidenced-based practice must be incorporated into the unfolding case during development. Elements in the case are based on high-quality research, evidence-based theory, and input from clinical leaders or specialists who are content experts. Student preparation for the unfolding cases may include having them reading protocols, standards of care, and research articles provided by faculty. For a more complex learning experience, students could be required to search for evidence to bring to the simulations as they care for a patient and family.

An assessment or evaluation plan should be part of the development of an unfolding case. Students should have formative or summative evaluation as part of the simulation. Feedback provides information to the students about their performance during the simulation. It is as important to identify errors in the participants' thinking and practice as it is to identify and commend strong performance. Creating an evaluation plan from the outset of the development of the unfolding case will help validate that all desired elements have been included and ensure the desired objectives can be met. Before using any new simulation, always pilot test it with people who are new to the case; people who have not participated in the development of the unfolding case will be able to uncover questions

---

[2] http://sirc.nln.org/mod/forum/discuss.php?d=83

or inconsistencies that the developers may not have considered as the case evolved. Problems related to the content or flow will be revealed. Issues that can negatively impact the students' experience and deter from a successful implementation of the simulation can be discovered during the pilot and the case presentation. A pilot will also allow the timing of the unfolding simulation to be practiced, although it is difficult to predict how the students will react during the simulation. Each time it is run will present a different experience.

Tables 10.1 and 10.2 provide examples for how unfolding cases could be used to reinforce specific content in nursing courses.

TABLE 10.1

Unfolding Cases Using Simulations

Topic of Study	Course	Point of Care in Patient Story	Focus of Scenario
Health promotion older adult	Fundamentals or medical/surgical	• Independent living facility • Senior center	• Learning needs assessment related to medication • SPICES assessment
Health promotion child	Fundamentals	• School • Clinic	• Vision and developmental screen • Assess immunization status and administer required immunizations • Collect data and plot on growth chart
Type 1 diabetes	Pediatrics	Initial hospitalization and diagnosis	Nurses assess child and assist parent with insulin administration Interprofessional education; role discussion
		Discharge from hospital	Nurses review patient teaching and assess continued learning needs
		Home visit in one week	Nurses review blood glucose records, carbohydrate intake, and family's adjustment to child's condition
Depression	Psych/mental health	Acute care unit after suicide attempt	Nurses assess patient and current safety risks

(continued)

TABLE 10.1

Unfolding Cases Using Simulations (*Continued*)

Topic of Study	Course	Point of Care in Patient Story	Focus of Scenario
		Psychiatric unit: transfer from acute care when physically stable	Nurses assess and communicate therapeutically with patient and family
Myocardial infarction	Med/surg nursing	Acute care unit: postop bariatric patient with pain	Nurses assess chest pain, notify provider, and follow initial orders (ECG, labs, MONA)
		Postcardiac catheterization	Nurses assess and support patient and family
		Hospital discharge	Nurses assess patient and learning needs

SPICES, **S**leep disorders, **P**roblems with eating and feeding, **I**ncontinence, **C**onfusion, **E**vidence of falls, **S**kin breakdown; ECG, electrocardiogram; MONA, **M**orphine, **O**xygen, **N**itrates, and **A**spirin.

TABLE 10.2

Unfolding Cases Beginning in a Classroom

Topic of Study	Course	Point of Care in Patient Story	Unfolding Case
High-risk pregnancy	Maternity nursing	Prenatal visit at 30 weeks, patient in early labor	Classroom study/ discussion of patient/ history/symptoms
		Home visit at 32 weeks, patient on bedrest	Nurses make home visit, assess and support patient
		Admission to labor and delivery at 34 weeks	Nurses assess and support patient through contractions, potentially through delivery
			Interprofessional team training
Congestive heart failure	Care of older adult	Provider office visit, patient unsure of medications	Classroom study/ discussion of patient/ history/symptoms
		Hospitalization for acute exacerbation	Nurses assess, administer meds and treatments

IMPLICATIONS FOR NURSING EDUCATION

Unfolding cases can be used in nursing education in numerous ways and are appropriate to use in multiple settings to enhance learning. As a teaching or learning strategy, the unfolding case provides a unique opportunity that allows students to develop clinical reasoning and problem-solving skills in a learner-centered environment. Components of newer national initiatives in nursing education such as QSEN, interprofessional education, the American Association of Colleges of Nursing's "Essentials" documents, and the NLN's Competencies for Nursing Education are being incorporated into the curriculum in prelicensure nursing programs. Unfolding case studies allow students to apply these concepts in simulation.

Additionally, unfolding cases are a creative way to integrate active learning strategies into the curriculum, and they have the following advantages:

- *Flexibility.* Each case can be designed with a flexible methodology and timing can evolve at the discretion of the faculty member.

- *Evidence-based practice.* Integration of national standards and guidelines throughout a case can help learners understand the concept of evidence-based practice and how it is put into practice.

- *Clinical reasoning.* Incorporating different learning strategies such as the use of open-ended questions, presenting unstructured problems with missing information, and guided reflection supports the development of clinical reasoning skills.

- *Engagement.* Unfolding cases use active learning strategies appropriate for teaching in the classroom, lab, and online. Learners work together to solve complex issues.

- *Classroom/clinical/practice bridge.* Unfolding cases based on current clinical practice can help bridge the gap from classroom learning into clinical and practice settings.

- *Interprofessional education.* Health care professionals from medicine, social work, physical therapy, respiratory therapy, pharmacy, and other areas can be integrated into the case to allow learners the opportunity to collaborate with various members of the health care team.

- *Teamwork/teambuilding.* Unfolding cases can incorporate teamwork to help learners develop team skills.

- *Good teaching practices.* An unfolding case follows the "Seven Principles of Good Practice in Undergraduate Education" by Chickering and Gamson (1987) and integrates principles of learner-center teaching. The "Seven Principles" include:
  1. Interaction between students and faculty
  2. Collaboration among students
  3. Active learning
  4. Prompt feedback
  5. Time on task

BOX 10.1 THE UNFOLDING CASE OF HENRY AND ERTHA WILLIAMS

Overview

Henry Williams is an 80-year-old African American man, a retired rail system engineer who lives in a small apartment with his wife, Ertha. Henry and Ertha had one son who was killed while serving in the military 10 years ago. They have a daughter-in-law, Betty, who is a nurse, and one grandson, Ty. Henry is concerned about Ertha because she is experiencing frequent memory lapses.

Monologue

Henry was admitted to the hospital last night after he called the doctor complaining of difficulty catching his breath. Henry has several medical problems including COPD, hypertension, and high cholesterol. Henry provides important details of how he views his current life situation.

Simulation Scenarios 1, 2, and 3

The simulation scenarios focus on the physical and psychosocial changes that Henry encounters over the next few weeks. His failing health and his concern for his increasingly forgetful wife lead him through various transitions that affect his family and his living situation. The objectives focus on assessment and appropriate use of evidence-based assessment tools. The objectives also focus on psychosocial issues with Henry's wife and their daughter-in-law's concern for their living arrangements; the proper use of the multiple assessment tools, and making appropriate community referrals.

Reprinted with permission from the National League for Nursing. Advancing care excellence for seniors. Retrieved from http://www.nln.org/facultyprograms/facultyresources/aces/index.htm.

6. High expectations
7. Respect for diverse ways of learning

As nursing education continues to transform, educators must begin to integrate learner-centered, evidence-based teaching and learning strategies into all settings. The unfolding case of Henry and Ertha Williams, from the NLN's ACES website, is described in Box 10.1 with examples of how the case can be integrated across the curriculum, in the traditional simulation laboratory, in the classroom, and online or in hybrid educational settings.

UNFOLDING CASES ACROSS THE CURRICULUM

A primary benefit of unfolding cases is the opportunity for the educator to use flexibility with the timing of the case. The case can be presented to students over a single day, over several weeks, over the length of the course, or over the duration of the entire educational program. Presentation of the entire case over a single day may meet the needs of more advanced students as they work through all of the scenarios in a short period of time. Careful planning of the day by the educator is essential to ensure that the students have quality prebriefing, simulation, and debriefing experiences with each scenario. Additionally, learners need guidance to adequately prepare for the demands of the case.

Cases may also be presented over several weeks or over the duration of a single course. Using course learning outcomes, a case can be designed to allow learners to apply content from the classroom and meet these outcomes. As the case unfolds, additional layers of complexity are added as learners progress through the course.

Lastly, unfolding cases are very amenable for use across a curriculum of study. Learners are introduced to the case early in their coursework. The first scenarios may focus on more basic concepts with a high degree of scaffolding through the purposeful use of embedded cues. As learners progress to more advanced courses, the scaffolding gradually decreases to promote development of clinical reasoning and problem-solving abilities. For example, a case could be introduced in a fundamentals of nursing course focused on the concept of pain assessment in an acute care setting. Cues would be planned to support the learner's assessment and intervention for pain. In a subsequent course, the same patient could be used with additional components added to increase the complexity of the scenario. The learner now must work with the patient who has chronic pain and family issues. As the case progresses, the learners identify community resources and consider the other health care professionals appropriate for the increasingly complex situations in the scenarios. In the final scenario of the case, learners may lead an interdisciplinary care conference for the patient as a component of a capstone leadership course. Table 10.3 provides suggestions for integrating the NLN's Henry and Ertha ACES Unfolding Case across a nursing curriculum.

TABLE 10.3

Use of an Unfolding Case Across the Curriculum: Henry Williams

First Nursing Course	Second Nursing Course	Third Nursing Course
Monologue: Students listen to Henry's audio monologue and engage in discussion of patient perspective to understand the case.

Scenario 1: Henry Williams is admitted to the hospital with an exacerbation of his chronic obstructive pulmonary disease. The case is complicated by his wife Ertha's confusion. | Scenario 2: Henry is being discharged from the hospital to a rehabilitation center. He will need teaching, medication reconciliation, and a plan of care for his wife Ertha until an assisted living apartment is located and available for both of them. | Scenario 3 takes place 15 days later as Henry is awaiting discharge from the rehabilitation center. He and Ertha will need assistance with the transition to new living arrangements and education regarding ongoing care. |

UNFOLDING CASES IN THE CLASSROOM AND ONLINE

The use of unfolding cases is not limited to the traditional simulation laboratory. Innovative use of unfolding cases has the potential to transform the traditional teacher-centered classroom into an active, engaging learning environment that supports the new flipped classroom concept (Educause Learning Initiative, 2012). The flipped classroom is garnering support in the higher education community as a strategy to integrate active learning and is designed with the learner preparing for class through the study of online resources, typically short prerecorded lectures, prior to attending class. The class time is devoted to active learning activities. The flexibility of the unfolding case fits very well with the flipped classroom.

The ACES Unfolding Cases can be easily used in the classroom. These cases each have an introductory prerecorded monologue recorded in the first person to introduce students to the primary patients in each case. These are available online for students to listen to prior to class. After listening to the monologue, learners may consider these questions to guide their thinking about the case: (1) What are your concerns for the patient/family? (2) What is the cause of your concern? (3) What else do you need to know about the patient/family? (4) What are you going to do about it? (adapted from Benner, Stutphen, Leonard, & Day, 2010). These questions can be discussed as part of prebriefing during class.

The simulation scenarios can then be presented to the class in several ways. A live or prerecorded video of the scenario could be shown to the class. The scenario could be conducted live in front of the class, with the simulator or standardized patient brought into the classroom and students from the class serving as the nurses in the scenario. This can also be accomplished in an online class as many online courses have synchronous audio and video capabilities allowing students to observe a live simulation. However, in

BOX 10.2 USE OF SIMULATION IN THE CLASSROOM, ONLINE, AND TRADITIONAL SIMULATION LABORATORY SETTING

Classroom or Online
- Class or online presentation of medical issue(s) evident in scenario
- Monologue
- Discussion questions
- Small groups discuss appropriate assessment tools to use in this scenario
- Scenario at front of classroom or shown as video
- Debriefing as a group/online, may use discussion boards or chat

Simulations Lab
- Prebriefing with monologue and discussion questions.
- Traditional scenario with simulator/standardized patient

Debriefing

an asynchronous class, students can listen to the monologue, post their thoughts about the questions on discussion boards, watch the prerecorded scenario, and debrief again using discussion boards. Box 10.2 offers suggestions for the use of simulation in classroom, online, and in the laboratory setting.

SUMMARY

Unfolding cases offer the nurse educator many options to bring active learning into the curriculum. These strategies can be used in all types of settings: the classroom, online, or in the simulation lab. Because of the unfolding nature of this type of case, the timeframe over which the case unfolds can be easily customized to the needs of the course or educational program. Unfolding cases are a useful tool for educators to use because this type of case promotes the development of context-based clinical reasoning and problem-solving skills necessary to prepare graduates for demanding, complex health care environments.

■ Key Concepts

- An unfolding simulation case evolves over time in a manner that is unpredictable to the learner and has elements and new situations that develop and are revealed with each encounter. It incorporates the power of storytelling with the experiential nature of simulation scenarios. Students develop problem-solving skills, critical-thinking skills, and increased clinical decision-making skills to address the complex health care needs of a patient and the support system or families of the patient.

- Unfolding cases take clinical situations and issues that students might face and put them into a realistic learning experience that will evolve over time. Unfolding cases as a teaching or learning strategy are supported by learning theory and easily allow for national standards and competencies to be integrated into the case. They can also be used to expose participants to experiences or situations they will likely encounter in the first months of practice. Unfolding simulation cases can follow the progression of a patient from a basic health assessment through a chronic condition or an acute situation to meet the learning objectives. In recent years, unfolding cases have advanced and evolved into various learning environments.

- Unfolding cases are very flexible and can be implemented in a classroom, online, or in a traditional skills lab setting. Standardized patients or high- to moderate-fidelity simulators may be used in the scenarios. Begin with the end in mind.

- The curricular objective(s) to be met should be identified first. Unfolding cases can be developed to meet a need that has been recognized in a course or program. Objectives should be related to the cognitive, affective, and psychomotor domains of learning to be inclusive providing dimensions of learning.

- An assessment or evaluation plan should be a part of the development of an unfolding case. Unfolding cases are appropriate to use in multiple settings to enhance learning, and students should have formative or summative evaluation as part of the simulation and with use of an unfolding case. Creating an evaluation plan from the outset of the development of the unfolding case will help ensure that all desired elements have been included and the desired objectives can be met.

References

Benner, P., Stutphen, M., Leonard, V., & Day, L. (2010). *Educating nurses: A call for radical transformation.* San Francisco: Jossey-Bass.

Brandon, A. & All, A. Constructivism theory analysis and application to curricula. *Nursing Education Perspectives, 31*(2), 89–92.

Bransford, J. D., Brown, A. I., & Cocking, R. R. (2000). *How people learn: Brain, mind, experience, and school.* Washington, DC: National Academy Press.

Chickering, A., & Gamson, Z. (1987). Seven principles of good practice in undergraduate education. *AAHE Bulletin, 39*(7), 5–10.

Educause Learning Initiative. (2012). Seven things you should know about flipped classrooms. Retrieved from http://net.educause.edu/ir/library/pdf/eli7081.pdf

Giddons, J. (2007). The neighborhood: A web-based platform to support conceptual teaching and learning. *Nursing Education Perspective, 28*(5), 251–256.

Glendon, K., & Ulrich, D. (2001). *Unfolding case studies: Experiencing the realities of clinical nursing practice.* Upper Saddle River, NJ: Prentice-Hall.

Jonnasen, D. H. (1994). Thinking technology: Toward a constructivist design model. *Educational Technology, 34*(4), 34–37.

Karani, R., Leipzig, R. M., Callahan, E. H., & Thomas, D. C. (2004). An unfolding case with a linked objective structured clinical examination (OSCE): A curriculum in inpatient geriatric medicine. *Journal of the American Geriatric Society, 52*(7), 1191–1198.

11

Developing a Research Focus in Simulations

Suzan Kardong-Edgren, PhD, RN, ANEF, CHSE
Joan Roche, PhD, RN, GCNS-BC

■ Learning Objectives

1. Review key elements to consider prior to beginning a research study.
2. Review key considerations when designing a study.

■ Key Terms

- Correlational research design
- Descriptive research design
- Experimental design
- Quasi-experimental design
- Research
- Theory

GETTING STARTED: KNOW THE CURRENT STATE OF THE SCIENCE

"[R]esearch is the diligent, systematic inquiry or investigation to validate and refine existing knowledge and generate new knowledge. The concepts *systematic* and *diligent* are critical to the meaning of research because they imply planning, organization, and persistence" (Burns & Grove, 2009, p. 2). Simulation researchers have only recently begun to diligently and systematically study simulation. Much of the early nursing simulation **research** was not rigorous. However, Shneider (2011) suggested the initial work in any emerging field is done by scientists who are willing "to be somewhat imprecise and even somewhat inaccurate" (p. 218). We are moving into the second stage of research in the discipline of simulation, characterized by Shneider as establishing the accepted techniques in the field and the language of the emerging discipline.

It is imperative that nursing simulation researchers be immersed in the simulation literature and regularly read medical and interdisciplinary education, clinical and simulation journals, such as *Simulation in Healthcare* and *Clinical Simulation in Nursing,* along with other health professions journals to be fully versed in all of the literature that could spark the next big idea in simulation. We recommend regularly searching the Cumulative Index to Nursing and Allied Health Literature (CINAHL), Medline, Psychinfo, and Google Scholar for simulation articles or other articles that might suggest research ideas. Another place to search regularly to maintain your simulation knowledge is the ProQuest listing of the latest dissertations. ProQuest may contain the first reports of new research that are yet to be processed into a manuscript, undergo review, and ultimately appear in the press list and final publication.

The First Educational Research Consensus Summit monograph issue (Issenberg, Ringsted, Ostergaard, & Dieckmann, 2011) of the *Society for Simulation in Healthcare* thoroughly covered the state of the science at the time and suggested research questions in topics of interest to nursing such as procedural skills (Nestel, Groom, Eikeland-Huesbo, & O'Donnell, 2011), team training (Eppich, Howard, Vozenilek, & Curran, 2011), factors affecting human performance (LeBlanc et al., 2011), instructional design and pedagogy (Schaeffer et al., 2011), the assessment of learning outcomes (Boulet et al., 2011), debriefing (Raemer et al., 2011), and simulation for assessment (Holmboe, Rizzolo, Sachdeva, Rosenberg, & Ziv, 2011). Manuscripts reporting the outcomes of the year-long review of the literature surrounding the National League for Nursing's (NLN) Jeffries Framework also provide suggestions for research studies (Groom, Henderson, & Sittner, in press; Hallmark, Thomas, & Gantt, in press).

There are a growing number of literature reviews on various topics in simulation that could also prove useful to build an initial understanding of what is known about a particular aspect of simulation (Foronda, Liu, & Bauman, in press; Ross, 2013; Foronda, Godsali, & Trybulski, 2013; Gunberg-Ross, 2012; Norman, 2012; Paige & Morin, in press; Shearer, 2013; Shinnick, Woo, & Mentee, 2011; Yuan, Williams, & Fang, 2012).

Ideas for research in nursing education abound. Teaching psychomotor skills and their retention and transfer to the clinical environment is a neglected area that is very amenable to simulation research (Nestel et al., 2011). Coupled with a deliberate repetitive practice framework, this one idea alone could provide years of research studies (Clapper & Kardong-Edgren, 2012; Ericsson, 2004). Evaluating the use of video playback in debriefing is also understudied with equivocal results at present. The use of expert modeling before simulation practice is awaiting a full evaluation and could enhance the time spent in the simulation lab. The evaluation of health care provider competency has been ignored by recent national research policy papers and agencies (McGaghie, Draycott, Dunn, Lopez, & Stefanidis, 2011) but remains of prime interest and importance to nursing and simulation researchers. The cost-effectiveness of simulation is rarely studied or reported in the literature (Nestel et al., 2011).

THEORY USE IN SIMULATION RESEARCH

The use of **theory** in simulation research has been sparse at best (Schaeffer et al., 2011) and not well understood by many researchers. Using a specific theory to guide a research study will provide a set of predefined vocabulary, concept definitions, logical structure, and relational statements between the concepts that provide links with other studies using the same theory (Burns & Grove, 2009). This also increases the usability for other researchers in the future. Theory use suggests hypotheses and a set of assumptions that predict what one may expect to find. Thus, study findings may validate the theory and its assumptions. "Linking studies is facilitated, and at times only possible, if the theoretical background is described" (Dieckmann et al., 2011, p. S4). Models are sometimes called midrange theories and are also used as guides for nursing research. Jeffries and Rizzolo (2006) developed a model of simulation education that could be used to guide simulation research.

The theories most commonly used in simulation research include the NLN's Jeffries Framework (Jeffries, 2005), Bandura's (1986) social learning theory, thinking on action (Schon, 1983), novice to expert (Benner, 1984), and experiential learning theory (Kolb, 1984). Deliberate practice, mastery learning, and skill decay and retention are all inter-related and could provide a low-cost but fruitful program of research (Arthur, Bennett, Stanush, & McNelly, 1998; Clapper & Kardong-Edgren, 2012; Ericsson, 2004). Cognitive load theory (Van Merriënboer & Sweller, 2005) has been virtually ignored by the nursing educa-tion community but could also provide a rich body of research for improving clinical teaching.

Becoming an expert in one aspect of the simulation, using all of the available research literature, is one astute way to build expertise and move research in an area forward. This approach may be appealing to someone who has a passion for a particular aspect of simulation. This would help one to learn key terms and find or read all research literature each month on a topic, at least at this point in time. The publications about simulation are increasing exponentially. It is becoming more challenging to stay current and know the state of the science intimately.

INDIVIDUAL OR TEAM RESEARCH

It takes amazing persistence to go it alone as a nursing education researcher. Some peo-ple working alone may eventually wear out and give up. A better approach is to find at least one kindred spirit to bounce ideas off of when thinking about or planning a research study. This can be done with a phone call, through Skype, or in a face-to-face meeting. It is wise to search out like-minded individuals from other on-campus pro-grams, other schools, or a simulation center in a clinical setting (Cooper et al., 2011; Roche, Schoen, & Kruzel, 2013) to build a research team. Consider reaching out to other disciplines for partners in simulation studies, for example, speech pathology (Potter & Allen, in press) and communications (O'Shea, Pagano, Campbell, & Caso, 2013). Willhaus (2010) provided multiple ideas for finding nontraditional campus programs to share health-based simu-lations. Many colleges have psychology or engineering departments with human factors' researchers, a large area of simulation research that nursing has barely tapped.

FUNDING

Nursing education research takes time and resources. Because of the promise of human patient simulation (HPS) technology, external funding has become available. If applying for this funding, through such programs as the NLN, you will be much more competi-tive with a team or multisite approach. For federal funding, a multidisciplinary team is frequently required. Multiple researcher or multisite studies bring with them new challenges, not the least of which is dealing with the division of credit and indirect funds to departments, colleges, or programs. If you have an office of research at your school, meet with them early and often to proactively tackle the challenges that certainly await you and your team.

EVALUATION RESEARCH

HPS has produced a new and sustained model for the evaluation of nursing education. The purpose of simulation research is ultimately the improvement of patient care outcomes through better-educated and prepared practitioners. In the early nursing simulation research, self-reports of satisfaction and feelings of competency were easy to glean and probably overused. This research was important to establish simulation into the nursing literature but not necessarily useful, in light of research that demonstrates the low-level correlation between reported self-confidence and actual ability (Baxter & Norman, 2011). This level is known as Kirkpatrick Level 1 evaluation (Kirkpatrick, 1994). This early level satisfaction research was followed thereafter by a flurry of Kirkpatrick Level 2 research focused on evaluating changes in knowledge postsimulation. Much of this research showed no change in knowledge level. If we had also considered the newness of the simulation environment itself (cognitive load theory; Artino, 2008) and the lack of training of the faculty in simulation and debriefing, these early stage designs and findings might have been anticipated. Knowledge appears to indeed be improved by simulation (Shinnick & Woo, in press). In addition, faculty are also more familiar with simulation and are better trained in debriefing, and many students are increasingly familiar with the simulation learning environment.

Further substantiation of a change in knowledge is warranted, because nursing licensing is based on a computerized exam. However, the more important research to be done is now Kirkpatrick Level 3, a change in behavior, and in the long term, Level 4, a change in outcomes for patients (Kirkpatrick, 1994). These studies are difficult to conduct for any health education providers. Meyer, Connors, Hou, and Gajewski (2011) provided an excellent model for how to evaluate a change in practice in nursing students using simulation.

METHODS

Ethical Conduct of Research

Federal law (U.S. Department of Health and Human Services, 2009) requires that research be voluntary and that the rights of the subjects are protected. Once the research team has determined the design and is planning the study, they need to obtain approval from the institutional review board or ethics committee. HPS offers additional challenges in the realm of ethics. In order to ensure consistency of interventions, and simulation fidelity, research studies are designed using the same simulation scenario with multiple students, often in the same school or same class. If students share any aspect of the scenario, it will contaminate the results obtained from future subjects. Consequently, in addition to obtaining written informed consent from each subject, researchers are encouraged to have all students sign a nonshare agreement stating that they will not share anything about the scenario with any other nursing students.

Research Question or Hypotheses

The focus of an HPS research study should combine the interest of the researchers and the current state of the science. Once the researchers complete the review of the literature in the area of interest, they formulate a question or hypothesis for a study. The research focus for simulation can also follow the four Kirkpatrick (1994) levels: (1) learner perceptions (satisfaction and confidence), (2) knowledge, (3) behavior/performance, and (4) clinical outcomes. As the level of the study increases, the researchers move from simple questions to complex hypotheses. The design is based on the question or hypothesis, and it also increases in strength and complexity as the level increases.

Designs

The purpose of a good design choice is to use the best and most realistic research method to accurately answer the question or test the hypothesis, while minimizing bias and threats to validity (Burns & Grove, 2009). It can be challenging to develop the best research design. A research team member who is a design expert is helpful in this step. The design expert does not need to be an expert in simulation but can advise the team specifically on design issues.

Descriptive Research Designs

Descriptive research designs answer simple questions such as, Are nursing students satisfied with HPS? There are several types of descriptive designs, including time series or comparative, answering questions such as, Does HPS increase nursing students' confidence in complex clinical situations? Because HPS research is a new area for nursing, much of the existing research is descriptive at Kirkpatrick Level 1 (Jeffries & Rizzolo, 2006; Weaver, 2011; Yuan et al., 2011) focused on learner perceptions of satisfaction and confidence or self-efficacy. Although there are many current studies in these areas, rigorous replication with valid and reliable measures in a variety of settings with large samples can strengthen the existing research. A rich body of descriptive research is important to support the development of more complex HPS research. These descriptive studies of learner perceptions can be qualitative (Dreifuerst, 2009) or quantitative survey research (Jeffries & Rizzolo, 2006; Szpak & Kameq, 2013). Given the existing body of research in these areas, it is wiser to replicate existing studies with tested questions and instruments rather than create new untested ones. Contact the authors for permission to use survey instruments, and request the most up-to-date results on reliability and validity.

Correlational Designs

The purpose of a **correlational research design** is to examine the relationship between variables. This can be descriptive correlational (Fountain & Alfred, 2009). Correlational designs can also be predictive correlation, using mathematical modeling to determine which variables (number of simulation scenarios) predict outcomes (student performance). However, the current state of measurement of HPS outcomes is in the developmental stage. Predictive correlation requires established reliable and valid measurement of variables and large multisite samples. It is beyond the scope of a single school or simulation center to conduct a solid predictive correlational study on HPS without external support.

Quasi-Experimental Designs

The purpose of a **quasi-experimental design** study is to examine the effect of one variable (simulation) on another variable (knowledge or performance). These studies compare a group (experimental group) with a clearly defined intervention (HPS) with a control group. The control group may have a traditional intervention (written case studies) or no intervention. The dependent variable or outcome measure should be measured before and after the intervention. The researchers compare the change in the pre–posttest scores and use appropriate statistical tests to determine if the difference between the two groups is significant. These studies require a predetermined sample size (determined by power analysis). There are several nurse researchers who have developed pilot quasi-experimental studies (Adamson & Kardong-Edgren, 2012; Radhakrishnan, Roche, & Cunningham, 2007; Roche et al., 2013). Quasi-experimental designs with adequate sample sizes can begin to develop evidence on which aspects of simulation are the most effective. Solid quasi-experimental designs with large sample sizes will provide strong contributions to the current state of research on simulation. Quasi-experimental research, however, does not determine causality. Fully randomized experimental studies are required to examine causality.

Experimental Designs

The purpose of **experimental designs** research is to study the effect of an independent variable (HPS) on a dependent variable (performance). The standard experiment design is the randomized controlled trial (RCT). This includes random selection of subjects, two group (experimental and control groups) with randomization into groups, and pre–posttests. It is usually beyond the scope of a single school or single simulation center to conduct a well-designed RCT. As HPS research grows, it is the role of large professional organizations to coordinate the development and implementation of large experimental studies. An example of this is the ongoing National Council of State Boards of Nursing study.

Sample and Setting

Generally speaking, simulation researchers start with single-site studies at their location. This is a good plan to get started in research. However, for nursing to develop higher-level studies with large samples, multisite research is needed. Multisite research has many challenges (Oermann et al., 2012). To bridge this gap, some research teams conduct research projects with a few schools working on one study (Powell-Laney, Keen, & Hall, 2012). This model allows researchers to increase the sample size in a local region.

Another strategy to get a larger sample size is to collect data over more than one year in the same school (Ashcraft et al., 2013).

Measurement

Simulation has spawned a plethora of new evaluation instruments for all aspects of the experience (Kardong-Edgren, Adamson, & Fitzgerald, 2010; Adamson, Kardong-Edgren, & Willhaus, 2013). Using a simulation evaluation instrument that matches the research question and participant population will greatly enhance the value of the research. Take time to review existing instruments and, if necessary, validate the use of an instrument that must be adapted for use in a particular population. Consulting with a statistician or methodologist to accomplish this may be a wise use of time and resources. Once an instrument has been chosen and validated, it is important to document the rater training for the use of the evaluation instrument and then to document interrater and intrarater reliability (Adamson & Kardong-Edgren, 2012). To measure interrater reliability, have two trained raters use the instrument for some of the same measurements and calculate the correlation of these scores. Intrarater reliability requires the correlation between instrument measures of the same rater of the same scenarios at different times. These provide significant support for the reliability of this instrument for a study.

The use of multiple sites for conducting research makes the validation of raters even more challenging. However, it is a necessary step. Using standardized training methodologies including technology will assist with this (Adamson & Kardong-Edgren, 2012).

Data Collection and Analysis

As with all worthwhile endeavors, the devil is in the details. The process of data collection, entry of data into computer programs, and transcription of qualitative interviews takes time and needs careful attention. This aspect of research is an ideal opportunity for graduate students and research assistants to participate in the research process. This adds valuable resources to the team and provides mentoring for future HPS experts. Collaboration with a statistician is important to ensure that the appropriate statistical tests are use on quantitative data. Social studies faculty can be excellent collaborators to interpret qualitative results. Nursing faculty report that time constraints are a major barrier in implementing both HPS and research. Engaging other team members for data collection and analysis can facilitate this important step of the process.

DISSEMINATION OF RESULTS

In order for nursing researchers to build an effective body of research on HPS, we all need to build on the existing work. This can only happen when researchers share the results of their work through professional journals and professional meetings. Peer-reviewed publications reach more future HPS researchers. Presentation of research results at regional, national, and international professional simulation conferences creates opportunities to network with potential research partners and explore new design and instrument possibilities. We recommend sharing all research results in both venues.

SUMMARY

There are many challenges to integrating a program of research into an already time-consuming HPS program. This will take time and organization. However, the benefits are worth the effort. If nursing educators are to use HPS effectively to improve the education of our students and the care of our patients, it is important that simulations be based on scientific evidence rather than opinion. An effective program of research can position a nursing program for external funding. Creating an interdisciplinary research team can enrich and expand the curriculum for students and the research capacity for faculty.

■ Key Concepts

- Start all research studies with a comprehensive review of the research literature on the area of interest and maintain an ongoing updated database of HPS research.
- Base individual HPS research studies or programs of research on a theoretical framework or model.
- Develop a research team with other simulation experts or users, including other disciplines or settings, research and statistical experts, and a librarian.
- Replicate simple solid designs based on the research literature.
- Use existing surveys, instruments, or performance measures with reported reliability and validity rather than developing new ones.
- Disseminate your results through professional and interprofessional journals and conferences.
- Build a program of research with your team, building each new study on the previous results and the updated current research evidence.

References

Adamson, K. A., & Kardong-Edgren, S. (2012). A method and resources for assessing the reliability of simulation evaluation instruments. *Nursing Education Perspectives, 33*(5), 334–339.

Adamson, K. A., Kardong-Edgren, S., & Willhaus, J. (2013). An updated review of published simulation evaluation instruments. *Clinical Simulation in Nursing, 9*(9), e393–e405.

Arthur, W., Bennett, W., Stanush, P. L., & McNelly, T. L. (1988). Factors that influence skill decay and retention: A quantitative review and analysis. *Human Performance, 11*(1), 57.

Artino, A. R. (2008). Cognitive load theory and the role of learner experience: An abbreviated review for educational practitioners. *Association for the Advancement of Computing in Education Journal, 16*(4), 425–439.

Ashcraft, A. S., Opton, L., Bridges, R. A., Caballero, S., Veesart, A., & Weaver, C. (2013). Simulation evaluation using a modified Lasater Clinical Judgment Rubric. *Nursing Education Perspectives, 34*(2), 122–126.

Bandura, A. (1986). *Social foundations of thought and action: A social cognitive theory.* Upper Saddle River, NJ: Prentice-Hall.

Baxter, P., & Norman, G. (2011). Self-assessment or self deception? A lack of association between nursing students' self-assessment and performance. *Journal of Advanced Nursing, 67*(11), 2406–2413.

Benner, P. (1984). *From novice to expert: Excellence and power in clinical nursing practice.* Menlo Park, CA: Addison-Wesley.

Boulet, J. R., Jeffries, P. R., Hatala, R. A., Korndorffer, D. M., & Roche, J. P. (2011). Research regarding methods of assessing learning outcomes. *Simulation in Healthcare, 6*, S48–S51.

Burns, N., & Grove, S. (2009). *The practice of nursing research: Appraisal, synthesis, and generation of evidence.* St. Louis: Saunders Elsevier.

Clapper, T., & Kardong-Edgren, S. (2012). Using deliberate practice and simulation to improve nursing skills. *Clinical Simulation in Nursing, 8*(3), e109–e113.

Cooper, D., Wilbur, L., Milgram, L., Ellender, K., Huffman, G., & Bowers, C. (2011). Can interprofessional simulation improve physician—nurse communication and error reporting confidence? *Simulation in Healthcare, 6*(398), abst 444.

Dieckmann, P., Phero, J. C., Issenberg, S. A., Kardong-Edgren, S., Ostergaard, D., & Ringsted, C. (2011). The first research consensus summit of the Society for Simulation in Healthcare. *Simulation in Healthcare, 6*, S1–S9.

Dreifuerst, K. T. (2009). The essentials of debriefing in simulation learning: A concept analysis. *Nursing Education Perspectives, 30*(2), 109–114.

Eppich, W., Howard, V., Vozenilek, J., & Curran, I. (2011). Simulation-based team training in healthcare. *Simulation in Healthcare, 6*, S14–S19.

Ericsson, K. A. (2004). Deliberate practice and the acquisition and maintenance of expert performance in medicine and related domains. *Academic Medicine, 79*(10 Suppl), S70–S81.

Foronda, C., Liu, S., & Bauman, E. (In press). Evaluation of simulation in undergraduate nurse education: An integrative review. *Clinical Simulation in Nursing.*

Foronda, C., Godsali, L., & Trybulski, J. (2013). Virtual clinical simulation: The state of the science. *Clinical Simulation in Nursing, 9*(8), e279–e286.

Fountain, R. A., & Alfred, D. (2009). Student satisfaction with high-fidelity simulation: Does It correlate with learning styles? *Nursing Education Perspectives, 30*(2), 96–98.

Groom, J., Henderson, D., & Sittner, B. J. (In press). National League for Nursing—Jeffries simulation framework state of the science project: Simulation design characteristics. *Clinical Simulation in Nursing.*

Gunberg-Ross, J. (2012). Simulation and psychomotor skills acquisition: A review of the literature. *Clinical Simulation in Nursing, 8*(9), e429–e435.

Hallmark, B., Thomas, C., & Gantt, L. (In press). The education practices construct of the NLN/Jeffries simulation framework. *Clinical Simulation in Nursing.*

Holmboe, E., Rizzolo, M. A., Sachdeva, A. K., Rosenberg, M., & Ziv, A. (2011). Simulation-based assessment and the regulation of healthcare professionals. *Simulation in Healthcare, 6*, S58–S62.

Issenberg, B., Ringsted, C., Ostergaard, D., & Dieckmann, P. (2011). Setting a research agenda for simulation-based healthcare education: A synthesis of the outcomes from an Utstein style meeting. *Simulation in Healthcare, 6*(3), 155–157.

Jeffries, J. (2005). A framework for designing, implementing, and evaluating simulations used as teaching strategies. *Nursing Education Perspectives, 26*(2), 96–103.

Jeffries, P. R., & Rizzolo, M. A. (2006). *Designing and implementing models for the innovative use of simulation to teach nursing care of ill adults and children: A national multi-site, multi-method study.* New York: National League for Nursing.

Kardong-Edgren, S., Adamson, K. A., & Fitzgerald, C. (2010). A review of currently published evaluation instruments for human patient simulation. *Clinical Simulation in Nursing, 6*(1), e25–e35.

Kirkpatrick, D. L. (1994). *Evaluating training programs: The four levels.* San Francisco, CA: Bernett-Koehler.

Kolb, D. (1984). *Experiential learning: Experiences as the source of learning and development.* Upper Saddle River, NJ: Prentice-Hall.

LeBlanc, V. R., Manser, T., Weinger, M. B., Musson, D., Kutzon, J., & Howard, S. (2011). The study of factors affecting human and systems performance in healthcare using simulation. *Simulation in Healthcare, 6,* S24–S29.

McGaghie, W. C., Draycott, T. J., Dunn, W. F., Lopez, C. M., & Stefanidis, D. (2011). Evaluating the impact of simulation on translational patient outcomes. *Simulation in Healthcare, 6*(Suppl), S42–S47.

Meyer, M. N., Connors, H., Hou, Q., & Gajewski, B. (2011). The effect of simulation on clinical performance. *Simulation in Healthcare, 6,* 269–277.

Nestel, D., Groom, J., Eikeland-Huesbo, S., & O'Donnell, J. M. (2011). Simulation for learning and teaching procedural skills. *Simulation in Healthcare, 6,* S10–S13.

Norman, J. (2012, Spring). Systematic review of the literature on simulation in nursing education. *ABNF Journal, 28,* 24–28.

Oermann, M., Hallmark, B., Haus, C., Kardong-Edgren, S., Keegan McColgan, J., & Rogers, N. (2012). Conducting multisite research studies in nursing education: Brief practice of CPR skills as exemplar. *Journal of Nursing Education, 51*(1), 23–28.

O'Shea, E. R., Pagano, M., Campbell, S. H., & Caso, G. (2013). A descriptive analysis of nursing student communication behaviors. *Clinical Simulation in Nursing, 9*(1), e5–e12.

Paige, J. B., & Morin, K. H. (In press). Simulation fidelity and cueing: A systematic review of the literature. *Clinical Simulation in Nursing.*

Potter, N., & Allen, M. (In press). Clinical swallow exam for dysphagia: A speech pathology and nursing simulation experience. *Clinical Simulation in Nursing.*

Powell-Laney, S., Keen, C., & Hall, K. (2012). The use of human patient simulation to enhance clinical decision-making of nursing students. *Education for Health, 25*(1), 11–15.

Radhakrishnan, K., Roche, J., & Cunningham, H. (2007). Measuring clinical practice parameters with human patient simulation: A pilot study. *International Journal of Nursing Education Scholarship, 4*(1), 1–11.

Raemer, D., Anderson, M., Cheng, A., Fanning, R., Nadkarnai, V., & Savoldelli, G. (2011). Research regarding debriefing as part of the learning process. *Simulation in Healthcare, 6,* S52–S57.

Roche, J., Schoen, D., & Kruzel, A. (2013). Human patient simulation vs. case studies

for new graduate nurses in nursing orientation: A pilot study. *Clinical Simulation in Nursing, 9*(6), e199–e205.

Schaeffer, J. J., Vanderbilt, A. A., Cason, C., Bauman, E. B., Glavin, R. J., Lee, F. W., & Navedo, D. D. (2011). Instructional design and pedagogy science in healthcare simulation. *Simulation in Healthcare, 6,* S30–S41.

Schon, D. A. (1983). *The reflective practitioner: How professionals think in action.* New York, NY: Basic Books.

Shearer, J. E. (2013). High-fidelity simulation and safety: An integrative review. *Journal of Nursing Education, 52*(1), 39–45.

Shinnick, M. A., & Woo, M. A. (In press). The effect of human patient simulation on critical thinking and its predictors in prelicensure nursing students. *Nurse Education Today.*

Shinnick, M. A., Woo, M. A., & Mentee, J. C. (2011). Human patient simulation: State of the science in prelicensure nursing. *Journal of Nursing Education, 50*(2), 65–72.

Shneider, A. M. (2011). Four stages of a scientific discipline; four types of scientist. *Trends in Biochemical Sciences, 34*(5), 217–223.

Szpak, J. L., & Kameq, K. M. (2013). Simulation decreases student anxiety prior to communication with mentally ill patients. *Clinical Simulation in Nursing, 9*(1), e13–e19.

U.S. Department of Health and Human Services. (2009). Code of Federal Regulations: Title 45 Part 46 Protection of Human Subjects. Retrieved from www.hhs.gov/ohrp/humansubjects/guidance/45cfr46.html

Van Merriënboer, J. J. G., & Sweller, J. (2005). Cognitive load theory and complex learning; Recent developments and future directions. *Educational Psychology Review, 17*(2), 147–177.

Weaver, A. (2011). High fidelity patient simulation in nursing education: An integrative review. *Nursing Education Perspectives, 12*(1), 37–20.

Willhaus, J. (2010). Interdepartmental simulation collaboration in academia: Exploring partnerships with other disciplines. *Clinical Simulation in Nursing, 6*(6), e231–e232.

Yuan, H. B., Williams, B. A., & Fang, J. B. (2012). The contribution of high-fidelity simulation to nursing students' confidence and competence: A systematic review. *International Nursing Review, 59*(1), 26–33.

Evaluation Tools and Metrics for Simulations

Katie A. Adamson, PhD, RN

■ Learning Objectives

1. Describe the essential criteria for producing valid and reliable data about participant performance for observation-based evaluations.
2. Outline a process for simulation evaluation.
3. Describe evaluation strategies and instruments for each level of evaluation: reaction, learning, behavior, and results.
4. Select appropriate evaluation strategies and instruments based on the intended purpose of an evaluation.
5. Apply the concepts of validity and reliability as qualities of simulation evaluation data.
6. Outline a process for creating simulation evaluation instruments.
7. Apply logic modeling to the evaluation of simulation programs.
8. Describe trends in the use of simulation evaluation including high-stakes and licensure exam testing.

■ Key Terms

- Formative evaluation
- Reliability
- Summative evaluation
- Validity

Simulation, whether manikin or computer based, provides a unique lens through which observers can view how participants might perform in an actual clinical encounter. These performances demonstrate participants' knowledge, skills, and attitudes and provide important data about participants' clinical abilities. In order to capture these rich data for the purpose of evaluation, educators must equip themselves with tools and metrics that reflect participants' learning from and performance in simulation activities. This chapter highlights the importance of valid and reliable evaluation data for establishing the evidence base for simulation as a teaching and learning strategy and for optimizing the potential uses of simulation.

CRITERIA FOR VALID AND RELIABLE DATA SIMULATION PERFORMANCE

Figure 12.1 lists the three essential criteria needed for valid and reliable data simulation performance. When using simulation for evaluation, one must examine the **reliability** and **validity** of the simulation activity itself, the psychometric properties of the tools or metrics used to evaluate the participant, and, when applicable, the objectivity and ability of the observer evaluating the performance.

Although this chapter is primarily about the tools and metrics, qualities of the simulation should also be addressed. The International Nursing Association for Clinical Simulation and Learning Board of Directors (INACSL, 2011) established the "Standards for the Evaluation of Expected Outcomes" that reflect the essential qualities of the simulation itself:

- The simulation-based evaluation should be conducted in an environment that is familiar to the participant.
- The content of the simulation should contain evidence-based content.
- The appropriate level of simulation fidelity should be employed.

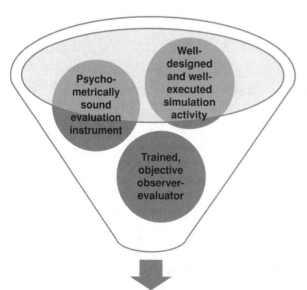

FIGURE 12.1 Essential criteria for producing valid and reliable data about participant performance for observation-based evaluations.

Valid and reliable data about participant performance for observation-based evaluations

- The simulation should encompass specific objectives that the participant is expected to meet, guidelines for appropriate participant responses or behaviors, and parameters for termination of the simulation should be established a priori.
- Observers or evaluators should be consistent in their coaching or prompting of participants.

Like INACSL, the National League for Nursing (NLN, n.d.a) includes the "Recommendations to Achieve a Fair Testing Environment" in their "Fair Testing Guidelines for Nursing Education." These standards and guidelines reflect criteria that must be met to provide a valid and consistent (reliable) testing environment for simulation participants. No performance evaluation instrument, however well developed or psychometrically sound, will provide useful data if the simulation that participants are exposed to is poorly designed or executed. Further, for observation-based simulation evaluations, the objectivity and ability of the observer who evaluates the simulation participant is paramount.

This chapter will focus on the tools and metrics for evaluating the effectiveness of simulation, from the participant experience to the final results of simulation activities, including patient care outcomes. The chapter concludes with ideas for using these concepts and associated metrics to communicate the value of a simulation program and a synopsis of trends in the use of simulation evaluation.

THE PROCESS OF EVALUATION

Simulation evaluation should be integrated into the larger process of planning, implementing, assessing, and revising simulation-based educational experiences. Starting with the end in mind and identifying the purpose of the evaluation early in this process will help ensure that the evaluation is relevant and that it addresses the objectives for which it was undertaken. Further, using this "backward design" process could also help guide the planning and implementation of simulation activities to best address the desired learning outcomes (Wiggins & McTighe, 2008). Building on steps suggested by Bourke and Ihrke (2009), consider the following for the process of simulation evaluation:

1. Determine the purpose, content, and stakes of the evaluation including whether it will be formative or summative.
2. Plan for the logistics of the evaluation including the timing, instrumentation, and training of evaluators for observation-based evaluations.
3. Collect and interpret the evaluation data.
4. Report and respond to the evaluation findings and consider the costs and intended or unintended consequences of the evaluation (pp. 392–393).

The purpose of the evaluation will guide all of the subsequent steps in the planning process. In determining the purpose of the evaluation, the evaluator should consider what questions the evaluation will be designed to answer and whether the evaluation is formative or summative. **Formative evaluations** help answer the question, Is this teaching strategy working?, while **summative evaluations** help answer the question, Did this

TABLE 12.1

Uses of Formative and Summative Evaluation Data

Choose Formative Evaluation	Choose Summative Evaluation
When you want to provide data for the participant or instructor about the participant's comprehension and ability to apply what he or she is learning	When you want to evaluate participants' performance or what he or she has learned to make decisions such as whether participants progress to the next level or to assign scores
When you want to measure the effectiveness of in-progress teaching and learning strategies	When you want to measure the effectiveness of completed teaching and learning strategies
When you want to identify whether participants need additional instruction or remediation	When you want to identify areas of potential improvement to completed simulation activities
When you want to answer the question, Is this teaching/learning strategy working and are the participants achieving success?	When you want to answer the question, Did this teaching and learning strategy work and did the participants achieve success?

Adapted with permission from Scheckel (2009).

teaching and learning strategy work? (Scheckel, 2009). A review of the uses of formative and summative evaluation data is provided in Table 12.1.

Questions to consider when determining the purpose, content, and stakes of the evaluation include: Is the evaluation meant to guide participants and identify actual or potential problems during the formative stages of learning? Is the evaluation meant to make a determination about participants' abilities or assign grades during the formative stages of learning? If the evaluation is addressing a simulation program, will the data it generates be used to reflect and guide implementation, make resource and management-related decisions, or determine the effectiveness of the program? Regardless of how these questions are answered, all stakeholders should be made aware of the purpose of the evaluation.

If the purpose includes anything in the realm of program evaluation or research that may be suitable for publication, it is essential to acquire approval from the appropriate institutional review board or ethics committee at this stage of the planning process. Internal evaluation data that are not meant to be generalizable to a wider population may not need ethics approval. However, evaluations frequently produce findings that are valuable for wider dissemination, so it is wise to leave this possibility open by getting approval before moving ahead with the evaluation.

After identifying the purpose, content, and stakes, it is time to plan for the logistics of the evaluation including the timing, instrumentation, and training of evaluators for observation-based evaluations. Formative evaluations can take place at any time during the course of the simulation-based activities, whereas summative evaluations will likely

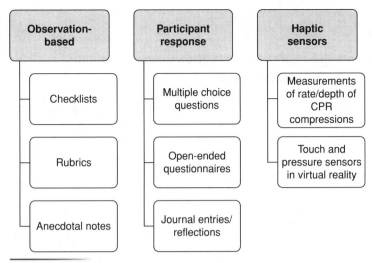

FIGURE 12.2 Three basic types of simulation evaluation instruments. (Adapted with permission from McGaghie et al., 2010.)

occur at the end of the activities. Next, selecting an appropriate instrument that will generate useful data to serve the intended purpose of the evaluation can be a challenge. There is often a temptation to develop a unique evaluation tool for each evaluation need. However, establishing the validity and reliability of data from a new instrument can be a daunting task. Recognize that no single instrument is likely to meet all of your evaluation needs. There will be a tradeoff when it comes to the resources expended on data gathering and the value of the data gathered.

Simulation evaluation instruments can be divided into three categories: observation-based, participant-response, and haptic sensors (McGaghie, Issenberg, Petrusa, & Scalese, 2010). Selection of the appropriate type of evaluation instrument will depend on the needs and resources available for a specific evaluation. Figure 12.2 and Table 12.2 illustrate various categories of simulation evaluation instruments and some of their strengths and weaknesses.

Additional questions to consider when selecting an evaluation instrument include: Is the proposed instrument specific to and comprehensive of the aspects of participant performance you seek to evaluate? Is it accessible and simple to use? What are the costs (both time and resource) associated with its use? Are there existing data about the reliability and validity of data produced using the instrument for a similar purpose? (Bourke & Ihrke, 2009). If an observation-based instrument is selected, rater training, interrater reliability assessment, and careful scheduling or video recording simulations will be essential. Further discussion of this is included later in the chapter.

After planning the work, it is time to work the plan and collect the evaluation data. The specific logistics of the data collection will depend on many of the decisions made earlier in the evaluation planning process. However, it is important to maintain consistent practices for the duration of the data collection activities. This consistency will facilitate appropriate and accurate analyses. For example, if you want to compare

TABLE 12.2

Categories of Simulation Evaluation Instruments and Their Strengths and Weaknesses

Category	Instrument	Strengths	Weaknesses
Observation based	Checklists	Highly standardized, comprehensive checklists provide objective reflections of what participants did or did not do	In order to capture all relevant actions, checklists may be long and cumbersome
	Rubrics	Well-designed rubrics can capture the essential elements of a simulation performance and provide objective data	Evaluators may interpret rubric criteria differently, leading to low reliability
	Anecdotal notes	Informal notes help instructors capitalize on every observation as an opportunity to provide feedback; well-organized notes can give a perspective over time of participants' progress	The subjectivity of these notes makes them difficult to defend. Summative or high-stakes evaluations should not be based solely on anecdotal notes.
Participant response	Multiple choice questions	Published resources including NCLEX-like exam questions have established content-specific reliability and validity	May not capture the complex learning that takes place in simulation, including critical thinking and psychomotor skills
	Open-ended questionnaires	Allow participants to demonstrate their thinking and decision making	Scoring may be time consuming and subjective
	Journal entries/ reflection	In addition to producing evaluation data, reflection may help participants develop their critical thinking abilities (Marchigiano, Eduljee, & Harvey 2010)	Subjective self-report of the participant's experience may not accurately reflect reality (Mudumbai, Gaba, Boulet, Howard, & Davies, 2012; Paul, 2010; Sadosty et al., 2011)

TABLE 12.2

Categories of Simulation Evaluation Instruments and Their Strengths and Weaknesses (Continued)

Category	Instrument	Strengths	Weaknesses
Haptic sensors	Measurements of rate/ depth of CPR compressions	Objective ratings of skill performance	Costs may be prohibitive and data may not capture the complexity of task performance
	Touch and pressure sensors in virtual reality	Objective ratings of skill performance	Costs may be prohibitive and data may not capture the complexity of task performance

CPR, cardiopulmonary resuscitation; NCLEX, National Council Licensure Examination.

pre- and postsimulation exam scores, it is important that all participants complete the same pre- and postsimulation exams. Likewise, it is important that the simulation and testing environments are consistent for all participants. These and other considerations are included in the INACSL's "Standards for the Evaluation of Expected Outcomes" and the NLN's "Fair Testing Guidelines for Nursing Education." Make sure the elements that will be evaluated are embedded in the simulation. Once the data are collected, analysis and interpretation might simply mean reading through participants' reflections or require the assistance of a biostatistician. Regardless of the scope of the analyses and interpretation, it is important that they are completed as soon after the data collection as possible and that they adhere to the highest of ethical standards.

The evaluation process is not over once the data are collected and analyzed. At this point, it is important to report findings to stakeholders, including simulation participants. This reporting, like the simulation debriefing, provides an opportunity for stakeholders to react and respond to the findings. When appropriate, data about individual performance may be shared with individuals to allow for appropriate progression or remediation. Likewise, aggregate data should be reported and responded to appropriately. Finally, it is important to rally the evaluation team and consider the costs and intended or unintended consequences of the evaluation.

Ideally, the process of evaluation should be a continuous cycle. In addition to providing information about participant performance, simulation evaluation data may be useful for appraising the effectiveness of instructional strategies (McDonald, 2014). The evidence produced from these evaluations should be implemented in order to facilitate evidence-based practices in simulation-based teaching and learning. In addition to making adjustments to local simulation practices, findings should be widely disseminated for others to learn from and build upon. This cycle will help advance simulation science.

WHAT CAN BE MEASURED AND WHY IT SHOULD BE MEASURED: THE VALUE OF EACH TYPE OF DATA

To paraphrase an often-cited quote, not everything that can be measured is worth measuring and not every attribute that is important to know about is measurable (Cameron, 1963). Among the challenges that simulation evaluation presents are identifying which evaluation data may be useful and then figuring out meaningful ways to capture these data. The nursing literature is flooded with reports about participants' satisfaction with simulation activities. This is due, in large part, to the fact that participant satisfaction is an easy metric to acquire. Although participant satisfaction is not wholly unimportant, it is not as important as, for example, whether learning from simulation-based training transferred into the clinical setting where the simulation participants provided improved patient care that resulted in superior patient outcomes.

The following subsections use Kirkpatrick's (1998) "Levels of Evaluation" to describe a framework for categorizing evaluations reflecting the range of data from participants' reactions to simulation activities to patient and organizational outcomes that result from simulation-based training. Kirkpatrick's "Levels of Evaluation" are: Level 1: Reaction; Level 2: Learning; Level 3: Behavior; and Level 4: Results. Evaluations are typically more complex and the data they produce more meaningful as you progress from Level 1 to Level 4.

Reaction

Level 1 evaluations reflect participants' reactions to a simulation activity. Evaluation strategies at this level are sometimes referred to as "smile tests." They provide data about how satisfied participants were with the simulation experience and their perception of how the activities affected their learning and confidence. Although this is considered the lowest level of evaluation, some value can be ascertained from Level 1 evaluation data. Frick, Chadha, Watson, Wang, and Green (2009) suggested that subjective measures of participants' satisfaction or perception of learning activities are highly correlated with their actual learning. Additionally, this type of evaluation can shed light on what participants enjoyed about the simulation and how they perceived that it met or did not meet their learning preferences. Kirkpatrick (1998) provided the following guidelines for Level 1 evaluations: (1) identify the purpose of the evaluation; (2) use an instrument that will quantify participants' reactions; (3) provide a space for participants to write comments and suggestions; (4) strive for 100 percent participation; (5) get immediate and honest responses; (6) decide upon reasonable standards or a comparison/reference for interpretation; (7) communicate results and respond appropriately (paraphrased from guidelines on p. 26).

Learning

Level 2 evaluations reflect participants' learning in the cognitive, affective, and psychomotor domains. These evaluations can reflect what participants learned from a simulation activity or their ability to apply what they learned through various instructional means in the context of a simulation activity. Cognitive and affective learning are often evaluated using paper-based participant response instruments such as multiple choice or open-ended questions, whereas psychomotor learning is often evaluated using observation-based performance evaluation instruments. Kirkpatrick (1998) provided the following guidelines for Level 2 evaluations: (1) if appropriate, use a comparison group; (2) evaluate cognitive, affective, and psychomotor learning pre- and postsimulation; (3) use a participant response instrument to evaluate cognitive and affective learning; (4) use an observation-based or haptic sensor instrument to evaluate psychomotor learning; (5) strive for 100 percent participation; (6) use the evaluation results to take appropriate action (paraphrased from p. 40).

Behavior

Level 3 evaluations reflect the degree to which participants' learning from simulation activities results in behavior change in the actual clinical environment. Behaviors that reflect cognitive, affective, and psychomotor learning are ideally evaluated using observation-based evaluation instruments. Because such observations can be difficult in the actual clinical environment, simulation is often used as a proxy for such observations.

There is a lack of agreement in the literature about whether simulation is an adequate proxy for observing clinical behavior. If simulation is used to evaluate behavior, special attention should be paid to the fidelity of the simulated environment because, theoretically, the more realistic the simulation is, the more likely it is to elicit the same behaviors that would be demonstrated in the clinical environment. This will enhance the validity of simulation evaluation (Gaba, 2009). Ideally, learning from simulation will be evaluated in the actual clinical setting. An example of this may be found in Meyer, Connors, Hou, and Gajewski's (2011) study about nursing students' clinical performance after participation in a pediatric simulation curriculum. Their results indicated that students who participated in the simulation activities received significantly higher clinical evaluations than those who did not.

Kirkpatrick (1998) provided the following guidelines for Level 3 evaluation: (1) if appropriate, use a comparison group; (2) recognize that behavior change takes time, so allow adequate time for it to take place; (3) if appropriate, conduct pre- and postintervention evaluations; (4) get a 360-degree picture of participants' behavior by soliciting evaluation data from the participants, their supervisors, subordinates, and others who observe their behavior; (5) strive for 100 percent participation; (6) repeat the evaluation when appropriate; (7) consider the cost–benefit ratio of the evaluation (paraphrased from p. 49).

Results

Level 4 evaluations reflect the results of simulation activities. These evaluations are done outside the simulation lab and reflect metrics such as patient and organizational outcomes. An example of a Level 4 evaluation may be found in Cohen et al. (2010). These authors completed a cost–benefit analysis to estimate the cost savings from a reduction in catheter-associated blood infections following the implementation of simulation-based central venous catheter insertion training. Another example of Level 4 evaluation is described in Draycott et al. (2008), where simulation-based training is shown to have resulted in improved shoulder dystocia management.

Kirkpatrick (1998) provided the following guidelines for Level 4 evaluation: (1) if appropriate, use a comparison group; (2) recognize that results take time, so allow adequate time for them to be achieved; (3) measure indicators of the results of pre- and postintervention; (4) repeat the evaluation when appropriate; (5) consider the cost–benefit ratio of the evaluation; (6) identify appropriate indicators of success and be satisfied when finding "proof" of success is not feasible (paraphrased from p. 61).

Although evaluations at each level—reaction, learning, behavior, and results—are valuable, nurse educators should strive to move beyond participant satisfaction ratings (reaction) and evaluate how simulation contributes to learning, behavior, and results. Tanner (2011) argued that within a practice discipline such as nursing, "content knowledge is a necessary but insufficient condition for safe practice" (p. 491) and simulation offers opportunities for "situated cognition" (Wooley & Jarvis, 2007) where students' abilities to recall and apply knowledge can be observed and evaluated.

In order to optimize the value of the data collected, work backward from the objectives of the evaluation and consider the following question: Is your objective to produce participants who are satisfied with the simulation (reaction), participants who achieve specific cognitive, affective, and psychomotor learning outcomes (learning), participants whose clinical behaviors demonstrate their learning (behaviors), or participants who provide care that impacts patient and organizational outcomes (results)? With this question in mind, consider the following examples of tools and metrics for evaluation at each level.

TOOLS AND METRICS FOR EVALUATION AT EACH LEVEL

The literature reflects a general sentiment of dissatisfaction with the tools and metrics available for simulation evaluation (Adamson, Kardong-Edgren, & Wilhaus, 2012; Kardong-Edgren, Adamson, & Fitzgerald, 2010; Tanner, 2011). Indeed, many nursing education programs employ "in-house" evaluation instruments supported by limited validity and reliability evidence. Further, the nursing literature is crowded with author-designed instruments and an overrepresentation of studies that employ lower-level evaluations such as participant-reported self-confidence and learning (Smith & Barry, 2013). But take heart, this disappointing trend is slowly changing course.

There is an increasingly robust body of literature highlighting tools and metrics for simulation evaluation. This trend will likely encourage the use and testing of existing measures, which will add to the body of knowledge about the validity and reliability of the data they produce. Below is a list of recent review articles that provide a wide selection of simulation evaluation instruments from the fields of pharmacy (Bray, Schwartz, Odegard, Hammer, & Seybert, 2011), nursing (Adamson et al., 2012; Davis & Kimble, 2011; Foronda, Liu, & Bauman, in press; Kardong-Edgren et al., 2010; Yuan, Williams, & Fang, 2011), and medicine (Foronda et al., in press; Ilgen, Sherbino, & Cook, 2013; Kogan, Holmboe, & Hauer, 2009; Yuan et al., 2012):

- Bray et al. (2011) provided examples of 11 evaluation strategies used in pharmacy education and categorized them according to the domain, topic, and design/method of assessment.
- Davis and Kimble (2011) reviewed evaluation instruments that reflect the American Association of Colleges of Nursing's "Baccalaureate Essentials."

- Foronda et al. (in press) reviewed over 100 articles and identified five themes including: confidence/self-efficacy, satisfaction, anxiety/stress, skills/knowledge, and interdisciplinary experiences.

- Ilgen et al. (2013) conducted a systematic review and meta-analysis about the effectiveness of technology-enhanced teaching and learning strategies used in emergency medicine training programs. Their literature review and references include a wide variety of simulation evaluation options.

- Kardong-Edgren et al. (2010) reviewed evaluation instruments from the health sciences literature and categorized them according to the learning domain they addressed. They also included a section on instruments designed for team performance evaluation. An update of this review was recently published (Adamson et al., 2012).

- Kogan et al. (2009) identified 55 instruments designed to evaluate medical trainees. The table in their article provides helpful information about the instruments including validity evidence.

- Yuan et al. (2012) reviewed studies from medicine and nursing education and provided a listing of the instruments used in each study.

Table 12.3 provides additional examples of simulation evaluation instruments for each level of evaluation.

VALIDITY AND RELIABILITY OF DATA

One of the challenges associated with observation-based evaluations is variability in how raters perceive participants' performances. Observer bias can introduce additional error into the evaluation. For this reason, it is especially important to assess the reliability and validity of data produced from observation-based simulation evaluation instruments. Reliability has to do with consistency and whether the instrument provides consistent data when administered by multiple raters (interrater), on multiple occasions (test–retest), or when compared with ratings from other evaluations designed to measure the same construct (interinstrument). Validity has to do with how well the data reflect the construct the instrument is supposed to measure. Simply put, reliability assessment answers the question: Are the data consistent? and validity assessment answers the question: Do the data reflect what they are intended to reflect?

There are several types of evidence that can be used to demonstrate the reliability and validity of data from an evaluation instrument. The most widely used measures of reliability are interrater, test–retest, and intrainstrument. The most common measures of validity include face-, content-, construct-, and criterion-related validity. However, these commonly used measures of validity have been updated with five types of validity evidence: (1) evidence based on test content, (2) evidence based on response processes, (3) evidence based on internal structure, (4) evidence based on relationships to other variables, and (5) evidence based on the consequences of testing (American Educational Research Association, American Psychological Association, & National Council on Measurement in Education, 1999). Table 12.4 provides an overview of each type of reliability and validity evidence and how each can be assessed.

TABLE 12.3

Simulation Evaluation Instruments for Each Level of Evaluation

Level of Evaluation	Instrument Description	Reference
Reaction	Simulation Effectiveness Tool (SET) designed to measure the effectiveness of the simulated clinical experience	Elfrink Cordi, Leighton, Ryan-Wegner, Doyle, & Ravert, 2012
	National League for Nursing Student Satisfaction and Self-Confidence in Learning Scale measures participants' satisfaction with the simulation activity and self-confidence	NLN, n.d.b
	Emergency Response Confidence Tool designed to evaluate participant's confidence in emergency response	Arnold et al., 2009
	Simulation Design Scale designed to evaluate five features the simulation activity including objectives/information, support, problem solving, feedback, and fidelity	NLN, n.d.b
Learning	Health Sciences Reasoning Test (Insight Assessment, 2011) designed to evaluate participants' reasoning skills and Heart Failure Clinical Knowledge Pre- and Post-Tests designed to evaluate participants' knowledge	Shinnick & Woo, in press
	Oral exam about the management of shock designed to evaluate participants' abilities to "explain key elements of patient evaluation in crises, invasive monitoring, and the pathophysiology and management of shock" (p. e1004)	Littlewood, Shilling, Stemland, Wright, & Kirk, 2013
Learning and behavior in simulation	Simulation Team Assessment Tool (STAT), a team performance assessment tool for pediatric resuscitation simulations designed "to evaluate key components of all pediatric resuscitations" (p. 880)	Reid et al., 2012
	OSCE for pediatric medication administration designed to evaluate participants' performance of specific skills	Cazzell & Howe, 2012
	Nursing Performance Profile (NPP) 41-item instrument including 9 competency categories of safe practice	Hinton et al., 2012; Randolph et al., 2012

TABLE 12.3

Simulation Evaluation Instruments for Each Level of Evaluation (*Continued*)

Level of Evaluation	Instrument Description	Reference
	The combat performance evaluation instrument used to evaluate participants' "ability to assess, intervene, and evaluate care given to simulated patients using the HPS" (p. 1131)	Johnson, Corrigan, Gulickson, Holshouser, & Johnson, 2012
Learning and behavior in virtual reality	Web-SP semiautomatic assessment system designed to evaluate participants' "interactions with virtual patients and their answers regarding diagnoses, caring procedures and their justifications" (p. 757)	Forsberg, Georg, Ziegert, & Fors, 2011
Learning and behavior	Performance checklists for CPR, ACLS, and PALS designed to evaluate participants' performance of specific skills	American Heart Association
	Self-assessment of performance using a rubric and the teamwork activity inventory in nursing scale (TAINS) designed to assess participants' nontechnical skills	Abe et al., 2013
Behavior	BSN student clinical evaluations designed to evaluate participants' performance, preparation, student-client communication, clinical judgment, therapeutic skills, interprofessional communication, and documentation	Meyer et al., 2011
Results	Cost-savings calculation done by comparing costs associated with bloodstream infections before and after the implementation of the simulation-based CVC insertion training intervention	Cohen et al., 2010
	Management of shoulder dystocia and neonatal injuries pre- and postsimulation-based training using intra- and postpartum records	Draycott et al., 2008

CVC, central venous catheter; CPR, cardiopulmonary resuscitation; ACLS, advanced cardiovascular life support; PALS, pediatric advanced life support; OSCE, objective structured clinical examination.

TABLE 12.4

Types of Validity and Reliability Evidence for Observation-Based Evaluation Instruments and Examples of Strategies for Assessing Each

Type of Reliability or Validity Evidence	Examples of Strategies for Assessing the Each Type of Evidence
Interrater reliability	Use video-recorded simulation vignettes and have raters independently score the vignettes. Then, compare scores for interrater reliability.
Intrarater (test–retest) reliability	Using a video-recorded simulation vignette, ask individual raters to view and score the vignette once, then, several weeks later, ask the same rater to view and score the same vignette. Then, compare scores for intrarater reliability.
Interinstrument reliability	Ask raters to view and score a simulation using multiple evaluation instruments that are designed to measure the same construct (clinical judgment ability, psychomotor skill, etc.) and compare ratings across instruments.
Evidence based on test content (content-related validity)	Does the content of the evaluation instrument represent the aspect of performance you are trying to measure? Ask experts to analyze the content of the instrument for relevance, representativeness, and clarity.
Evidence based on response processes (construct-related validity)	Are there systematic differences between different groups of individuals completing the evaluation instrument or being evaluated with it? Ask raters how they arrived at scores they assign and assess whether this is in line with the intentions of the evaluation.
Evidence based on internal structure (construct-related validity)	Look at the correlations between items on the instrument. Do they align with the construct the instrument is designed to assess? Analytic strategies such as factor analysis may be useful for assessing evidence based on internal structure.
Evidence based on relationship to other variables (criterion-related, concurrent, and predictive validity)	Assess the relationship between scores on the evaluation and other related variables such as grade point average, year in school, or clinical performance or whether scores on the evaluation accurately predict future performance.
Evidence based on relationship to other variables (construct validity)	Assess for convergent and discriminant validity. For example, participants' scores on the simulation evaluation rubric should be highly correlated with scores of clinical performance (convergent) but not necessarily with the day on which they completed the evaluation (discriminant).
Evidence based on consequences of testing	Assess whether the intended benefits of the evaluation are being realized and whether there are any negative, unintended consequences of the evaluation.

Adapted from SIRC; source: Goodwin, 2002.

Designing simulations and using appropriate videography for observation-based evaluations can also enhance the validity and reliability of evaluation data. When designing a simulation activity, whether computer or manikin based, it is essential to include opportunities for participants to demonstrate the knowledge, skills, and abilities they are going to be evaluated on. Likewise, the positioning of observers or cameras must allow for the viewing of evaluated behaviors.

Selecting an existing instrument with existing reliability and validity data is usually preferable than creating a new one. However, existing reliability and validity data are specific to the context in which it was generated. Just because an instrument has been "validated" for one purpose with one type of participant does not mean that it will produce data that are valid and reliable for another type of participant or with another group of raters. For example, a ruler may provide reliable and valid data about an infant's length, but it would not provide valid or reliable data about an infant's weight. Or, a skills checklist might provide valid data about a participant's ability to perform a technical skill, but it may not provide valid data about his critical thinking skills. Although it is recommended to select an existing instrument that will suit your needs, consider assessing the reliability and validity of the data within the context and for the purposes for which you intend to use it.

CREATING YOUR OWN TOOLS AND METRICS

Instrument development is a specialty of its own, and this chapter cannot provide a comprehensive examination of this art. However, this section will provide a starting point. If you choose to develop your own simulation evaluation instrument, the first step is defining your construct. Before you can decide how you are going to measure, you have to decide what you are going to measure. If you are creating a skills checklist, this may be as simple as identifying the skill. If you intend to develop a scale or rubric for evaluating a more complex construct such as critical thinking, establishing an appropriate theoretical foundation and the scope for your instrument are essential first steps.

After defining your construct, DeVellis (2003) suggested generating a pool of potential items for measuring that construct, determining a format for the measurement instrument, and having a group of content experts review these selections. Using feedback from the content experts, you can then construct a draft instrument to pilot test within the environment you wish to employ the finished instrument, which will help assess the appropriateness of items as well as clarify what revisions are needed.

Finally, using the suggestions from Table 12.4, assess the reliability and validity of the data produced using the instrument for its intended purposes. After you have gone to all the effort to develop an evaluation instrument, it is important to disseminate it so that others can not only benefit from it, but where it could also contribute to the body of knowledge about the reliability and validity of the data it produces.

USING A LOGIC MODEL TO EVALUATE AND DESCRIBE THE VALUE OF YOUR SIMULATION PROGRAM

This chapter is primarily focused on participant evaluation. However, simulation programs require extensive resources, and evaluations may also be undertaken to demonstrate how a program uses those resources and whether the program is achieving its intended goals.

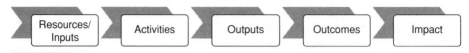

FIGURE 12.3 Basic components of a logic model.

In order to provide information about the value of a simulation program, it may be useful to draw a logic model representing the resources and inputs, activities, outputs, outcomes, and impact of the program. Figure 12.3 presents the basic components of a logic model.

A program logic model is a "visual representation of the structure of the program that describes and explains the intended cause-and-effect linkages connecting resources, activities, and results" (McDavid, Huse, & Hawthorn, 2013, p. 47). Figure 12.4 provides a logic model for a hypothetical simulation program.

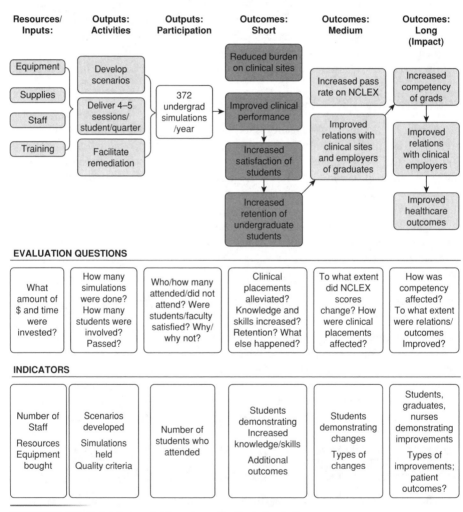

FIGURE 12.4 Logic model for a hypothetical simulation program.
(Source: www.uwex.edu/ces/pdande/evaluation/evallogicmodel.html.)

The key to using logic models for simulation program evaluation is to identify evaluation questions and develop indicators and the associated metrics to communicate the *value* (or challenges) for your program (W.K. Kellogg Foundation, 2013).[1]

TRENDS IN SIMULATION EVALUATION INCLUDING HIGH-STAKES AND LICENSURE EXAM TESTING

Although the use of simulation is growing rapidly in nursing education, it has been slower to catch on as a platform for high-stakes evaluation (Bensfield, Olech, & Horsley, 2012). According to the INACSL's "Standards of Best Practice," high-stakes evaluation refers to "An evaluation process associated with a simulation activity and that has a major consequence or is the basis for a major grading decision, including pass/fail implications. High stakes refers to the outcome or consequences of the process" (p. S5). These implications may relate to academic progress, initial licensure, or continuing competency and require policymakers to give thoughtful consideration to the reliability and validity of the entire evaluation process.

Internationally, simulation-based evaluations are increasingly being used by regulatory bodies for licensure (Holmboe, 2011) and remediation (Hinton et al., 2012; Randolph et al., 2012). Although many would agree with Tanner (2011) that "content knowledge is a necessary but insufficient condition for safe practice" (p. 491), the United States has adhered to the tradition of granting nursing licensure based on a knowledge-centered exam (e.g., the National Council Licensure Examination for Registered Nurses). Simulation offers an enticing alternative to this tradition. Levine, Schwartz, Bryson, and Demaria (2012) described five driving forces that will likely lead to the increased use of simulation evaluation for licensure and health care provider competency assurance:

> (1) the public's demand for a safer healthcare industry; (2) the identification of core competencies and the recognition that simulation-based tools can be effectively used to assess them; (3) time-limited board certification and recertification standardization; (4) the use of computer-based examinations for licensure; and (5) processes to promote excellence and standardization of simulation programs. (p. 141)

CONCLUSION

These forces underscore the importance of simulation-based evaluation and the unique lens simulation provides for viewing how participants will likely perform in actual clinical encounters. Optimizing simulation's applications for evaluation requires careful consideration of the evaluation process, instrumentation, and types, qualities of interpretations of evaluation data. Further, it requires the ability to articulate the value of simulation programs through program evaluations such as logic models. This chapter provided an overview and resources for the intermediate and advanced simulation practitioner.

---

[1]Additional resources for developing a logic model for your own program can be found at: http://www.uwex.edu/ces/pdande/evaluation/evallogicmodel.html; http://www.wkkf.org/knowledge-center/resources/2006/02/wk-kellogg-foundation-logic-model-development-guide.aspx.

■ Key Concepts

- ■ Essential criteria for producing valid and reliable data about participant performance for observation-based evaluations includes well-designed and -executed simulation activities, psychometrically sound simulation evaluation instruments, and trained, objective observer evaluators.
- ■ The process of simulation evaluation includes determining the purpose of the evaluation, planning for the logistics of the evaluation, collecting and interpreting the evaluation data, and reporting and responding to findings from the evaluation.
- ■ Kirkpatrick's (1998) four levels of evaluation include reaction, learning, behavior, and results.
- ■ Evaluation strategies and instruments should be used based on the intended purpose of a proposed evaluation.
- ■ Validity and reliability should be applied as qualities of simulation evaluation data.
- ■ Simulation evaluation instruments can be created by defining a construct, generating a pool of potential items for measuring that construct, determining a format for the measurement instrument, having a group of content experts review these selections, and disseminating the instrument for use.
- ■ Logic models can be applied the evaluation of simulation programs in order to communicate the value of a simulation program to stakeholders.
- ■ Simulation evaluation has been slower to catch on as a platform for high-stakes evaluation, but simulation-based evaluations are increasingly being used for licensure exam testing.

References

Abe, Y., Kawahara, C., Yamashina, A., & Tsuboi, R. (2013). Repeated scenario simulation to improve competency in critical care: a new approach for nursing education. *American Journal of Critical Care, 22*(1), 33–40.

Adamson, K. A., Kardong-Edgren, S., & Willhaus, J. (2012). An updated review of published simulation evaluation instruments. *Clinical Simulation in Nursing, 9*(9), e393–e405.

American Educational Research Association, American Psychological Association, & National Council on Measurement in Education. (1999). *Standards for educational and psychological testing.* Washington, DC: American Educational Research Association.

American Heart Association. (N.D.). Resources accessible via: http://www.heart.org

Arnold, J. J., Johnson, L. M., Tucker, S. J., Malec, J. F., Henrickson, S. E., & Dunn, W. F. (2009). Evaluation tools in simulation learning: Performance and self-efficacy in emergency response. *Clinical Simulation in Nursing, 5*(1), e35–e43.

Bensfield, L. A., Olech, M. J., & Horsley, T. L. (2012). Simulation for high-stakes evaluation in nursing. *Nurse Educator, 37*(2), 71–74.

Bourke, M. P., & Ihrke, B. A. (2009). The evaluation process. In D. M. Billings, & J. A. Halstead (Eds.), *Teaching in nursing: A guide for faculty* (3rd ed., pp. 391–408). St. Louis, MO: Saunders Elsevier.

Bray, B. S., Schwartz, C. R., Odegard, P. S., Hammer, D. P., & Seybert, A. L. (2011). Assessment of human patient simulation-based learning. *American Journal of Pharmaceutical Education, 75*(10), 208.

Cameron, W. B. (1963). *Informal sociology: A casual introduction to sociological thinking.* New York: Random House.

Cazzell, M., & Howe, C. (2012). Using objective structured clinical evaluation for simulation evaluation: Checklist considerations for inter-rater reliability.

Clinical Simulation in Nursing, 8(6), e219–e225.

Cohen, E. R., Feinglass, J., Barsuk, J. H., Barnard, C., O'Donnell, A., McGaghie, W. C., & Wayne, D. B. (2010). Cost savings from reduced catheter-related bloodstream infection after simulation-based education for residents in a medical intensive care unit. *Simulation in Healthcare, 5*(2), 98–102.

Davis, A. H., & Kimble, L. P. (2011). Human patient simulation evaluation rubrics for nursing education: Measuring the essentials of baccalaureate education for professional nursing practice. *Journal of Nursing Education, 50*(11), 605–611.

DeVellis, R. F. (2003). *Scale development.* Thousand Oaks, CA: Sage.

Draycott, T. J., Crofts, J. F., Ash, J. P., Wilson, L. V., Yard, E., Sibanda, T., & Whitelaw, A. (2008). Improving neonatal outcome through practical shoulder dystocia training. *Obstetrics and Gynecology, 112*(1), 14–20.

Elfrink Cordi, V. L., Leighton, K., Ryan-Wenger, N., Doyle, T. J., & Ravert, P. (2012). History and development of the Simulation Effectiveness Tool (SET). *Clinical Simulation in Nursing, 8*(6), e199–e210.

Foronda, C., Liu, S., & Bauman, E. B. (In press). Evaluation of simulation in undergraduate nurse education: An integrative review. *Clinical Simulation in Nursing.*

Forsberg, E., Georg, C., Ziegert, K., & Fors, U. (2011). Virtual patients for assessment of clinical reasoning in nursing—A pilot study. *Nurse Education Today, 31*(8), 757–762.

Frick, T. W., Chadha, R., Watson, C., Wang, Y., & Green, P. (2009). College participant perceptions of teaching and learning quality. *Educational Technology Research and Development, 57*(5), 705–720.

Gaba, D. M. (2009). Do as we say, not as you do: using simulation to investigate clinical behavior in action. *Simulation in Healthcare, 4*(2), 67–69.

Goodwin, L. D. (2002). Changing conceptions of measurement validity: An update on the new standards. *Journal of Nursing Education, 41*(3), 100–106.

Hinton, J. E., Mays, M. Z., Hagler, D., Randolph, P., Brooks, R., DeFalco, N.,

Kastenbaum, B., Miller, K. & Weberg, D. (2012). Measuring post-licensure competence with simulation: The nursing performance profile. *Journal of Nursing Regulation, 3*(2), 45–53.

Holmboe, E., Rizzolo, M. A., Sachdeva, A. K., Roesnberg, M., & Ziv, A. (2011). Simulation-Based Assessment and the Regulation of Healthcare Professionals. *Simulation in Healthcare, 6,* S58–S62.

Ilgen, J. S., Sherbino, J., & Cook, D. A. (2013). Technology-enhanced simulation in emergency medicine: a systematic review and meta-analysis. *Academic Emergency Medicine, 20*(2), 117–127.

International Nursing Association for Clinical Simulation and Learning (INACSL) Board of Directors. (2011). Standard VII: Evaluation of expected outcomes. *Clinical Simulation in Nursing, 7*(4S), s18–s19.

Johnson, D., Corrigan, T., Gulickson, G., Holshouser, E., & Johnson, S. (2012). The effects of a human patient simulator vs. a CD-ROM on performance. *Military Medicine, 177*(10), 1131–1135.

Kardong-Edgren, S., Adamson, K., & Fitzgerald, C. (2010). A review of currently published evaluation instruments for human patient simulation. *Clinical Simulation in Nursing, 6*(1), e25–e35.

Kirkpatrick, D. L. (1998). *Evaluating training programs: The four levels* (2nd ed.). San Francisco, CA: Berrett-Koehler.

Kogan, J. R., Holmboe, E. S., & Hauer, K. E. (2009). Tools for direct observation and assessment of clinical skills of medical trainees. *Journal of the American Medical Association, 302*(12), 1316–1326.

Levine, A. I., Schwartz, A. D., Bryson, E. O., & Demaria, S. J. (2012). Role of simulation in U.S. physician licensure and certification. *The Mount Sinai Journal of Medicine, New York, 79,* 1.

Littlewood, K. E., Shilling, A. M., Stemland, C. J., Wright, E. B., & Kirk, M. A. (2013). High-fidelity simulation is superior to case-based discussion in teaching the management of shock. *Medical Teacher, 35*(3), 1003–1010.

Marchigiano, G., Eduljee, N., & Harvey, K. (2010). Developing critical thinking skills from clinical assignments: A pilot study on nursing students' self-reported perceptions. *Journal of Nursing Management, 19*(1), 143–152.

McDavid, J. C., Huse, I., & Hawthorn, L. R. L. (2013). *Program evaluation & performance measurement: An introduction to practice* (2nd ed.). Thousand Oaks, CA: Sage.

McDonald, M. (2014). *The nurse educator's guide to assessing learning outcomes.* Burlington, MA: Jones & Bartlett Learning.

McGaghie, W., Issenberg, S., Petrusa, E., & Scalese, R. (2010). A critical review of simulation-based medical education research: 2003–2009. *Medical Education, 44,* 50–63.

Meyer, M. N., Connors, H., Hou, Q., & Gajewski, B. (2011). The effect of simulation on clinical performance. *Simulation in Healthcare, 6,* 269–277.

Mudumbai, S. C., Gaba, D. M., Boulet, J. R., Howard, S. K., & Davies, M. F. (2012). External validation of simulation-based assessments with other performance measures of third-year anesthesiology residents. *Simulation in Healthcare, 7*(2), 73–80.

National League for Nursing (NLN). (n.d.a). NLN fair testing guidelines for nursing education. Retrieved from www.nln.org/facultyprograms/facultyresources/fairtestingguidelines.PDF

National League for Nursing. (n.d.b). Research & grants. Descriptions of available instruments. Retrieved from www.nln.org/researchgrants/nln_laerdal/instruments.htm

Paul, F. (2010). An exploration of student nurses' thoughts and experiences of using a video-recording to assess their performance or CPR during a mock objective OSCE. *Nurse Education in Practice, 10*(5), 285–290.

Randolph, P. K., Hinton, J. E., Hagler, D., Mays, M. Z., Kastenbaum, B., Brooks, R., … Weberg, D. (2012). Measuring competence: collaboration for safety. *Journal of Continuing Education in Nursing, 43*(12), 541–547.

Reid, J., Stone, K., Brown, J., Caglar, D., Kobayashi, A., Lewis-Newby, M., … Quan, L. (2012). The Simulation Team Assessment Tool (STAT): Development, reliability and validation. *Resuscitation, 83*(7), 879–886.

Sadosty, A., Bellilio, M. F., Laack, T., Luke, A., Weaver, A., & Goyal, D. (2011). Simulation-based emergency medicine resident self assessment. *Journal of Emergency Medicine, 41*(6), 679–685.

Scheckel, M. (2009). Selecting learning experiences to achieve curriculum outcomes. In D. M. Billings, & J. A. Halstead (Eds.), *Teaching in nursing: A guide for faculty* (3rd ed., pp. 154–172). St. Louis, MO: Elsevier.

Shinnick, M. A., & Woo, M. A. (In press). The effect of human patient simulation on critical thinking and its predictors in prelicensure nursing students. *Nurse Education Today.*

Smith, S. J., & Barry, D. G. (2013). The use of high-fidelity simulation to teach home care nursing. *Western Journal of Nursing Research, 35*(3), 297–312.

Tanner, C. (2011). The critical state of measurement in nursing education research. *Journal of Nursing Education, 50*(9), 491–492.

Wiggins, G. P., & McTighe, J. (2008). *Understanding by design.* Alexandria, VA: Association for Supervision and Curriculum Development.

W.K. Kellogg Foundation. (2013). Logic model development guide. Retrieved from www.wkkf.org/knowledge-center/resources/2006/02/wk-kellogg-foundation-logic-model-development-guide.aspx

Wooley, N., & Jarvis, Y. (2007). Situated cognition and cognitive apprenticeship: A model for teaching and learning clinical skills in a technologically rich and authentic learning environment. *Nurse Education Today, 27,* 73–79.

Yuan, H. B., Williams, B. A., & Fang, J. B. (2011). The contribution of high-fidelity simulation to nursing students' confidence and competence: A systematic review. *International Nursing Review, 59,* 26–33.

13

Implementing Clinical Simulations in the Clinical Practice Arena

Jennifer Dwyer, MSN, RN-BC, CNRN, FNP-BC

■ Learning Objectives

1. Identify how simulation can be applied in a variety of clinical service settings from orientation to continuing education.
2. Describe strategies where simulation can be integrated across one or more disciplines.
3. Discuss the benefits of interprofessional education simulations to the learner and ultimately the patient.
4. Differentiate the advantages and disadvantages between in situ and in center simulations.
5. Apply one of the examples cited in this chapter to a program curriculum in a clinical setting.

■ Key Terms

- Certification
- Competencies
- Continuing education
- Handoffs
- In situ
- Interprofessional
- Orientation
- Staff development

Simulation in medical and nursing education began in the second half of the 21st century (Wallace, 1997). In the clinical practice arena, simulation methodology is in its infancy. Interprofessional education is gaining momentum as a foundational methodology to enhance communication across disciplines and is a mechanism endorsed by the Institute of Medicine to improve the overall quality of health care. The Institute of Medicine (2003) clearly states that patients receive safer, high-quality care when health care professionals work effectively in a team, communicate productively, and understand one another's roles.

Construction of simulation centers across the country has accelerated over the past decade. Most are located on college campuses aligned with a school of medicine or nursing. A few have associations with health care institutions, and even fewer have the privilege of becoming partners as a triad where those in medicine, nursing, and acute care work and learn side by side in a simulation environment.

Through case examples, various clinical concepts are interwoven across roles and within a variety of programs to offer a snapshot of how simulation is realized. Cases are available for purchase or written to meet the outcomes desired (Jeffries, 2005). A variety of learners can benefit from these cases in a single simulation or in combination with others for an interprofessional experience. This chapter will present clinical simulations and explain how they are being used in the clinical practice setting. Uses range from orientation to staff development to continuing education, with the use of clinical simulations increasing to meet the needs of patients in an ever-evolving complex health care environment (Nagle, McHale, Alexander, & French, 2009). The use of simulation in competency assessment and certification programs will also be discussed.

SIMULATION USE IN ON-BOARDING OR ORIENTATION PROGRAMS

In the clinical setting, simulations are being created and implemented as a retention strategy for new nurses through **orientation** to reduce stress and to increase confidence, lessen unmet expectations, and improve job satisfaction, creating an environment where patient outcomes are enhanced and errors are minimized (Olejniczak, Schmidt & Brown, 2010; Nursing Executive Center, 2003). This provides a safe and supportive environment, socialization, and opportunities for role development and fosters retention of new nurses (Ackermann, Kenny, & Walker, 2007). These principles apply to other roles, associated responsibilities, and expectations for various health care providers and professionals. These roles are described below as well as how simulations are being used for the initial educational training.

Pairing Licensed and Unlicensed Staff

The use of simulation in on-boarding programs provides a rich environment to practice communication with health care providers. A case titled "Safety Simulation" allows three health care providers to participate in a patient encounter where the new RN and nurse assistive personnel collectively identify patient safety concerns and utilize delegation skills. The RN calls the physician to give an overview of the safety concerns through the use of a situation, background, assessment, and recommendation. Relationship building among the various health care team members is crucial to establish an environment of trust and mutual respect. The report the RN receives from the off-going nurse is incomplete and places the RN and patient at risk for gaps in the care needed for the patient. A crucial conversation between the two nurses occurs during the subsequent handoff. The learners self-identify that there is an increase in their stress during this encounter. The debriefing is rich with discussion.

The following exemplar illustrates the impact this simulation had on the learners, the units where they are practicing, and the leadership feedback on new hire performance:

> "Simulation training builds mind muscle and skills. It is one method [of] improving nursing confidence and skill which strongly affects patients' safety and outcomes. A pre- and postevaluation of the Safety Simulation, following a three-year use of the case, shows a reduction in incident reports that are directly linked to new nurses as noted by the clinical managers. Individual unit performance is benchmarked against the National Database of Nursing Quality Indicators. The system critically reviews the number of falls and other safety concerns to ensure patient safety." This particular simulation is modified as needed to continue to address organizational initiatives, learner's needs and the changes in health care as a whole. (D. Bennett, personal communication, May 21, 2013)

Nurse assistive personnel and their course facilitator, who have been involved in the "Safety Simulation" for the past year, provided the following comments regarding their experiences. "By participating in the SIM program, I feel that I now know what to actually expect and being able to see and review myself helps me know what I need to work on" (N. Gerard, personal communication, May 21, 2013). A. Green-Jones stated: "Just watching them interact with this life-like talking, breathing and interactive manikin, the real setup of the room, and the realism that is transcended throughout the experience opens up a door to a meaningful learning opportunity" (personal communication, May 21, 2013).

Multitasking

Another area where clinical simulations are being incorporated into the clinical practice setting includes the development and training of various health professionals and ancillary nonhealth professionals who work in the clinical environment. These roles of nonhealth professionals may include unit clerks, certified nursing assistants, transportation personnel, and visitors. Clinical simulations are set up to immerse the new employees into multitasking events and encounters.

To practice the skills of multitasking, a unit secretary (US), an RN, transportation personnel, and a visitor come together to create a busy nurses' station where the US is admitting patients, directing visitors, sending lab tubes, answering telephone calls, and coordinating procedural transports off the unit. This simulation is a summative experience for the new US following a three-day training course. The learners appreciated the opportunity to practice multiple tasks prior to doing so for the first time in their unit. The debriefing is energy filled with active discussion by those directly and indirectly involved in the scenario. D. Mohr, course team-facilitator, summarizes the experience in this way:

> "During the debriefing session the learner has felt overwhelmed with all the tasks, comfortable with the computer skills, however, did not have time to enter the orders or put the new admission chart together. This is a critical piece of their learning during the simulation. The learner realizes they have just started to learn the role and how much they do not know. A learner can be lectured in the classroom on the activity level, but actually experiencing it firsthand in a safe environment is a sample of reality." (Personal communication, May 21, 2013)

Electronic Medical Record

Across the nation, clinical practice organizations are adopting new electronic medical record systems and devices, which is essentially a new way of documentation for health and nonhealth professionals. To conduct the training, clinical simulations are important to replicate the actual environment in which learners will be working. A model of partnering informatics and clinical education together provides new staff members the unique opportunity to connect concepts of care and the importance of documentation through the use of a training domain and education facilitators. The training domain contains simulated electronic charts, and the facilitators guide the staff through caring for the patient via a case study. The author identified that implementing this approach, at a large Midwestern multicampus health care system, recently has been well received by the new hires, clinical staff, educators, and managers. Overall response themes include comments such as: this helps to connect the dots between patient care content and the computer documentation system before I begin orientating on the unit; I can now navigate the chart to find needed information; I am more confident to start my time with a preceptor knowing what to do and how to document.

SIMULATION USE IN COMPETENCY ASSESSMENT

Competencies vary across professions, although all of them have the primary focus on patient care and quality outcomes (Beyea, Von Reyn & Slattery, 2007). The Quality and Safety Education for Nurses graduate-level competencies include quality improvement, safety, teamwork and collaboration, patient-centered care, evidence-based practice, and informatics (American Association of Colleges of Nursing, 2012; Cronenwett, Sherwood, Pohl, Barnsteiner, et al., 2009). The Accreditation Council for Graduate Medical Education (2013) expects residents to obtain competency in the following six areas to the level expected of a new practitioner: patient care, medical knowledge, interpersonal and communication skills, professionalism, practice-based learning and improvement, and systems-based practice. The American Association of Critical Care Nurses (2013) "Synergy Model" depicts eight areas of nursing competencies: clinical judgment, advocacy and moral agency, clinical practice, collaboration, systems thinking, response to diversity, facilitation of learning, and clinical inquiry (Table 13.1).

Nursing competencies in the clinical practice arena are conducted on site in a location on or near the unit and facilitated by a clinical educator, clinical nurse specialist, or unit leadership. These competencies are based on nurse-sensitive indicators or low-frequency, high-risk skills for a specific patient population. Competency evaluations throughout the year, with a quarterly focus, may include one unit or multiple units partnering together on common skills and practices. For example, one unit's yearly nurse-sensitive indicators focus may relate to reducing pressure ulcer prevalence, whereas another unit may focus on catheter-associated urinary tract infections or an entire campus may direct its attention to addressing central line–associated bloodstream infections. Competencies for physicians could include those that are skills based, such as central line insertion or laparoscopic techniques. Communication and teamwork skills may comprise the focus for one profession or multiple professionals in an interprofessional competency encounter.

TABLE 13.1

Competencies Across the Disciplines of Nursing and Medical Education and Nursing Practice

Quality and Safety Education for Nurses	Accreditation Council for Graduate Medical Education	American Association of Critical Care Nurses SYNERGY Nurse Characteristics
Quality improvement	Patient care	Clinical judgment
Safety	Knowledge	Advocacy: moral agency
Teamwork and collaboration	Interpersonal and communication skills	Clinical practice
Patient-centered care	Professionalism	Collaboration
Evidenced-based practice	Practice-based learning and improvement	Systems thinking
Informatics	Systems-based practice	Response to diversity Facilitation of learning Clinical inquiry

Diagnosis or Intervention Cases

Regulatory agencies that accredit programs such as the Joint Commission and the American Heart Association identify standards for institutions to meet on their journey to excellence. ST segment elevation myocardial infarction (STEMI) and the primary stroke center are two examples where simulation is a component to assess competency of the RN staff in caring for these patients alongside physicians and chaplains. Because of the required standards by the American Heart Association, M. Wallace offers the following:

"We decided providing STEMI simulations on random units, at random times, would provide the education, evaluation of process, and uncover barriers preventing the patient from getting to the cath lab in a timely manner. Tracking of time and monitoring of key events and barriers to the process are in the notes taken during the simulations. Participation by the rapid assessment team, operator, cath lab, unit charge nurse, and the cardiac interventionalist and the availability of an open bed for our "patient" set the stage to make our first STEMI simulation a huge success. The nursing staff stated they could easily identify atypical symptoms after the simulation and begin the Level I STEMI process. The subsequent STEMI simulations were beneficial in identifying gaps in training for the operators, nursing staff, and the critical care unit staff in using the rapid assessment team. Health care team members, resistant to the new process, changed their perceptions of the increased work load as they moved through the actual process. This was a positive and unexpected result of the STEMI simulations." (Personal communication, May 24, 2013)

Equipment and Standardized Patients

Another unique area where clinical simulations are being used in clinical practice organizations includes ancillary services, such as the environmental and nutrition services. Clinical simulations are set up so departmental managers from these areas can assess how well their staff perform greetings and closures with patients through the use of cameras to capture verbal and nonverbal aspects of communication with standardized patients. "Initial training and retraining of 60 percent of the room services ambassadors to department standards and expectations provide opportunities for coaching by the management team and performance improvement. Over time the processes and procedures were altered, and this retraining put those back in alignment with the department's goal" (W. Boyd, personal communication, May 24, 2013).

Standardized patients are individuals who are trained to perform the role of patients or family members and use scripts to portray the roles. Typically used for taking medical histories or conducting physical examinations, they are expanding their use with psychosocial skills related to communication and relationship building (Weaver & Erby, 2012; Hodge, Martin, Tavemier, Perea-Ryan, Alcala-Van-Houten, 2008). Physical therapy uses the simulation center annually to assess the interpersonal and technical skill level of the therapists through the use of standardized patients as patients and family members. According to one standardized patient, "in some small way I hope my contributions to the development of students and staff makes a lasting impression as they gain confidence in their important role as healthcare professionals" (M. Dwyer, personal communication, May 22, 2013).

SIMULATION USE IN CERTIFICATION PROGRAMS

Simulation-based assessments can make a meaningful and positive difference in credentialing, licensing, and **certification** programs (Holmboe, Rizzolo, Sachdeva, Rosenberg, & Ziv, 2011). The use of simulation for board certification, training requirements, and quality assurance of educational programs and professional competence may soon become a standard for performance assessment (Steadman & Huang, 2012). Simulation centers can be a resource for agencies, organizations, and certifying bodies who seek regional sites for provider certification. Centers who complete an extensive, rigorous application process and demonstrate excellence in simulation education serve as regional areas for credentialing. Some examples include the Center for Medical Education at Harvard in Boston, Massachusetts, and the Peter M. Winter Institute for Simulation Education and Research at the University of Pittsburgh in Pennsylvania which offers Maintenance of Certification in Anesthesiology courses. Other credentialing resources include a National Skills Curriculum available from the American College of Surgeons and the program offered by the Association of Program Directors in Surgery (Scott & Dunnington, 2007).

Advanced Life Support

In the clinical institution, many health professionals, including physicians, nurses, and respiratory therapists, are required to go through the Advanced Life Support program to provide care to patients in rapidly changing physiologic states and environments. Current Advanced Life Support programs including Advanced Cardiac Life Support,

Pediatric Advanced Life Support, and Neonatal Resuscitation Programs are well suited to the simulation environment where a variety of health care providers are engaged in patient care. Flight staff, respiratory therapists, physicians, and nurses who are colleagues during transport and simulation activities together allow the reality of everyday work processes to continue for a more realistic environment. Advanced Life Support programs bring prehospital, emergency room staff, allied health providers, nurses, physicians, and surgeons together to work side by side in an ambulance or helicopter shell. Wireless manikins allow simulation to occur at remote locations, enhancing the realism and offering a look into the prehospital setting that fellow health care workers seldom experience.

B. Hidde began using the simulation center when the American Academy of Pediatrics announced its new simulation-based Neonatal Resuscitation Program. Hidde shares:

> "I knew I wanted to utilize the center for implementation of this new program. With the encouragement and assistance of the Clinical Education Department, and leaders from Nursing, Respiratory Care and Lifeline, we merged multiple unit/hospital/discipline-based programs into one program at the Simulation Center. Staff were no longer in class with members of their unit; people they knew. They are in learning groups with, in many cases, strangers . . . requiring direct and specific communication. I think the most important lesson I have learned in implementing this program with several disciplines from different environments is remembering it is not about the individual performer (learner, team member), but the performance (team work and communication of all members) for the sake of the baby." (Personal communication May 23, 2013)

Skills

Skills training in the simulation arena is crucial to ensure quality and safety in caring for patients in a variety of clinical settings. Providing this skills' training prior to assuming care for patients offers opportunities to practice and to dialogue clinical situations requiring critical thinking. Task trainers come in many varieties, ranging from simple to complex, and provide the learner with the opportunity to become immersed in the moment when performing skills demonstrations. Simple devices created by simulation technicians such as heel or finger stick trainers and ostomies to high vascular access and needle decompression manikins allow the learner to experience the skill prior to performing the actual procedure in the clinical setting. Sophisticated cardiac catheterization lab models, laparoscopic simulators, anesthesia gas-driven high-fidelity manikins, to piston-driven extracorporeal membrane oxygenators all provide a rich learning environment to practice and evaluate skills' performance. Automatic drug dispensing cabinets combined with electronic medication records offer health care providers the opportunity to see patient safety mechanisms in action and to partner with pharmacists in safe medication practices.

A safe medication administration simulation is in use as an alternative to the traditional math and pharmacology examination tools. "This simulation is bringing to the surface many before-hidden knowledge gaps in the use of certain high-alert medications and calculation deficits not seen with the previously used written format. Sharing this simulation across the Indiana University Health system of hospitals is helping to bridge knowledge and practice gaps and address safety concerns identified by the Institute for Safe Medication Practice" (J. Dwyer, personal communication, May 15, 2013). Another unique feature designed for the Simulation Center at Fairbanks Hall, located in Indianapolis, Indiana, on the campus of Indiana University Health, is a simulated laboratory tube transportation system that allows maintenance workers and engineers to contaminate, clean, release, and repair a network of tubes without hindering the function of the active patient care environment. The actual lab tube system is used in the clinical setting by ward clerks, nurses, pharmacists, and lab technicians to efficiently send and receive patient records, medications, and lab results via a channel housed beneath a monorail track connected to a network of three campuses.

SIMULATION USE IN STAFF DEVELOPMENT

For **interprofessional** or intraprofessional teamwork, using clinical simulations to practice and enhance these skills is very important. Clinical simulations are set up to focus on teamwork, crisis management, and communication skills. Professional competencies in high-risk, low-volume settings among practicing nurses and high-fidelity simulation should be considered a strategy for **staff development** (Merchant, 2012). Frengley et al. (2011) found that the use of simulation-based and case-based learning seemed to provide an effective teaching strategy for practice-based learning with established multidisciplinary teams. Leadership, teamwork, and self-confidence among established advanced practitioners are enhanced with the use of human patient simulator training (Pascual et al., 2011).

The use of interprofessional partners is increasing as disciplines become aware of the benefits of shared experiences in enhancing the relationship building. Indiana University Health was host to a statewide interprofessional event in the fall of 2012 with pharmacy, physician assistant, nursing, radiography, and respiratory therapy students. Cases included gastrointestinal bleed, pulseless electrical activity, oversedation, hypokalemia, and angina and response from students was positive with overall scores of 4.5 on a five-point Likert scale. L. Wolford provides this exemplar: "I have noticed usually quiet or nervous nurses become empowered nurses who take 'charge' of the scenario such as leading a code, delegating care to other members of the time, or questioning inappropriate orders" (personal communication, May 23, 2013).

Handoffs

An area of concern in promoting quality and safety in patient care environments is **handoffs**, which contain timely and accurate information regarding a patient's plan of care, current condition, and changes in condition or treatment regimen. The level of acuity, variability in one's skill development, and multiple caregivers interacting with patients in the acute care setting lead to an increase risk of gaps in safe patient care. The notion of a safe handoff has been further explored by Brown, Rasmussen, Baldwin, and Wyeth (2012) through the development of a virtual world training simulator for intensive care unit first-hour handover processes. Using analytical skills, on the job training, remote learning, flexible learning times, and recordable session responses offers a supplemental training option in the complex world of hospital wards. Including handoffs in simulated or in situ settings offers the health care provider opportunities to create safe environments for patients and provides effective communication to support staff and health care providers in a variety of settings.

Preceptor and Charge Nurse Training

Preparing quality nurses and health professionals for the unit's skills sets such as delegation, prioritization, coordination, communication, and critical thinking is necessary for success. Simulations used to reinforce these skill sets and create an environment in which the professionals can benefit from missteps in their decision making in a nonthreatening setting with others is essential in preparing the nurse leader for the complexities that exist in our current health care environment. Preceptor and charge nurse training is a natural pairing with simulation. Numerous licensed, unlicensed, and supportive roles paired together offer a rich environment to practice decision making, critical thinking, advocacy, and leadership skills. In the fast-paced acute care settings of today's hospitals, with the high acuity of patients, on-the-job training of preceptors and charge nurses is the typical approach taken to train staff for the role of preceptor or charge nurse. Using simulated settings allows for variation in the approach to the situation posed for those learning new leadership skills. Delegation and relationship building are two common skills health care providers use, though they often need refinement. A technique to promote professional growth is to immerse the learner in situations where his or her skill level is revealed. Self-reflection during debriefing is an effective strategy to foster the next level of learning for the health care professional.

Advancing Mentoring Skills

In situ simulation use within the clinical units provides a level of patient safety when work hours and exposure to live codes by residents is less within an environment in which health care professionals are comfortable, where finding equipment is second nature, and where professional growth thrives. Placing experienced preceptors into simulated or in situ settings with new or early career staff creates a dual learning environment for both individuals. Taking simulation to the bedside offers a natural setting to observe behaviors where the health care team practices daily. Staff members who participate in either setting verbalize how effective these mixed learner sessions are to the health care team. An exemplar from an outreach program sees the benefits of monthly in situ simulations, which include increased comfort level in working together among health care team members in their own environment and decreased time spent covering shifts to attend the education and identification of workflow gaps. "The in situ setting allows identification, discussion, and resolution of latent safety threats in a professional manner with those participating in the simulation" (C. Weidman, personal communication, May 23, 2013). "One lesson that is learned from in situ simulations is that the attitude of leadership greatly affects the attitudes of the learners. For the neonatal simulation team, the time spent writing scenarios, organizing simulations, and traveling with equipment is well worth the experience when it means improving care to the tiniest of patients in the hospital" (L. Mayer, personal communication, May 23, 2013).

SIMULATION USE IN CONTINUING EDUCATION

In clinical organizations, **continuing education** is required for health care professionals to renew licensure, credentials, or certification in one's specialty. Continuing education consists of short or part-time courses that promote knowledge, skills, and professional attitudes. Surcouf, Chauvin, Ferry, Yang, and Barkemeyer (2013) described the use of simulation-based training and high receptivity to in situ settings along with gains in confidence and observed competency-related abilities. Simulation allows integration of priorities for improvement in health care practice with the training goals of individuals.

Human factors as a scientific discipline is focused on human performance in complex environments and how people interact with one another and with technology. Human factor techniques can benefit health care simulation by designing better feedback and task guidance cases, differentiating levels of expertise where performance is essentially perfect, and in developing task-relevant fidelity for simulations (Seagull, 2012). Lansdowne, Machin, and Grant (2012) identified the need for team and human factor skills when working with complex technology to mitigate adverse events, which can lead to significant morbidity and mortality.

TeamSTEPPS

TeamSTEPPS® (Team Strategies and Tools to Enhance Performance and Patient Safety) is a teamwork system developed jointly by the U.S. Department of Defense and the Agency for Healthcare Research and Quality (2011) to improve the culture of safety within an organization. The concepts of communication, leadership, situation monitoring, and mutual support paired with performance, knowledge, and attitudes provide the foundation for the system. These concepts can be integrated into simulation, offering the health care team the opportunity to practice communication teamwork skills to improve patient safety.

KNOWLEDGE OF TECHNIQUES, EQUIPMENT, AND EVALUATION

Simulations are continually being used to enable physicians and other health care professionals to practice and prepare on the newest equipment being used in the clinical setting. "Evidence is mounting that long-established approaches to surgical training are no longer acceptable in the current ethical and professional climate" (Kneebone, Scott, Darzi, & Horrocks, 2004). Task-based surgical learning that takes place within skills laboratories alongside clinical practice is the current recommendation for situated learning. In an effort to promote excellence and patient safety in physician training while reducing risk to patients, the interventional cardiologists at Mayo Clinic in Arizona have acquired the Samantha endovascular simulator. John P. Sweeney, director of the Cardiac Catheterization Laboratory at the Mayo Clinic (2013) in Arizona stated: "Fellows learn basic cardiac catheterization techniques and face common scenarios before ever touching an actual patient." "Nurses and radiology technologists will update their skill sets and learn new techniques using this system. Orientation of new staff will start with simulation training instead of with patients" (Mayo Clinic, 2013).

A recent use of simulation is practicing complex skills using extracorporeal membrane oxygenation and continuous venovenous hemofiltration. Both pediatric and adult patients are benefiting from these therapeutic modalities, which rely on complex filtration and pulsatile flows in which clinicians need technical training. Reliance on these machines is high, and backup procedures are exercised to ensure their effectiveness. Little effort has been made to simulate these scenarios because of the complexity and expense of modifying extracorporeal circuits. In the development of simulations that could test the knowledge of extracorporeal clinicians, we looked to create scenarios that they encounter on a regular basis, such as kinked tubing, plugged filters, low venous/arterial pressure, air embolism, and circuit leaks.

To create these scenarios, actuator valves were implemented to remotely control pressures at different points on the extracorporeal membrane oxygenation/continuous venovenous hemofiltration circuit. Encasing the valves in a discreet aluminum enclosure and hiding them from plain view, this extracorporeal simulator is remotely operated behind one-way glass to meet current simulation practices. The benefits of a remote-controlled simulator include allowing the clinician to be tested without the help of others and examining his or her critical-thinking skills. Testing of this nature in the recent past would have been done with the instructor in the room. Now, up to 15 different scenarios that an extracorporeal clinician would encounter can be tested without affecting patient outcome (P. Curtis, personal communication, May 23, 2013).

SUMMARY

This chapter is rich with cited evidence, personal experience, innovative approaches, technical expertise, and summaries of simulation practice examples important to help professionals to orient, adapt, and advance their knowledge, maintain their certification, and enhance collaborative relationships with patients entrusted to their care. Learning the importance of teamwork, communication, and role clarity to keep patients safe along the journey in a complex health care environment is the hallmark of the Institute of Medicines (2003) report. Exemplars have been provided to show how simulations have been used by professionals and nonhealth professionals with the intent of creating safe, quality care environments.

■ Key Concepts

- ■ The clinical practice arena is rich with learning experiences for the new and experienced health care provider.
- ■ Opportunities to practice the skills needed to safely care for patients are available in virtual hospitals and in situ settings. Pairing nursing, medicine, allied health, and others together in these settings provides an environment where orientation, competency assessment, certification, staff development, and continuing education, individually or collectively, can occur.
- ■ Innovation by simulation technicians partnered with the creativity of practitioners creates a rich learning environment.

- The safe passage of patients through a complex health care system is the responsibility of all providers. Simulation settings offer staff the ability to practice skills before performing on a patient.
- Building confidence, enhancing communication and teamwork, promoting professionalism, and practicing safely all contribute to positive outcomes for our patients.

References

Accreditation Council for Graduate Medical Education. (2013). Home page. Retrieved from www.acgme.org/acgmeweb/

Ackermann, A., Kenny, G., & Walker, C. (2007). Simulator programs for new nurses' orientation. *Journal for Nurses in Staff Development, 23*(3), 136–139.

Agency for Healthcare Research and Quality. (2011). TeamSTEPPS. Retrieved from http://teamstepps.ahrq.gov/

American Association of Colleges of Nursing. (2012). *Graduate-level QSEN competencies knowledge, skills and attitudes.* Retrieved from www.aacn.nche.edu/faculty/qsen/competencies.pdf

American Association of Critical Care Nurses. (2013). The AACN synergy model for patient care. Retrieved from www.aacn.org/wd/certifications/content/synmodel.pcms?menu=

Beyea, S. C., Von Reyn, L. K., & Slattery, M. J. (2007). A nurse residency program for competency development using human patient simulation [Online exclusive]. *Journal for Nurses in Staff Development, 23*, 77–82.

Brown, R., Rasmussen, R., Baldwin, I., & Wyeth, P. (2012). Design and implementation of a virtual world training simulation of ICU first hour handover processes. *Australian Critical Care, 25*(3), 178–187.

Cronenwett, L., Sherwood G., Pohl, J., Barnsteiner, J., Moore, S., Sullivan, D.,…Warren, J. (2009). Quality and safety education for advanced nursing practice. *Nursing Outlook, 57*, 338–348.

Frengley, R. W., Weller, J. M., Torrie, J., Dzendrowskyj, P., Yee, B., Paul, A. M.,…Henderson, K. M. (2011). The effect of simulation-based training intervention on the performance of established critical care unit teams. *Critical Care Medicine, 39*(12), 2605–2611.

Hodge, M., Martin, C., Tavemier, D., Perea-Ryan, M., & Alcala-VanHouten, L. (2008). Integrating simulation across the curriculum. *Nurse Educator, 33*(5), 210–214.

Holmboe E., Rizzolo, M. A., Sachdeva, A. K., Rosenberg, M., & Ziv, A. (2011). Simulation-based assessment and the regulation of healthcare professionals. *Simulation in Healthcare, 6*(Suppl), S58–S62.

Institute of Medicine. (2003). *Health professions education: A bridge to quality.* Washington, DC: National Academies Press. Retrieved from www.nap.edu/openbook.php?record_id=10681&page=R1

Jeffries, P. (2005). A framework for designing, implementing, and evaluating simulations used as teaching strategies in nursing. *Nursing Education Perspectives, 26*(2), 96–103.

Kneebone, R. L., Scott, W., Darzi, A., & Horrocks, M. (2004). Simulation and clinical practice: Strengthening the relationship. *Medical Education, 38*(10), 1095–1102.

Lansdowne, W., Machin, D., & Grant, D. J. (2012). Development of the Orpheus perfusion simulator for use in high-fidelity extracorporeal membrane oxygenation simulation. *Journal of Extra-Corporeal Technology, 44*(4), 250–255.

Mayo Clinic. (2013). New simulation training in the Cardiac Catheterization Laboratory at Mayo Clinic in Arizona. Retrieved from www.mayoclinic.org/medicalprofs/simulation-training-cardiac-catheterization.html

Merchant, D. C. (2012). Does high fidelity simulation improve clinical outcomes? [Review] *Journal for Nurses in Staff Development, 28*(1), E1–E8; quiz E9–E10.

Nagle, B., McHale, J., Alexander, G., & French, B. (2009). Incorporating a scenario-based simulation into a hospital nursing education program. *Journal of Continuing Education in Nursing, 40*(1), 18–25.

Nursing Executive Center. (2008). *Bridging the preparation-practice gap.* Volume 1: *Quantifying new graduate nurse improvement needs.* Washington, DC: Advisory Board Company.

Olejniczak, E. A., Schmidt, N. A., & Brown, J. M. (2010). Simulation as an orientation strategy for new nurse graduates: An integrative review of the evidence. *Society for Simulation in Healthcare, 5,* 52–57.

Pascual, J. L., Holena, D. N., Vella, M. A., Palmieri, J., Sicoutris, C.,. .. Schwab, C. W. (2011). Short simulation training improves objective skills in established advanced practitioners managing emergencies on the ward and surgical intensive care unit. *Journal of Trauma-Injury Infection & Critical Care, 71*(2), 330–338.

Scott, D. J., & Dunnington, G. L. (2008). The new ACS/APDS Skills curriculum: Moving the learning curve out of the operating room. *Journal of Gastrointestinal Surgery, 12*(2), 213–221.

Seagull, F. J. (2012). Human factors tools for improving simulation activities in continuing medical education. *Journal of Continuing Education in the Health Professions, 32*(4), 261–268.

Steadman, R. H., & Huang, Y. M. (2012). Simulation for quality assurance in training, credentialing, and maintenance of certification. Best practice & research. *Clinical Anaesthesiology, 26*(1), 3–15.

Surcouf, J. W., Chauvin, S. W., Ferry, J., Yang, T., & Barkemeyer, B. (2013). Enhancing residents' neonatal resuscitation competency through unannounced simulation-based training. *Medical Education Online, 18,* 1–7.

Wallace, P. (1997). Following the threads of an innovation: The history of standardized patients in medical education. *Caduceus, 13*(2), 5–28.

Weaver, M., & Erby, L. (2012). Standardized patients: a promising tool for health education and health promotion. *Health Promotion Practice, 13*(2), 169–174.

14

Incorporating Simulations into the Curriculum: Undergraduate and Graduate

Andrea Parsons Schram, DNP, CRNP, FNP-BC
Diane S. Aschenbrenner, MS, RN

▇ Learning Objectives

1. Examine how simulation can be strategically embedded within the curriculum to achieve program outcomes.
2. Utilize Bloom's Taxonomy of Learning to increase the complexity of simulations within the curriculum.
3. Describe how simulation can be used in a variety of educational settings including classrooms, online, and in the simulation lab.

▇ Key Terms

- Bloom's Taxonomy of Learning
- Curriculum development
- Objective structured clinical experiences

Simulation can be used in nursing education to provide a variety of innovative educational activities to promote active and engaged learning, as well as a means of formative and summative evaluation. There is ample evidence demonstrating that simulation is not only effective in health profession education but also is associated with small to moderate positive effects for knowledge, skills, and behavior learning outcomes when compared with other instructional methods (Cook et al., 2011, 2012). Further, evidence of clinical performance improvement has been demonstrated with the use of both high-fidelity simulation and low-fidelity simulation (Norman, Dore, & Grierson, 2012). Simulations can be used within the classroom or within the simulation lab or employed for synchronous or asynchronous online learning. In order to gain the most from any simulation, faculty must consider the overall curriculum to determine how and where to best employ this pedagogy.

The nursing curriculum identifies learning activities that allow students to achieve the desired program outcomes (Billings & Halstead, 2009). Faculty must consider how simulation will fit into the theoretical or conceptual framework adopted by their school, which serves as a model in **curriculum development**. It may be useful to explore the use of a framework that incorporates simulation, such as Jeffries's Simulation Framework (Jeffries, 2005), to guide best practice for the development of simulation into the curriculum (Irwin, 2011).

To make the best use of simulation, faculty should take a purposeful, planned, and organized approach to appraise the curriculum to determine how this pedagogy will support the acquisition of desired course and clinical competencies as well as to meet program outcomes. Simulations can be used in a variety of ways to meet different learning goals, ranging from knowledge acquisition, to application of a theoretical concept, to professional role development, to evaluation of student competency (Anderson, Aylor, & Leonard, 2008; Hyland, Weeks, Ficorelli, & Vanderbeek-Warren, 2012; Irwin, 2011). With the understanding that student knowledge and experience build throughout the curriculum to help students achieve the desired program outcomes, simulation experiences can be incorporated into each level to promote cognitive, psychomotor, and affective domains of learning (Jeffries et al., 2011; Lapkin, Levett-Jones, Bellchambers, & Fernandez, 2010; Wamsley et al., 2012).

Bloom's Taxonomy of Learning domains can be helpful as faculty consider how to appropriately "level" simulations throughout prelicensure and graduate curricula (Bloom, 1956; Krathwohl, 2002; Wu & Osisek, 2011). The complexity of the simulation should match the expected knowledge and skills defined at a given point of the curriculum. Faculty should mark out simulation objectives for each level of the curriculum to clearly identify increasing levels of complexity throughout the entire curricula. To assist in this process, faculty will want to prioritize key learning outcomes for each level of learner (Jeffries, 2005). Once these outcomes have been identified, faculty can then best determine how simulation can be used so students meet these outcomes. Box 14.1 lists examples of issues faculty should consider.

BOX 14.1 ISSUES TO CONSIDER WHEN IDENTIFYING LEARNING OUTCOMES FOR SIMULATION

- Will the simulations focus on high-risk but low-exposure situations?
- Will they focus on common clinical situations?
- Is the goal to provide key identical experiences for all students?
- Is the goal to enrich the basic clinical learning experience with opportunities not normally provided to students?
- Will there be several common threads that will recur throughout various simulations such as teamwork, communication, and patient safety?
- Will the simulations cover core clinical concepts such as fluid imbalance, pain, and grief and loss?
- Are there skills, knowledge, attitudes, or communication techniques that have been difficult to master where students need additional experience?
- Are there key safety issues that need further emphasis within the program of study?

BOX 14.2 USING SIMULATION TO EVALUATE STUDENT COMPETENCY: QUESTIONS TO CONSIDER

- What is the purpose of the evaluation?
- Do students know precisely how they will be evaluated?
- Is it a pass/fail experience where the stakes are limited, as students may repeat until they can pass?
- Is it a high-stakes experience where failure to pass the simulation on the first attempt may mean failure in a course, a semester, or the entire program?
- How will the simulation experiences be evaluated? By individual faculty or teams of faculty?
- Will faculty watch students as they perform in the simulation or will they review a videotape of the simulation at a later time?
- What tool will be used for the evaluation? Is there evidence of interrater reliability?

SOURCE: Jeffries, P., Dreifuerst, KT., Aschenbrenner, DS., Adamson, KA., & Schram, AP. (2013). Clinical Simulations in Nursing Education: Overview, Essentials, and the Evidence. In M. Oermann (Ed.), *Teaching in Nursing: The Complete Guide.* New York: Springer Publishing, Co.

After these issues have been determined, specific simulations in particular courses can be created. Course faculty will determine the specific simulations for their course as well as the manner in which the simulation will be delivered.

If the educational institution has decided to use simulation as a mechanism of student evaluation, there are some caveats to keep in mind. Because of the high level of student anxiety associated with simulation (Cordeau, 2010), faculty should incorporate simulation in teaching and learning activities prior to using it for formative and summative evaluation. The evaluative use of simulation should mimic the manner in which students learned from a simulation. For example, if students learned the simulation through use of a high-fidelity manikin, they should be tested using the high-fidelity manikin. Faculty should identify the purpose of the evaluation, specific outcomes to be measured, and how the evaluation will take place. Guiding questions are shown in Box 14.2. All of these questions must be considered prior to using simulation as a method to evaluate student progression.

Schools of nursing should spend time considering how to best use simulation in the curriculum to promote student learning. Understanding the pedagogical component of simulation is crucial to implement simulation successfully within the curriculum and should be of equal priority as creating simulation space, establishing a budget, and purchasing equipment.

SIMULATION WITHIN NURSING EDUCATION

The most common use of simulation is to create a clinical experience that replaces part or all of a clinical experience normally spent outside the school. Faculty might need to use simulation to provide sufficient clinical experiences with a particular patient population, such as pediatrics, if there are limited clinical sites for students, or they may wish to broaden the clinical experience for students via simulation. Nursing students at clinical practice sites are frequently prohibited from performing certain skills or interacting with certain types of patients because of law or institutional policies; simulation can be used very effectively in these cases to provide a clinical experience not generally available. In simulation, it is important for students to portray their future role, whether it is a registered nurse or an advanced practice registered nurse (APRN), in order to experientially learn the responsibilities of their future role upon graduation.

Creating an Environment for Learning

Simulations frequently take place in a simulation lab that has been staged to resemble a hospital room, a clinic, a home, or some other specified environment. The simulation can be with high-fidelity manikins, with a standardized patient, or a hybrid of low- and high-fidelity technology. Beyond the simulation lab, simulation can also be incorporated into the classroom for theoretical courses to assist students in recognizing how theory and practice intersect. This strategy is an effective method for a large number of students to participate in a simulation at one time. Students are provided with a simulation scenario that defines two or three key course or clinical outcomes, background on the patient and clinical situation, clinical environment, roles to be assigned (both active and observer), and learning activities that should be completed by students prior to the experience. Students should prepare for the simulation prior to the in-class activity and come prepared to play an active role. The simulation can be held within the classroom or the simulation lab if there is the capacity for live video streaming into the classroom so that all students can observe the simulation. Directly after the simulation, the faculty and students who played active roles during the simulation take their place at the front of the classroom for a live debriefing session.

There are benefits and drawbacks when using this simulation method. Faculty who have large classes where there is neither the time nor the resources to employ one-to-one or small group simulation experiences for each student can benefit from this resource's efficient method (Norman, Thompson, & Missildine, in press). This is particularly true if the simulation requires the use of a standardized patient (SP), which can be costly. Another benefit of this strategy is that it can be used to enhance active learning in the classroom where normally a more passive lecture format is employed.

This method is also beneficial to build capacity in nursing faculty who are then trained to be effective in the role of debriefing. A faculty member who has expertise in debriefing leads the debriefing session, thereby role modeling effective debriefing techniques to the nursing faculty observers. Over the course of several in-class simulations, faculty gain knowledge and experience in the process of debriefing that allows for a more active role in future debriefing exercises.

One drawback to this method is that although students express satisfaction with this type of simulation, those who play a more active role are more satisfied than those who are observers. Students who observe may not remain engaged during the simulation unless they are given specific tasks to guide their observations and are actively sought out to share their thoughts during the debrief.

In-class simulation may also be employed for distance learning. Educators may stream a live video of the simulation while distance learners observe. Using web conferencing programs, such as Adobe© Connect™, allows learners to actively participate in simulation and debriefing sessions.

This type of simulation can also occur online. Online simulation could be part of a fully online course or a blended course. A variety of media can be used in the online simulation. A live or prerecorded simulation using a high-fidelity manikin or an SP with other students serving as the active role participants could be posted or viewed remotely online by the students in the observer roles. A premade video file could be posted on a course management system such as Blackboard. Incorporating visual components into online learning, such as a video, adds value to the learning experience, as visualization will enhance learning and recall (Hartland, Biddle, & Fallacaro, 2008).

Online simulation could also include the creation of a virtual patient using software such as Second Life® or other gaming-type software. Faculty must select a software platform for their virtual patient and virtual environment that will allow students to comfortably navigate through simulation. Students should be able to quickly move through the virtual experience and gain the necessary information to meet the objectives (Horstmann, Renninger, Hennenlotter, Horstmann, & Stenzl, 2009). Creation of a virtual learning environment can be costly and usually requires the faculty to have partnerships with an instructional technologist, instructional designer, or the information technology department of their school to be successful. Posel, Fleiszer, and Shore (2009) offered several guidelines for faculty authoring virtual patient cases. Consider how the virtual patient will be used in a curriculum and what additional uses the virtual patient could serve in the future. If it can be anticipated that the virtual patient simulation might need to serve multiple purposes or repurposed at a later date, then plans should be made during the development phase to incorporate mechanisms that will meet those later needs. During the development phase, faculty also need to think ahead and determine all of the materials that will be needed by students in the virtual patient simulation or that must be linked to the virtual patient simulation (Jeffries et al., 2013).

CONSIDERATION OF BLOOM'S TAXONOMY

Because simulation provides such a rich learning environment, it is possible to incorporate a combination of cognitive, psychomotor, and affective learning domains within each simulation. As students progress throughout the program, simulations build in complexity and may add various elements of ambiguity so that advancing levels of critical reasoning must be employed in order to provide safe and effective care (Jeffries, Dreifuerst, Aschenbrenner, Adamson, & Schram, in press).

During the debriefing session, students have an opportunity to reflect on the experience. This reflection allows students to analyze and evaluate their behaviors and responses, synthesize new materials, and discover new ways to appreciate their patients and their families and team members and respond accordingly. Learning advances to a more complex level through the reflection process within the debriefing exercise in all domains of learning.

Another mechanism of meeting all domains of learning is to use an unfolding case to introduce increasing complexity. In the initial simulation, students are introduced to a particular patient. As they progress through the course or program, students are reintroduced to this same patient, but the clinical environment or particular problems may change, adding complexity not included in the initial simulation. As the complexity advances, students are required to engage at a higher level of learning in all three domains (Jeffries et al., in press).

Within the Prelicensure Program

For illustrative purposes, consider how a simulation related to congestive heart failure (CHF) could be leveled in a prelicensure curriculum, adding complexity and meeting various levels of Bloom's Taxonomy. In the initial courses of the curriculum, the student is learning the basic knowledge and skills needed to be a nurse, including how to perform basic physical assessment and basic psychomotor nursing skills, utilize the nursing process, recognize the nurse–patient relationship, and recall basic factual knowledge about various pathophysiologies.

Students have limited clinical experience. Based on the knowledge and skills that students have obtained at this point, the patient in the first simulation has just recently been diagnosed with CHF. The patient is located in a hospital bed on a general medical unit. The patient's spouse is at the bedside. A high-fidelity manikin is used to portray the patient. The manikin's lung sounds are set with bilateral crackles, respiratory rate of 18, pulse of 90, and the blood pressure is 140/90. Students play the roles of the primary nurse and spouse.

The first objective of this simulation is to use basic therapeutic communication principles to introduce themselves to the patient and family member (Bloom's Taxonomy of receiving phenomena in the affective domain). The second objective of the simulation is to perform a brief assessment including vital signs and cardiovascular and respiratory assessment (Bloom's Taxonomy of guided response for psychomotor skills). Students should recognize hypertension and identify respiratory crackles (Bloom's Taxonomy of understanding in the cognitive domain). The third objective of the simulation is to provide basic education about the pathophysiology of heart failure (Bloom's Taxonomy of understanding in the cognitive domain) after the patient provides a cue such as, "The doctor said my heart is failing. What does this mean?" During debriefing, students who played the role of the spouse will share the feelings and concerns they experienced as the family member. In this way, students also develop understanding of how the nurse should effectively and empathetically interact with the family member (Bloom's Taxonomy of understanding in the affective domain).

The next time students encounter this same patient, they are further along in the curriculum. They have taken a pharmacology course and are able to care for adults in the hospital with acute illnesses and who have more complex problems. Students are reintroduced to the same patient who is now admitted to the nursing unit with acute exacerbation of CHF. Again, a high-fidelity manikin portrays the patient. The manikin is essentially lying flat in the bed. The settings for the patient include coarse breath sounds with bilateral crackles extending throughout the lung fields, respiratory rate of 22, pulse of 120, and blood pressure of 150/92. When a pulse oximeter is attached, it will show an oxygen saturation of 90% on two liters of oxygen via nasal cannula. Moulage has been applied so that the lower extremities appear edematous and the lips are slightly blue tinged. An intravenous device has been inserted. Although the patient is on oxygen, the nasal prongs are not situated in the nares. Students again play the roles of the primary nurse and the spouse. The first objective of the simulation is to recognize acute exacerbation of heart failure and poor oxygenation to the tissues after conducting the initial patient assessment. Students should implement nursing measures to increase oxygenation by properly connecting the nasal cannula and elevating the head of the bed. As the simulation progresses, nursing measures to increase oxygenation are not effective, as evidenced by failure of oxygen saturation to improve and continued cyanosis of the lips. Students must recognize the potential causes of impaired oxygenation (lying flat, nasal cannula not in nares) from the true cause of impaired oxygenation (excess fluid volume in the heart and lungs) (Bloom's Taxonomy of analyzing in the cognitive domain). The second objective is to use appropriate communication techniques, such as the SBAR (Situation-Background-Assessment-Recommendation) technique, to inform the provider of a patient in acute distress and obtain an order for medication (Bloom's Taxonomy of applying in the cognitive domain). The next objective is to administer medication for acute exacerbation of heart failure. Students would be expected to show basic proficiency in giving an intravenous dose of medication such as furosemide (Bloom's Taxonomy of mechanism or basic proficiency in the psychomotor domain). The final objective is to demonstrate an awareness of a patient and family member in emotional distress and respond in a therapeutic manner (Bloom's Taxonomy of valuing in the affective domain).

The same patient could be introduced a third time in the prelicensure curricula toward the end of the program. Students are expected to synthesize content from a variety of courses, including caring for adults who are acutely or terminally ill. The simulation can take place using a home environment for students who are taking or have taken the public health nursing course. At this level, students should be capable of functioning relatively independently. The objective of this simulation is to conduct a home visit for a patient who is near the end of life and receiving hospice care. During this simulation, this same patient is now portrayed by an SP. The patient has moulage to show dusky skin tones and significant peripheral edema. The patient, who is on oxygen, is dyspneic, sitting up in a chair, exhausted, and has difficulty moving and speaking. He sleeps sitting up, when he can sleep. Simulation products that allow selected pathologic sounds to be heard in the heart and lungs (such as by radio frequency tags) could be placed on the SP so that realistic, abnormal sounds are heard on auscultation. Students play the roles of the visiting nurse and family member.

The first objective for the simulation is to evaluate the current health status of the patient. From the assessment findings, students should determine that the patient's health has deteriorated, his symptoms are not controlled, he is uncomfortable, and the goals of hospice are not currently being met (Bloom's Taxonomy of evaluating in the cognitive domain). The second objective is to collaborate with the health care provider to create a revised plan of care based on the patient's current status (Bloom's Taxonomy of creating in the cognitive domain as well as internalizing values by showing teamwork in the affective domain). This communication and collaboration could be via telephone or using handheld technology such as a smartphone or a tablet as a mechanism of telehealth (Bloom's Taxonomy of adaptation of a psychomotor skill). The third objective is to provide appropriate emotional support to the patient and family in their stage of grief (Bloom's Taxonomy of internalizing values in the affective domain).

Depending on the needs of each unique school or program, any of these above simulations could be completed in the simulation lab, in a classroom, or online. Faculty could add additional complexity and fidelity to the cases by turning the simulations into interprofessional educational experiences. More complexity can also be achieved using different levels of learners, such as first-semester students teamed with final-semester prelicensure students or prelicensure students teamed with graduate nursing students (Kaplan, Holmes, Mott, & Atallah, 2011). Another way to add complexity to a simulation is to create hybrid situations where a static model (such as an intravenous arm) is combined with an SP. Technology can be added in various ways such as using an electronic health record to document or receive or review orders, integrating handheld devices to access a drug database, or use bar code scanning or other software to decrease the risk of medication errors. Changing the patient variables can also add complexity, such as identifying the patient as hard of hearing or blind or someone who speaks little or no English or is from a different culture.

However complexity is added, the faculty must ensure that students have the requisite knowledge and skills based on their attained level in the curriculum and are able to be successful in the simulation.

Within Graduate Education

Unfolding case scenarios can also be effectively used in various graduate nursing programs. To carry the above illustrative example further, simulations involving a patient with CHF could be leveled for graduate curricula as well as to add complexity and meet various levels of Bloom's Taxonomy. For the initial graduate courses, APRN students are expanding their ability to conduct an organized and systematic history and physical examination and develop diagnostic reasoning skills including differential diagnosis. Because communication plays a major role in this encounter, an SP is best used to portray the patient. The patient is introduced in the initial simulation as an older established male patient who presents to an ambulatory clinic with the chief complaint of shortness of breath and leg edema with previous history of hypertension. The first objective of the simulation is to conduct an episodic history (Bloom's Taxonomy of remembering the cognitive domain) and physical examination (Bloom's Taxonomy of perception/awareness of the psychomotor domain).

Although an SP can provide appropriate answers during the solicitation of the history, the faculty will provide the student with abnormal physical examination findings that support the differential diagnosis of CHF. The faculty can provide the student with auditory crackles via an Internet site or use a hybrid simulation technique using a digital breath sound simulator and pictorial or video image depicting grade 2 or higher lower extremity edema. The student should recognize the presence of uncontrolled hypertension, bilateral crackles, and lower leg edema as the rationale for a differential diagnosis of CHF (Bloom's Taxonomy of applying in the cognitive domain). The third objective is to use therapeutic communication to understand the patient's self-management strategies for his hypertension (Bloom's Taxonomy of responding to phenomena in the affective domain).

Later in the curriculum, the student might have a second encounter with this same patient played by an SP. At this point, the student has had coursework in advanced pharmacology and additional clinical experience. Based on the knowledge and skills obtained at this point, the second simulation is the same patient who is now experiencing an acute exacerbation of CHF. The patient presents to the ambulatory clinic with increased dyspnea, weight gain, fatigue, and orthopnea. The patient could be portrayed by either an SP or a high-fidelity manikin. Moulage is applied to either the manikin or SP to create realism of the condition of acute exacerbation of heart failure with peripheral edema. Technology could again be used to create the altered heart and breath sounds. Students are expected to conduct the history and physical examination and present a case presentation that includes differential diagnoses and management plan.

The first objective is to detect an acute exacerbation of CHF (Bloom's Taxonomy of analyzing in the cognitive domain, and mechanism/basic proficiency in the psychomotor domain). The second objective is to develop a management plan that includes the prescription of appropriate drug therapy (Bloom's Taxonomy of applying in the cognitive domain). A third objective is to demonstrate concern for the patient and family (Bloom's Taxonomy of valuing in the affective domain). For APRN students who have an acute care focus, the simulation may include determining the need for hospitalization (Bloom's Taxonomy of analyzing in the cognitive domain). This simulation scenario could also be run as a joint simulation with prelicensure students, where the prelicensure students are caring for the patient in the hospital and contact the APRN provider for new medication orders (see the section "Within the Prelicensure Program").

The final simulation in this unfolding scenario occurs near the end of the curriculum for APRN students and the objective is to deliver bad news to the patient who is now in end-stage heart failure and terminally ill. The patient, played by an SP, would present to the clinic for posthospitalization follow up. The simulation objective is to use therapeutic communication to deliver bad news in an empathetic manner (Bloom's Taxonomy of internalizing values/characterization in the affective domain).

An alternative simulation for acute care APRN students is to conduct the simulation in the acute care hospital setting. A manikin would portray the patient while the role of the family and other health care professions would be portrayed by APRN or undergraduate students. The primary APRN student would lead the interprofessional family meeting to deliver bad news of a terminal condition and work with the patient and family member to determine their interest in hospice care. The objectives would be similar to those just described, but there might also be the objective of demonstrating professional and ethical practice for a patient who has a terminal illness (Bloom's Taxonomy of internalizing values/characterization in the affective domain).

Further complexity could be added to any of the above simulations by adding additional comorbidities to the case, increasing the number of medications the patient receives, adding technology, or adding challenging personality traits or life situations that impose threats to the patient's ability to self-manage his or her disease.

OBJECTIVE STRUCTURED CLINICAL EXPERIENCES

Some graduate nursing programs are using **objective structured clinical experiences** (OSCE) to teach and evaluate students (Katz et al., 2002; Rushforth, 2007; Vessey & Huss, 2002). The OSCE experience consists of multiple stations where an SP portrays a patient with a specific clinical complaint. Students are scheduled to rotate to each station for a specific period of time to conduct a history and physical examination. Students might also be

TABLE 14.1

Example of Objective Structured Clinical Experiences Schedule: Four Students, Four Different Simulation Encounters for Each Student

	Room 1 Patient 1	Room 2 Patient 2	Room 3 Patient 3	Room 4 Patient 4
8–8:45 am	Student 1a	Student 2a	Student 3a	Student 4a
8:50–9:35 am	Student 4b	Student 1b	Student 2b	Student 3b
9:40–10:25 am	Student 3c	Student 4c	Student 1c	Student 2c
10:30–11:15 am	Student 2d	Student 3d	Student 4c	Student 1d

asked to provide a case presentation of the encounter, including the differential diagnosis and rationale, along with the plan of treatment. The number of stations and clinical problems presented can vary depending on the resources available.

This type of experience takes a great deal of planning. A different simulation scenario must be developed for each station, and SPs must be trained to consistently portray the patient during each encounter so that every student has the same experience. This is particularly true if there is any formative or summative evaluation attached to the OSCE.

The number of OSCE stations will depend on the availability of simulation space, time allowed for the experience, and number of faculty and SPs available. For example, an OSCE experience may be developed to evaluate the clinical competency of a group of APRN students. The objective is to conduct an episodic encounter in the ambulatory care environment on four patients, each with a different chief complaint. For each encounter, students have 30 minutes to conduct the history and physical examination and 15 minutes to present the case (including differential diagnosis with rationale and management plan) and debrief with faculty. A sample schedule is shown in Table 14.1.

The OSCE can be modified to accommodate more students if each student has only one encounter, as shown in the example of a modified schedule in Table 14.2. It is evident that the OSCE can be quite costly when one considers the resources required.

Student evaluation during the OSCE experience can be challenging. It is important that a valid and reliable tool be used to evaluate the cognitive, psychomotor, and affective outcomes of student performance (Rushforth, 2007). Student evaluation can be conducted by either the clinical faculty or, if sufficiently trained, the SP (McLaughlin, Gregor, Jones, & Sylvain, 2006). However, in order for the SP to act as a student evaluator, faculty must make certain that the SP has the knowledge to evaluate and uses an evaluation tool that is valid and reliable for SP evaluation of student. Finally, educators need to understand that in order for the OSCE experience to be a reliable and valid means for summative evaluation, students must be familiar with and have had a sufficient number of prior simulation experiences to use the simulation pedagogy to evaluate student competency (Vessey & Huss, 2002).

TABLE 14.2

Example of Modified Objective Structured Clinical Experiences Schedule: 16 Students, One Simulation Encounter for Each Student

	Room 1 Patient 1	Room 2 Patient 2	Room 3 Patient 3	Room 4 Patient 4
8–8:45 am	Student 1	Student 2	Student 3	Student 4
8:50–9:35 am	Student 5	Student 6	Student 7	Student 8
9:40–10:25 am	Student 9	Student 10	Student 11	Student 12
10:30–11:15 am	Student 13	Student 14	Student 15	Student 16

Graduate nursing programs can also used video-recorded OSCEs for APRN distance programs for the purpose of teaching and reinforcing learning (Barratt, 2010). The OSCE can be developed to demonstrate either "best evidence care" or care with some type of deficiency, such as critical omissions in the history, incorrect physical examination technique, or ineffective communication or teamwork. Students are able to access the video-recorded OSCEs online, either on the university's virtual learning environment or on public access such as YouTube. Faculty can use this method to enable students to participate in a synchronized or asynchronized discussion or to reinforce learning.

Other Graduate Nursing Roles

The simulation lab can also be used to depict various clinical environments beyond the traditional patient care environment in order to help graduate nurse role development. Nurse educator programs use simulation to provide a safe environment for students to develop expertise in the teacher role (Shellenbarger & Edwards, 2012). A scenario could depict a clinical situation where the nurse educator is required to instruct a nurse on a particular skill, such as changing a Foley catheter. The simulation clinical environment is also used to develop leadership skills (Kaplan et al., 2011) and interprofessional teamwork (Wamsley et al., 2012). The simulation scenario could call for a clinical situation that includes a patient safety issue such as a near miss or failure to rescue. The desired behavioral outcomes require the use of effective communication, problem solving, leadership, teamwork, and understanding the knowledge and skills of each team member. The debriefing session should not only include whether the students were able to function in their role, but also to appreciate the unique strengths and challenges that comes with teamwork.

SUMMARY

There are a variety of ways to use simulation in innovative educational activities to promote active and engaged learning. Moreover, simulation will continue to play an increasingly important role in the formative and summative evaluation of clinical competency.

It is important to strategically embed simulation within the curriculum to help students achieve the desired program outcomes. Bloom's Taxonomy of Learning domains can serve as a guide as faculty consider how to appropriately "level" simulations throughout prelicensure and graduate curricula, adding complexity in order to achieve learning in the cognitive, psychomotor, and affective domains.

■ Key Concepts

- Faculty should take a purposeful, planned, and organized approach to appraise the curriculum to determine how simulation will support achievement of program outcomes.
- Bloom's Taxonomy of Learning domains can serve as a guide to level simulations within the program and to build complexity of learning.
- Simulation can be used in a variety of settings, including classroom, simulation labs, and OSCE, to help students achieve course and clinical outcomes.

References

Anderson, J., Aylor, M. E., & Leonard, D. T. (2008). Instructional design dogma: Creating planned learning experiences in simulation. *Journal of Critical Care, 23*(4), 595–602.

Barratt, J. (2010). A focus group study of the use of video-recorded simulation objective structured clinical examinations in nurse practitioner education. *Nurse Education in Practice, 10,* 170–175.

Billings, D., & Halstead, J. (2009). *Teaching in nursing: A guide for faculty.* St. Louis: Saunders Elsevier.

Bloom, B. S. (Ed.) (1956). *Taxonomy of Educational Objectives Book 1: Cognitive Domain.* New York: Longman.

Cook, D., Brydges, R., Hamstra, S. J., Zendejas, B., Szostek, J. H., Wang, A. T., Erwin, P. J., & Hatala, R. (2012). Comparative effectiveness of technology-enhanced simulation versus other instructional methods. *Simulation in Healthcare, 7*(5), 308–320.

Cook, D., Hatala, R., Brydges, R., Zendejas, B., Szostek, J. H., Wang, A. T., Erwin, P. J., & Hamstra, S. J. (2011). Technology-enhanced simulation for health professional education. *Jounal of the American Medical Association, 306*(9), 978–988.

Cordeau, M. (2010). The lived experience of clinical simulation of novice nursing students. *International Journal for Human Caring, 14*(2), 9–15.

Hartland, W., Biddle, C., & Fallacaro, M. (2008). Audiovisual facilitation of clinical knowledge: A paradigm for dispersed student education based on Paivio's Dual Coding Theory. *AANA Journal, 76*(3), 194–198.

Horstmann, M., Renninger, M., Hennenlotter, J., Horstmann, C. C., & Stenzl, A. (2009). Blended e-learning in a web-based virtual hospital: A useful tool for undergraduate education in urology. *Education for Health, 22*(2), 269.

Hyland, D., Weeks, B. H., Ficorelli, C. T., & Vanderbeek-Warren, M. (2012). Bringing simulation to life. *Teaching and Learning in Nursing, 7,* 108–112.

Irwin, R. (2011). The diffusion of human patient simulaton into an associate degree in nursing curriculum. *Teaching and Learning in Nursing, 6*(4), 153–158.

Jeffries, P. R. (2005). A framework for designing, implementing, and evaluating simulations used as teaching strategies in nursing. *Nursing Education Perspectives, 26*(2), 96–103.

Jeffries, P., Aschenbrenner, D. S., Dreifuerst, K. T., Hensel, D., Keenan, C., & Vazzano, J. (2013). Using simulation to enhance clinical reasoning and judgment. In K. Frith,

& Clark, D. J. (Eds.), *Distance education in nursing* (3rd ed.). New York: Springer.

Jeffries, P., Beach, M., Becker, S., Dlugasch, L., Groom, J., & O'Donnell, J. (2011). Multi-center development and testing of a simulation-based cardiovascular assessment curriculum for advanced practice nurses. *Nursing Education Perspectives, 32*(5), 316–322.

Jeffries, P., Dreifuerst, K. T., Aschenbrenner, D. S., Adamson, K. A., & Schram, A. P. (In press). Clinical simulations in nursing education: Overview, essentials, and the evidence. In M. Oermann (Ed.), *Teaching in nursing: The complete guide.* New York: Springer.

Kaplan, B., Holmes, L., Mott, M., & Atallah, H. (2011). Design and implementation of an interdisciplinary pediatric mock code for undergraduate and graduate nursing students. *Computers, Informatics, Nursing, 29*(9), 531–538.

Katz, D. A., Muehlenbruch, D. R., Brown, R. B., Fiore, M. C., Baker, T. B., & AHRQ Smoking Cessation Guideline Study Group. (2002). Effectiveness of a clinic-based strategy for implementating the AHRQ Smoking Cessation Guideline in primary care. *Preventive Medicine, 35,* 293–302.

Krathwohl, D. (2002). A revision of Bloom's Taxonomy: An overview. *Theory into Practice, 41*(4), 212–218.

Lapkin, A., Levett-Jones, T., Bellchambers, H., & Fernandez, R. (2010). Effectiveness of patient simulation manikins in teaching clinical reasoning skills to undergraduate nursing students: A systematic review. *Clinical Simulation in Nursing, 6*(6), e207–e222.

McLaughlin, K., Gregor, L., Jones, A., & Sylvain, C. (2006). Can standardized patients replace physicians as OSCE examiners? *BMC Medical Education, 6*(12), 1–5.

Norman, G., Dore, K., & Grierson, L. (2012). The minimal relationship between simulation fidelity and trasfer of learning. *Medical Education, 46,* 636–647.

Norman, J., Thompson, S., & Missildine, K. (In press). The 2-minute drills: Incorporating simulation into a large lecture format. *Clinical Simulation in Nursing.*

Posel, N., Fleiszer, D., & Shore, B. M. (2009). Twelve Tips: Guidelines for authoring virtual patient cases. *Medical Teacher, 31*(8), 701–708.

Rushforth, H. (2007). Objective structured clinical examination (OSCE): Review of literature and implications for nursing education. *Nurse Education Today, 27,* 481–490.

Shellenbarger, T., & Edwards, T. (2012). Nurse educator simulation: Preparing faculty for clinical nurse educator roles. *Clinical Simulation in Nursing, 8*(6), e249–e255.

Vessey, J., & Huss, K. (2002). Using standardized patients in advanced practice nursing education. *Journal of Professional Nursing, 18*(1), 29–35.

Wamsley, M., Staves, J., Kroon, L., Topp, K., Hossaini, M., Newlin, B., Lindsay, C., & O'Brien, B. (2012). The impact of an interprofessional standardized patient exercise on attitudes toward working in interprofessional teams. *Journal of Interprofessional Care, 26*(1), 28–35.

Wu, W., & Osisek, P. J. (2011). The revised Bloom's Taxonomy: Implications for educating nurses. *Journal of Continuing Education in Nursing, 42*(7), 321–327.

15

Certification in Clinical Simulations: The Process, Purpose, and Value Added

Sharon I. Decker, PhD, RN, ANEF, FAAN
Joseph O. Lopreiato, MD, MPH
Mary D. Patterson, MD, MEd

■ Learning Objectives

1. Discuss the process of developing a certification program.
2. Describe the process used to develop a certification program specific to simulation.
3. Determine the phases involved in developing a certification exam.
4. Identify resources available to prepare for certification specific to simulation.
5. Explore the value of certification to the individual, the professional society, and the public.
6. Identify the importance of marketing for a certification program.

■ Key Terms

- Certification
- Job analysis
- Portfolio
- Standards of practice
- Test blueprint

The concept of certification is embraced by many professions: dog trainers, financial planners, software specialists, and baristas. In health care, certification for nurses was first entertained around 1966, while the American Board of Medical Specialties (awarding "board certification") came into existence in 1933. Although licensure attests to basic competence, certification implies special expertise or competence in a particular domain (Barnum, 1997). Over time, there came to be an emphasis on the incorporation of adult education principles in health care, for example, the specialization of health care educators gained credibility with the accreditation of the

National League for Nursing's (NLN) Certification of Nurse Educator program in 2009 (NLN, 2011).

HISTORY AND DEFINITION OF CERTIFICATION

Certification is a voluntary process that validates an individual's obtainment of specific, predetermined qualifications and competencies (education, experience, knowledge, and skills) in a defined area of expertise. As a volunteer process, obtaining certification demonstrates an individual's commitment to his or her career development and professional attainment (Knapp & Knapp, 2002). Professional attainment is visible through an acronym after the individual's name to designate the obtainment of the specific achievement. Eligibility requirements and validation of the identified knowledge and skills are through a formalized process established by an organization. Individuals who meet the set qualifications are provided time-limited certification. Recertification or renewal of the certification requires the individual to demonstrate continued competence through a mechanism established by the organization.

A certification program is expected to have a national and international scope and be designed to recognize competency, promote professional achievement, and ultimately protect the consumer. Factors associated with an organization's efforts to develop a certification process include a desire to (1) establish professional standards of practice specific to an area of expertise, (2) elevate professional repetition and status, and (3) seek a form of nonmembership dues revenue (Knapp, Fabrey, Rops, & McCurry, 2006; Knapp & Knapp, 2002).

Standards of practice include the knowledge, skills, and practice identified by a professional society to describe a specialty's scope of practice (AOME, 2012). Standards are used as guidelines to assist individuals in developing career trajectories "to identify professional development needs, acquire new skills or develop existing skills to meet the specific requirements of new teaching and learning contexts" (AOME, 2012, p. 9).

OVERVIEW OF CERTIFICATION IN SIMULATION

Simulation in health care, as a professional domain, evolved over a number of years. Most practitioners of health care simulation initially developed competence and eventually proficiency through "on-the-job training," experience, and continuing education. The Society of Simulation in Healthcare (SSH) embarked on development of an accreditation process for simulation programs with the explicit intent of ensuring the quality of simulation-based educational experiences. The discussions for a certification process for simulation educators initiated from requests from members within the simulation community. These initial requests presented both personal and professional rationale, with individuals citing a need to validate professional credibility and fulfill position, tenure, or promotion criteria.

A review of the literature presented both intangible and tangible benefits of certification. For example, nursing literature indicated that nurses who are certified in their specialty perceive a higher level of self-confidence (Altman, 2011; Kaplow, 2011), demonstrate higher levels of knowledge and skills (Briggs, Brown, Kesten, & Heath, 2006; Wade, 2009), and obtain increased recognition from peers (Altman, 2011; ANCC, 2009). Certification provides evidence of excellence to the public (ANCC, 2009), and patient care provided by certified nurses has been correlated to increased patient satisfaction (Kaplow, 2010). Additionally, a national survey demonstrated managers prefer to hire nationally certified nurses (Stromborg et al., 2005). Therefore, the certification program for simulation educators was a logical step for the SSH in terms of ensuring the quality of the simulation educational experience as well as promoting the role and professionalism of the simulation educator.

Authorities caution that developing and maintaining a certification program need to be viewed as a business endeavor (Knapp & Knapp, 2002). Development of a valid certification program requires a financial commitment without guarantee of recoup and should not be endeavored until a strong business model, including a SWOT (Strengths, Weaknesses, Opportunities, and Threats) analysis, is established and critiqued. Recognizing the substantial financial and resource investment required, it is important to have preliminary discussions related to the proposed certification program to consider the program's potential value to the public, the organization, and its customers and the financial and time commitments required to develop and maintain the program.

When the development of a simulation educator certification program was initially discussed in 2008 and 2009, a number of controversial issues were openly discussed. These included who should be eligible to apply for certification based on experience, education, and demonstrated knowledge and skills. There were discussions within the SSH's leadership as well as the SSH's education committee and key stakeholders in health care education. These included international and national simulation organizations (the Society in Europe for Simulation Applied to Medicine, the Australian Society for Simulation in Healthcare, etc.). In addition, specific stakeholders in the discipline, such as the National League for Nursing (NLN), the Association of Standardized Patient Educators (ASPE), and the International Nursing Association for Clinical Simulation and Learning (INACSL), were consulted. These discussions identified three major concerns that required consensus among the stakeholders:

- The level of formal education and training required for simulation certification
- The levels of certification that would be offered (competent, competent and advanced, and master levels)
- The process for certification (test, portfolio, demonstration of skills)

The levels of education and formal training for simulation certification were the first issues addressed. There was considerable discussion as to whether simulation educators should be required to possess terminal degrees in order to qualify for certification. The position of the SSH's leadership was that the majority of simulation educators did not possess terminal degrees, and that setting this as a requirement would exclude large numbers of competent and practicing simulation educators.

Philosophically, the SSH viewed the certification process as a means to ensure competency and quality in the simulation experience as well as a means to advance professionalism in this domain. The discussions related to the levels of certification were directly tied to the first issue. Although consensus was eventually reached that the initial level of certification should be broadly inclusive and reflect competency, there were also strong feelings that an advanced level of certification would be desirable for many. It was believed that an advanced level of certification would also provide a higher and desirable goal for many simulation educators.

Finally, the actual logistics as to how certification would occur was contentious. For some stakeholders, simulation, as an experiential educational process, seemed to demand a practice-based evaluation of the applicant's skills. On the other hand, the logistics of such a process, including the cost, limited number of simulation "experts," and the time required to review individual portfolios, would have potentially resulted in severely limiting the number of educators who could be certified. Limiting certification to a small number of educators was counter to the goals of the SSH and to advancing the professionalism of simulation educators.

Historical Overview

A working group of simulation experts convened in London in November 2009 to summarize the work of the previous two years and develop a plan to move forward. At that meeting, the SSH established a certification subcommittee under the auspices of the Committee on Certification, Accreditation, Technology and Standards. This subcommittee was tasked by the SSH leadership to move the process of certifying simulation educators to the next level. To that end, the subcommittee on certification was constituted with members from medicine, nursing, and education backgrounds. Members were from North America, Europe, and Australia and represented several societies including the SSH, the ASPE, the International Nursing Association for Clinical Simulation and Learning, the Society for Education in Simulation as Applied to Medicine, and the Australian Society for Simulation in Healthcare. The London meeting ended with agreement that any new certification program would need to specify elements of knowledge, skills, and attitudes that were desirable in simulation educators. The subcommittee borrowed heavily from the Academy of Medical Educators in the United Kingdom (AOME, 2012), which had specified the elements necessary to be an effective educator. The subcommittee's work was to adapt these domains specifically to simulation education in its forthcoming work.

Over the next few months, the subcommittee met monthly and began to formulate a way to proceed. Early on, "certified simulation educator" was agreed upon as the title for newly certified individuals. This clarified the subcommittee's intent to certify educators and faculty members rather than other groups involved in simulation. This title was later revised to certified health care simulation educator (CHSE) to highlight the health care focus of the certification.

The subcommittee borrowed the definition from the SSH's accreditation program, which defined core instructors, educators, or faculty as "those individuals that are intricately and routinely involved in the simulation education curriculum and that are responsible for the content, implementation, and evaluation of the curriculum" (SSH, 2013a). The subcommittee's first document, developed in December 2009, was a statement of principles (Box 15.1) to guide these efforts. The subcommittee also defined the term certification as a voluntary process, initiated by an individual wanting to be recognized for special knowledge, skills, and attitudes in the field of health care simulation. The certification was to be time limited and renewable and a certificant had

BOX 15.1 CERTIFICATION SUBCOMMITTEE STATEMENT OF PRINCIPLES

Certification is a voluntary process of confirming the knowledge, skills, and attitudes essential to qualified individuals in the field of simulation. Health care simulation certification has benefits for learners, educators, health administrators, and funders to ensure standards in simulation educational delivery.

- Certification is a voluntary process.
- Certification will be seen as a service to our members and our communities of interest.
- Certification will confirm the knowledge, skills, and attitudes essential to instructors in the field of simulation.
- Certification, in order to maximize efficiency and impact, should be a cooperative effort between simulation and professional organizations.
- Certification will be time limited and renewable.

SOURCE: SSH, Certification Standards and Elements, 2012b.

to meet certain prerequisites before certification could be granted. The subcommittee had surveyed other certification programs in many related fields before deciding on a statement of principles.

In January 2010, a decision was made to conduct a worldwide survey of simulation educators to determine demographic information and interest in the certification process to help inform the subcommittee as it constructed certification prerequisites, elements, and value. The SSH agreed to provide administrative resources and funding to move the program forward and to conduct a survey. As the certification for simulation educators program was developing, the subcommittee sought guidance in creating a program that adhered to accepted standards for certification programs as put forth by the Institute for Credentialing Excellence (ICE) (ICE, 2005).

Three new working groups were formed within the subcommittee with the specific goals of (1) reviewing the proposed elements and standards, (2) developing the criteria for the professional portfolio, and (3) formulating business plans and marketing strategies. These committees met monthly throughout the year by telephone conference. The proposed business plan and budget allowed discussion and informed decision making related to the certification program. These documents provided data to assist the SSH board of directors in making informed decisions. The documents included the projected program profiles; timeline for inception and growth; projected number of individuals to be certified annually; potential sponsoring organizations; reviewers (cost and training); cost analysis for test development, delivery, and maintenance; and criteria for quality assessment and review. By the summer of 2010, a SWOT analysis had been conducted by the subcommittee and the results were presented to the board of directors of the SSH. The board approved moving forward with the certification project and assigned a budget for the following fiscal year.

In the summer and fall of 2010, a simple marketing survey (analysis) of simulation educators was sent to all members of the SSH. Based on the return rate, the number of simulation educators was estimated to be approximately 10,000 and growing. The survey

> ## BOX 15.2 THE FIVE DOMAINS FOR CERTIFICATION OF HEALTH CARE EDUCATORS
>
> - Professional values and capabilities
> - Scholarship-spirit of inquiry
> - Designing and developing learning activities
> - Implementing evaluating simulation-based educational activities
> - Effective management of the learning environment and educational activities

revealed that 71 percent of the respondents were interested in becoming certified. This translates into potentially 7,100 people having an interest in certification. Approximately 80 percent of respondents indicated they were at the basic or competent level. The results confirmed a need for a more formal practice analysis to be conducted.

A face-to-face meeting of the certification subcommittee was held in Washington, D.C., in September 2010. At that meeting, the initial survey results were reviewed, the task groups reported on their progress, and the five domains identified in Box 15.2 were accepted as the underlying framework for the certification process.

For each domain, standards and elements were written and examples provided of how the standards could be validated by an applicant (SSH, 2013b). In this way, applicants and reviewers could easily visualize which standards were required and how an applicant might demonstrate meeting the standards. At that same meeting, two different levels of certification were established: a base level defined as CHSE and an advanced level designated CHSE-A to recognize those individuals with more experience and leadership in the field. Initial standards for the five elements were developed for both levels.

The meeting concluded with a decision to hire a professional testing and analysis firm to conduct a formal practice or job analysis. A practice or **job analysis** is an in-depth study conducted to identify, validate, and update competency domains (performance activities and knowledge, skills, and abilities) of an identified specialty (Doyle et al., 2012). The practice analysis for the development of the certification process for health care simulation educators was patterned after a similar analysis done by the NLN as part of their nurse educator certification program (NLN, 2011). The practice analysis sought to define the demographics of "simulationists" worldwide and obtain information on the teaching and learning environment of simulation educators.

The original intent of the subcommittee was to develop the advanced program first with the idea that a small number of qualified people could then serve as reviewers for the base program called CHSE. The CHSE program was always envisioned as a review of credentials and successful passage of a multiple-choice knowledge based exam to ensure that simulation educators had a broad knowledge of the many methods used in simulation education. The advanced program was envisioned to include a demonstration of specific skills and curricula that a more experienced educator or leader develops through formalized education and experience to distinguish him- or herself from the baseline CHSE. For example, the eligibility criteria for the initial certification (CHSE) require a bachelor's degree or equivalent experience and two-year continued use of simulation; whereas, the advanced certification (CHSE-A) requires a master's degree or

TABLE 15.1

Comparing Elements for the Identified Certification for Simulation

Certified Simulation Educator	Certified Simulation Educator-Advanced
"Participates and contributes to a professional organization related to simulation."	"Advocates for simulation through active participation in national/international level organizations."

SOURCE: SSH, Certification Standards and Elements, 2012b.

equivalent and five years or more of experience using simulation in health care education (SSH, 2013b). During the fall of 2013, the pilot for the certification process for CHSE-A will be completed with appropriate modifications implemented from feedback from participants and reviewers.

Throughout the winter of 2010 and the spring of 2011, the task groups defined the elements to be considered for certification and a preliminary application and review process was constructed. Table 15.1 provides a proposed example demonstrating the difference between the suggested evidence for the domain: professional values and capabilities, standards/elements, leadership, and "demonstrates advocacy for simulation education" for the levels of certification.[1]

In the fall of 2011, a more detailed practice analysis was performed through a survey to SSH and all its affiliate members worldwide. A total of 1,239 responses were received and analyzed for content. The demographics of simulation educators suggested that most were in nursing or medical schools and had approximately one to five staff working to deliver simulation to between 500 and 1,000 learners per year. Simulation educators used a variety of modalities to teach, including full-body manikins, standardized patients, computer-based instruction, and task trainers. Most had been in the field only one to five years and had worked in the academic or acute care setting.

At that time, several members of the subcommittee agreed to submit mock applications and other members agreed to be reviewers in the first pilot of the certification process. Prerequisites, entry criteria, and review elements were highly influenced by the practice analysis data and the experience of similar educator simulation programs such as the Nurse Educator Program from the NLN. These templates helped immeasurably in constructing the new simulation certification program. The standards of ICE were kept in mind throughout the process.

In the summer of 2011, the board of directors of the SSH directed the subcommittee on certification to focus their efforts on the CHSE program first and then develop the CHSE-A program thereafter. The board reasoned it was easier to implement a base program in CHSE than a more sophisticated advanced program at the outset, given their experience with the accreditation program. The subcommittee agreed to this direction

---

[1]The document Certification Standards and Elements, providing the elements and standards for certification, is available at http://ssih.org/uploads/static_pages/PDFs/Certification/CHSE%20 Standards.pdf

TABLE 15.2

Certified Health Care Simulation Educator Exam Blueprint

Domain	Weight
Display professional values and capabilities	4%
Demonstrate knowledge of simulation principles, practice, and methodology	34%
Educate and assess learners using simulation	52%
Manage overall simulation resources and environments	6%
Engage in scholarly activities	4%

SOURCE: SSH, Certification and Elements, 2012b.

and began work on constructing the certifying exam for the CHSE level. In November 2011, a test writing committee was convened in Atlanta, Georgia, under the auspices of a test development company to write and validate questions for a future certification exam. Test writing authors were from many of the simulation societies that were affiliates of the SSH and represented nursing, medicine, and allied health.

Development of a certification exam is a complex process requiring test items be fair, psychometrically sound (valid and accurate), and legally defensible. The initial step in developing the written exam for CHSE was to develop the overall **test blueprint** and item weights (Table 15.2) based on the practice or job analysis and standards. A blueprint lists the domains of required knowledge and skills included in an exam. The item weight clarifies the value placed on each domain, identifying areas of knowledge valued more than others as identified through the practice analysis. A detailed outline of the blueprint is provided in the certification handbook available on the SSH's website (SSH, 2013b).

A panel of individuals with expertise in various simulation modalities, representing multiple organizations and several countries, met face to face to develop the test blueprint and begin writing test items. These experts were guided by a psychometrician with expertise in exam development. A set format was provided and items were expected to be based on best practices supported through literature, reflect difference simulation modalities, and have relevance to the international simulation community.

The second step of the test development process required each question to undergo a critique by an expert review panel. The reviewers evaluated each question for format, structure, authenticity, and relevance, resulting in an item being accepted as written, modified by the review panel, sent back to the test writer, or deleted from the test bank.

Meanwhile, the portfolio development team finished creating CHSE and CHSE-A application forms and a proposed certification process. This process specified that candidates seeking CHSE-A distinction would be required to initially obtain the CHSE. A detailed handbook for applicants was completed that walked applicants through the application process. The CHSE-A application form was put on hold pending the rollout of the CHSE program. The business plan team contracted with a company to deliver and validate the results of the certification exam and developed a marketing plan. The marketing subcommittee stressed the importance of creating awareness and consistent branding of the certification program. This included the development of a recognized logo for the certification program, brochures, and other products for certified individuals. A pin with the certification's acronym, certification plaque, and letter of congratulations were developed to promote visibility and recognition for individuals achieving the designation.

The certification standards for a CHSE applicant were published by the SSH on their website in early 2012 and distributed to affiliated societies. The test writing task force completed its work in the late spring of 2012, and together with the work of the other task forces, a decision was made to launch a CHSE certification program with 200 applicants starting in June 2012. These first 200 applicants would help set the standards for passing the certification exam and test the application process. Specific information related to the certification process included the application, certification standards and suggested evidence and the mechanism to validate, handbook, exam information, and references.

After completion of the pilot of CHSE and setting the cut score in fall of 2012, the focus of the CHSE component of the program shifted to marketing and sustainability. A modification in committee structure was required as the overall goals of the certification program expanded. Additional goals were established to review and complete the initial work related to the CHSE-A and to develop an additional exam for simulation technology specialists.

The CHSE-A subcommittee modified the previously developed application process of the advanced certification establishing the differences between CHSE and CHSE-A within each competency domain. Requirements for seeking the CHSE-A credential were accepted that include successful completion of the exam for CHSE followed by a portfolio review. A **portfolio** is a collection of materials that represents an individual's progress and achievements in an identified specialty. Portfolio development requires reflection and has been correlated to improved self-awareness (Buckley et al., 2009). The portfolio requires reflective statements addressing the domains of professional values and capabilities, knowledge of simulation principles, practice and methodology, education and assessment of learners using simulation, management of overall simulation resources and environments, and engagement in scholarly activities. An example of a learner-focused simulation-based education intervention created by the applicant that could be incorporated into the portfolio could include a media presentation, case study, or screen-based simulations.

The development process for the certification of Simulation Technology Specialists parallels that used for CHSE. This process includes completion of a job analysis, development of standards, designation of a blueprint, and writing and critique of test item. As these and other endeavors of the certification processes are completed, information will be available at the SSH's website.

PREPARATION FOR CERTIFICATION

Preparation for taking the certification exam specific for simulation educators includes the same process used for any exam. It is essential to review the eligibility criteria published at the SSH's website. Candidates should ask themselves if they qualify, and if the answer is yes, they should review the published standards and blueprint to identify any perceived

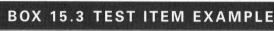

BOX 15.3 TEST ITEM EXAMPLE

What would be the appropriate verb according to Bloom's Taxonomy for an objective related to assessing competency of a procedure using a hybrid-simulated experience integrating standardized patients and a partial trainer?

A. Explain

B. Choose

C. Apply

D. Identify

Answer: B. Choose is a high-level action verb requiring an individual to make and defend his/her judgments.

SOURCE: Bloom's Taxonomy Action Verbs (n.d.). Retrieved from www.clemson.edu/assessment/assessmentpractices/referencematerials/documents/Blooms%20Taxonomy%20Action%20Verbs.pdf

area needing further review. For example, if they are not familiar with a specific simulation modality (for example, standardized patient), they would concentrate study time in this area. Remember, adult learning principles are integrated throughout the exam, requiring review of educational theorists such as Knowles, Kolb, and Levin. Box 15.3 provides an example of an item to assess an individual's understanding of Bloom's Taxonomy.

A recommended listing of articles and textbooks is available from the SSH's website. Other recommended online sites to assist studying include the NLN's Simulation Innovation Resource Center[2] and the Standards of Best Practice: Simulation through the INACSL website. Webinars providing an overview of the pedagogy and techniques of teaching with simulation are available through numerous organizations. For example, both SSH and INACSL provide and archive webinars, many of which are provided as a membership benefit. Additionally, programs are offered at various conferences to assist individuals in preparing for the certification exam for health care simulation educators. Additionally, review of test-taking strategies might be appropriate. Strategies are available from multiple reliable websites such as the testing site from the University of Minnesota–Duluth or the "Test Taking Strategies" from the Center for Academic Success at Southwestern University.[3]

If the candidates' answer to the eligibility question was no, they should develop a personalized "pathway to distinction" plan. This pathway should include a career trajectory with specific goals and a timeline to develop a personalized professional portfolio specific to simulation.

VALUE OF CERTIFICATION

Nursing and medical certification as a documentation of competence has existed for some time. (Although pharmacy and other types of health care providers have also

---

[2] www.nln.org/facultyprograms/simulation_tech.htm

[3] www.d.umn.edu/kmc/student/loon/acad/strat/test_take.html and www.southwestern.edu/offices/success/assistance/skilldevelopment/testtaking.php

developed certification processes, nursing and medicine have the longest history of certification and can therefore provide more lessons on the value of certification.) The creation of the American Board of Medical Specialties in 1934 was based on the premise that a physician who met certain established criteria in knowledge, skill, and experience would be a better specialist physician than those who did not meet the identified measures (Slogoff, Hughes, Hug, Longnecker, & Saidman, 1994). The American Board of Medical Specialties currently recognizes 24 medical boards and the American Board of Nursing Specialties (incorporated in 1991) recognizes 31 specialty nurse organizations.

Such widespread adoption of certification speaks to the perceived value of certification in health care. In fact, one nursing certification organization developed a "Perceived Value of Certification Tool" (PVCT), which has demonstrated validity and reliability (Byrne, Valentine, & Carter, 2004) and has been used in a number of nursing studies of certification (Haskins, Hnatiuk, & Yoder, 2011; Niebuhr & Biel, 2007; Sechrist, Valentine, & Berlin, 2006). Although the value of simulation educator certification has yet to be proven, it is likely that the same types of values that are attributed to nursing and medical certification are, or will be, attributable to simulation educator certification. In this section, the value of certification as described for nursing and medicine is extrapolated to the value of certification for a health care simulation educator.

A number of authors have characterized the value of certification in nursing and medicine. Indeed, some of the descriptions relate directly to elements of the PVCT. The descriptive terms include: intrinsic value, empowerment, enhanced collaboration, competence and expertise, (patient) satisfaction, (patient) outcomes or quality of care, employment and compensation (Kaplow, 2011; Miller & Boyle, 2008; Sechrist et al., 2006; Wade, 2009). Clearly, several of these classifications are defined clinically, but it is not much of a stretch to translate patient satisfaction and outcomes to learner satisfaction and outcomes.

Certainly the easiest area in which to draw parallels to simulation educator certification is that of intrinsic value to the individual attaining certification. In nursing studies using the PVCT, substantial majorities of certified and noncertified nurses participating in the study expressed strong agreement with statements about certification, such as:

- Enhances feeling of personal accomplishment
- Validates specialized knowledge
- Enhances professional credibility
- Indicates level of clinical competence
- Enhances personal confidence in clinical abilities (Haskins et al., 2011; Sechrist et al., 2006).

Although an equivalent tool for assessing the value of board certification among physicians does not exist, several surveys have reported on the value of certification for physicians. In these studies, a majority of responding physicians express that board-certified physicians are perceived as more competent by peers and patients or that certification was important to maintain a professional image (Culley, Sun, Harman, & Warner, 2013; Lipner et al., 2006). It is also likely that certification as a simulation educator will result in similar intrinsic value to the participant.

Empowerment and enhanced collaboration are cited in the nursing literature as benefits to certification. Wade (2009) described empowerment as related to the perceptions of formal and informal power on a nursing unit. In eight of nine studies that Wade reviewed, certification was positively associated with perceived nursing empowerment. Likewise, Wade found that seven of eight studies associated nursing certification with improvements in both team and physician–nurse communication and collaboration. Given that simulation can be viewed as an "extra" or an extravagance in some organizations, the professional certification designation is likely to result in similar degrees of empowerment and improvement in interdisciplinary interactions. This is particularly so as the vast majority of simulation educators are and will be nurses.

Improvement in patient satisfaction is one of the benefits ascribed to nursing certification, although only 25 percent or fewer internists associated certification with improved patient satisfaction (Kaplow, 2011; Lipner et al., 2006; Wade, 2009). In the case of simulation educator certification, it is likely that improvements in learner satisfaction will be of significant value to the participant. Ongoing evaluation of simulation-based education is a best practice for simulation and is typically a component of the individual educator's evaluation. It is frequently used as a means of evaluating the simulation program performance and determining program funding. Certification's emphasis on adult education and experiential learning and best practices for simulation education are likely to result in measurable improvements in learner satisfaction.

Competence and perceptions of competence are cited by nurses and physicians as a major value associated with certification. Most studies related to certification and competence address perceived competence or competence as related to test performance. In these types of studies, certification is typically associated with improved competence or improved test scores related to those who are not certified (including nurses and physicians) (Culley et al., 2013; Kaplow, 2011; Ramsey et al., 1989; Wade, 2009).

It is more difficult to demonstrate that certification is associated with better patient outcomes, but there are a few studies that show this. There is evidence that increasing proportions of certified staff nurses in intensive care units are inversely related to the number of falls, frequency of urinary tract infections, and medication administration errors (Kendall-Gallagher & Blegen, 2009). In one study, board-certified surgeons performing colon resections had significantly lower morbidity and mortality rates compared with noncertified surgeons (Prystowsky, Bordage, & Feinglass, 2002). Likewise, patients experiencing a myocardial infarction and cared for by board-certified internists and cardiologists had a 19 percent lower mortality rate compared with patients cared for by nonboard-certified physicians (Norcini, Lipner, & Kimball, 2002). In the case of simulation, the challenge will be to demonstrate a relationship between simulation-based education conducted by a certified educator and improved learner competence and translation to clinical settings. This will be difficult for several reasons. Simulation-based research is growing, and there are increasing numbers of examples of the relationship of simulation-based education to improvements in clinical outcomes. However, it is unlikely that a randomized controlled trial comparing the outcomes of a certified educator with those of a noncertified educator will be conducted. It may be that we will only be able to retrospectively identify programs or curriculum that use certified educators and are successful in accomplishing clinical translational research. This will be indirect evidence at best.

In practical terms, there is a belief that professional certification will be of value to employers (perhaps even a prerequisite for employment) as well as result in increased compensation for certified simulation educators. The nursing literature describes that

BOX 15.4 EVIDENCE-BASED PRACTICE: THE IMPACT OF NURSES' CERTIFICATION ON PATIENT OUTCOMES AND WORKPLACE SATISFACTION

Evidence-Based Practice

This study investigated (1) whether the ratio of certified nurses on a unit affected nurse-sensitive patient outcomes and (2) if certification influenced the nurses' perception of overall workplace employment.

Study

A nonexperimental, correlational, descriptive design surveyed 866 nurses working in intensive care units. Outcome data were collected using the Work Effectiveness Questionnaire-II and three nurse-sensitive outcomes.

Findings

No significant relationship was identified between the numbers of certified nurses on a specific unit to patient outcomes, but a positive, statistically significant relationship was identified between certification and the nurses' perception of overall workplace employment.

Nursing Considerations

The study identified the importance of specific work factors that promote overall workplace employment which could impact nurse retention.

SOURCE: Krapohl, G., Manojlovich, M., Redman, R., & Zhang, L. (2010). Nursing specialty certification and nursing-sensitive patient outcomes in the intensive care unit. *American Journal of Critical Care, 19*(6), 490–498.

nursing certification results in a perception of improved marketability among certified nurses, but the results for increasing compensation are mixed (Niebuhr & Biel, 2007; Sechrist et al., 2006). Although some hospitals report a 15 percent differential for certified nurses, others report no difference in salaries for certified and noncertified nurses (Kaplow, 2010). However, some hospitals do provide reimbursement for continuing education, paid time off, and career advancement opportunities for nursing certification (Niebuhr & Biel, 2007). See Box 15.4 for an evidence-based practice study.

Among physicians, board certification is often required as a condition of employment or insurance reimbursement and may be associated with improved compensation as well (Culley et al., 2013; Lipner et al., 2006). It is still early in the course of simulation educator certification and as such it is not yet clear if certification will be associated with improved employability and compensation. Given that currently there is no particular degree or training course that is required or associated with simulation education professionals, it is possible that the certification designation will serve as a proxy for completion of a particular degree or training program.

Although much of this section has examined the positive values associated with certification, physicians and nurses have also identified negative aspects of certification. For both groups, these are reflected in concerns about the cost of certification, inability to prepare for an exam, the process of test taking, and the inability to get to a location where the exam is offered or to get time off to take the exam (Haskins et al., 2011). In addition, physicians also voice concerns about the cost of certification as well as the ongoing requirements of maintenance of certification, viewed as confusing by many physicians (Culley et al., 2013; Lipner et al., 2006).

Certification of simulation educators is in its very early stages. Simulation educator certification has just begun to be awarded. Although there are lessons that can be adapted from certification in other health care fields, it is also clear that the value of simulation certification will likely include unique elements that we cannot even imagine at this time.

FUTURE PROJECTION

Continuous modification of the certification process, policies, and exams is mandatory for a certification program to be successful. An annual gap analysis is recommended to assess achievement of goals and identify strategies to close any identified gaps. For example, if goals were not met, the analysis should identify the cause and determine appropriate modification in the action plan to achieve the goals. Modification in the action plan might include extending the project timeline across several fiscal years to assist with financial feasibility, hiring additional personnel to promote customer satisfaction and efficiency of the certification process

Periodic review and update of the exams must be integrated into the timeline. This review should include a practice analysis to determine current professional practice. Test banks will need to be critiqued, modified, and increased by subject-matter experts to ensure current best practices are reflected in the exams. To ensure updates are appropriate, the practice analysis and test bank modifications are recommended to be conducted every three to five years. Continuous review and update might require periodic review of the practice analysis to reflect current professional practice and by subject-matter experts to ensure the exam reflects current accurate practice and measurement principles.

In the near future a commission on certification will need to be developed to govern the certification program. A commission would provide oversight of a certification program and be required to be legally and administratively autonomous for the organization. A governing body should be established to have authority to determine policies and procedures related to the certification program. In order for the commission to be accredited, guidelines by accreditation agencies will need to be followed as the commission is designed. These guidelines should reflect the practice standards for professional certification programs. For example, the National Commission of Certifying Agencies created by the ICE requires "demonstration of a valid and reliable process for development, implementation, maintenance, and governance of certification programs" (ICE, 2013).

SUMMARY

Education of health care professionals has changed during the past decade due to multiple contributing factors including a shortage of qualified faculty, insufficient clinical placement opportunities for student learning, and outdated curricula. Patient safety issues and mandates set by accreditation agencies demand a paradigm shift to evidence-based educational strategies. The proposed educational transformation required to prepare a workforce for the dynamic health care environment requires educators to (1) promote active learning strategies, (2) design supportive, collaborative, authentic learning environments, and (3) validate learning outcomes and competency attainment. Health care providers must be given the tools and experiences to provide safe, quality patient care.

Key Concepts

- Simulation has been identified by professional organizations, accreditation bodies, and funding agencies as one solution to these challenges.
- An evidence-based certification program specific to the pedagogy of simulation has been developed and validated by international experts representing multiple organizations. Certification allows health care simulation educators a mechanism to demonstrate their competency and be recognized for their unique knowledge and skills. Each certification available through the certification program has specific eligibility requirements, identified objectives and blueprint, and a specific assessment process.
- The identified value of obtaining certification identified by health care providers includes promoting (1) career advancement, (2) learner fulfillment, and (3) patient satisfaction and quality, safe patient care.

References

Academy of Medical Educators (AOME). (2012). *Professional standards*. London: Author.

Altman, M. (2011). Let's get certified: Best practices for nurse leaders to create a culture of certification. *AACN Advanced Critical Care, 22*(1), 68–75.

American Nurses Credentialing Center (ANCC). (2009). Nursing excellence. Your journey. Our passion. Retrieved from http://ancc.nursecredentialing.org/FunctionalCategory/AboutANCC/ANCC-Overview-Brochure.aspx

Barnum, S. B. (1997). Licensure, certification, and accreditation. *Online Journal of Issues in Nursing, 2*(3). Retrieved from www.nursingworld.org/MainMenuCategories/ANAMarketplace/ANAPeriodicals/OJIN/TableofContents/Vol21997/No3Aug97/LicensureCertificationandAccreditation.aspx

Briggs, L. A., Brown, H., Kesten, K., & Heath, J. (2006). Certification: A benchmark for critical care nursing excellence. *Critical Care Nurse, 26*(6), 47–53.

Buckley, S., Coleman, J., Davidson, I., Khan, K. S., Zamora, J., Malick, S., Pollard, D., Ashcroft, T., Popovic, C., & Sayer, J. (2009). The educational effects of portfolios on undergraduate student learning: A best evidence medical education (BEME) systematic review. BEME guide no 11. *Medical Teacher, 31*(4), 282–298.

Byrne, M., Valentine, W., & Carter, S. (2004). The value of certification—a research journey. *AORN Journal, 79*(4), 825–828, 831–835.

Culley, D. J., Sun, H., Harman, A. E., & Warner, D. O. (2013). Perceived value of board certification and the Maintenance of Certification in Anesthesiology Program (MOCA(R)). *Journal of Clinical Anesthesia, 25*(1), 12–19.

Doyle, E. L., Caro, C. M., Lysoby, L., Auld, M. E., Smith, B. J., & Muenzen, P. M. (2012). The national health educator job analysis 2010: Process and outcomes. *Health Education & Behavior, 39*(6), 695–708.

Haskins, M., Hnatiuk, C. N., & Yoder, L. H. (2011). Medical-surgical nurses' perceived value of certification study. *Medsurg Nursing, 20*(2), 71–77, 93.

Institute for Credentialing Excellence (ICE). (2005). National commission for certifying agencies standards for the accreditation of certification. Retrieved from www. credentialing excellence.org/p/cm/ld/fid=15

Institute for Credentialing Excellence (ICE). (2012). Certification vs. certification. Retrieved from www.credentialing excellence.org/p/cm/ld/fid=4

Institute for Credentialing Excellence (ICE). (2013). NCCA accreditation. Retrieved from www.credentialingexcellence.org/ncca

Kaplow, R. (2011). The value of certification. *AACN Advanced Critical Care, 22*(1), 25–32.

Kendall-Gallagher, D., & Blegen, M. A. (2009). Competitive and certification of registered nurses and safety of patients in intensive care units. Patient safety issue. *American Journal of Critical Care, 18*(2), 106–116.

Knapp, J., Fabrey, L., Rops, M., & McCurry, N. (2006). Basic guide to credentialing terminology. Retrieved from www.credentialingexcellence.org/p/cm/ld/fid=14

Knapp, L. G., & Knapp. J. E. (2002). *The business of certification a comprehensive guide to developing a successful program.* Washington, DC: American Society of Associate Executives.

Lipner, R. S., Bylsma, W. H, Arnold, G. K., Fortna, G. S., Tooker, J., & Cassel, C. K. (2006). Who is maintaining certification in internal medicine—and why? A national survey 10 years after initial certification. *Annals of Internal Medicine, 144*(1), 29–36.

Miller, P. A., & Boyle, D. K. (2008). Nursing specialty certification: A measure of expertise. *Nursing Management, 39*(10), 10–16.

National League for Nursing (NLN). (2011). *Certification for nurse educators.* Retrieved from www.nln.org/certification/index.htm

Niebuhr, B., & Biel, M. (2007). The value of specialty nursing certification. *Nursing Outlook, 55*(4), 176–181.

Norcini, J. J., Lipner, R. S., & Kimball, H. R. (2002). Certifying examination performance and patient outcomes following acute myocardial infarction. *Medical Education, 36*(9), 853–859.

Prystowsky, J. B., Bordage, G., & Feinglass, J. M. (2002). Patient outcomes for segmental colon resection according to surgeon's training, certification, and experience. *Surgery, 132*(4), 663–672.

Ramsey, P. G., Carline, J. D., Inui, T. S., Larson, E. B., LoGerfo, J. P., & Wenrich, M. D. (1989). Predictive validity of certification by the American Board of Internal Medicine. *Annals of Internal Medicine, 110*(9), 7197–7226.

Sechrist, K. R., Valentine, W., & Berlin, L. E. (2006). Perceived value of certification among certified, noncertified, and administrative perioperative nurses. *Journal of Professional Nursing, 22*(4), 242–247.

Slogoff, S., Hughes, F. P., Hug, C. C., Longnecker, D. E., & Saidman L. J. (1994). A demonstration of validity for certification by the American Board of Anesthesiology. *Academic Medicine, 69*(9), 740–746.

Society for Simulation in Healthcare (SSH). (2013a). Accreditation program. Accreditation information guide. Retrieved from www.ssih.org/uploads/static_pages/PDFs/Accred/2013

Society for Simulation in Healthcare (SSH). (2013b). Certification program. Standards and elements for CHSE. Retrieved from https://www.ssih.org/certification/handbook

Stomborg, M. F., Niebuhr, B., Prevost, S., Fabrey, L., Muenzen, P., Spence, C., Towers, J., & Valentine, W. (2005). More than a title. *Nursing Management, 36*(5), 36–46.

Wade, C. H. (2009). Perceived effects of specialty nurse certification: A review of the literature. *AORN Journal, 89*(1), 183–192.

16

Incorporating an Electronic Health Record and Other Technologies into Simulations

E. LaVerne Manos, DNP, RN-BC
Helen B. Connors, PhD, RN, DrPS (HON), FAAN
April J. Roche, MBA, CPEHR

■ Learning Objectives

1. Summarize the rationale for integrating the electronic health record and other technologies with simulation.
2. Discuss the organizational and pedagogical framework for technology integration.
3. Describe selected scenarios that integrate technology tools with simulation.

■ Key Terms

- Academic electronic health record
- Electronic health record
- Learning health system
- Nursing informatics
- Organizational culture
- Pedagogy

Use of information and communication technologies such as the **electronic health record** (EHR), simulation, and other related technologies should be integrated into the health professional's curriculum, not an add-on to an already over-crowded program of study. These technologies are increasingly prevalent in health care practice today, so it is beyond time to meaningfully use the technologies for teaching and learning in the curriculum for nursing and other health professionals. Haugen (2012) points out that the next logical step to achieving quality health care outcomes and improving patient care is to ensure that caregivers are using the technology consistently and accurately. What better way to accomplish this goal than to incorporate the various technologies, including an **academic EHR** (AEHR) with reality-based simulated experiences throughout the curriculum in an integrated fashion that engages the learner and advances desired competencies for practice. An AEHR is a reality-based clinical information system specifically designed to support the health professional curriculum by following education workflow and developing informatics competencies for nurses and other health professionals (Connors, 2006; Connors, Warren, & Weaver, 2007; Warren & Connors, 2007; Warren, Manos, Meyer, & Roache, 2013; Warren, Meyer, Thompson, & Roche, 2010).

OVERVIEW AND BACKGROUND

For over a decade, significant forces and resources have been directed at utilization of technology to improve the quality, safety, efficiency, and effectiveness of health care, yet the integration of the technology in practice has been slow to follow. The Health Information Technology for Economic and Clinical Health Act of 2009 provided the framework and financial incentives (approximately $20 billion) to drive the vision for the meaningful use of health information technology and to develop both a Nationwide Health Information Network and a learning health system.

Nursing Informatics and the AEHR

Health care is information intensive. Management of large amounts of data and information requires automation through use of technology. Every facet of health care and health care education is changing because of technology. At the core of this change are informaticians including nurse informatics specialists. **Nursing informatics** is one of the indirect care provider specializations that facilitates the integration of data, information, knowledge, and wisdom to support decision making in clinical areas. Nursing informatics also supports standardization to improve information management and secondary use of data and information.

Data, information, knowledge, and wisdom are the metastructures that support nursing practice. As the continuum of these metastructures unfolds, increased understanding is revealed. Successful secondary uses of health data by researchers is dependent on the ease in which the appropriate data can be located and harvested at the time of need (Waitman, Warren, Manos, & Connolly, 2011). Data utilization should not be restricted to operational need or to dissemination of knowledge to the care providers; it should also extend to the direct support of research and quality improvement (Piwowar, Becich, Bilofsky, & Crowley, 2008). Electronic data are being collected on patients in the context of health care interactions. These data are already being used by health care systems and practices for administrative and operational needs. They provide an opportunity for us to learn about what care interventions are best and how patients and populations will fare over time. In the past, research and practice have been separated because it was believed there were different interests at play. In reality there is a continuum where we are using data all the time and health care is always growing.

Creation of a **learning health system** is a national goal. The Institute of Medicine's report "Best Care at Lower Cost" advises the need to "[e]xpand commitment to the goals of a continuously learning health care system. Continuous learning and improvement should be a core and constant priority for all participants in health care—patients, families, clinicians, care leaders, and those involved in supporting their work" (Smith, Saunders, Stuckhardt, & McGinnis, 2013, p. 10). To reach this goal, there must be alignment of informatics, science, policy and incentives, health care guidelines, continuous improvement, and innovation.

The data from individual patients and documentation of care must be constantly gathered, analyzed, and transformed into information and knowledge with the end goal of utilization for the purposes of current care of the patient and for a secondary purpose of improving population health and health care (Grossman & McGinnis, 2011). A learning health care system is centric to patient and family needs and encourages the inclusion of patients, families, and caregivers as fundamental members of the continuously learning care team. According to the Institute of Medicine's report "Best Care at Lower Cost," "[p]atients and families should be given the opportunity to be fully engaged participants at all levels, including individual care decisions, health system learning and improvement activities, and community-based interventions to promote health" (Smith et al., 2013, p. 5).

The fundamental changes in health care create a need for better ways to manage information and demands and that health care and education embrace technology as a way to manage data and information. Because of increasing technology in practice and changing policy and drivers for technology, students must have the opportunity to learn about and embrace technology and informatics methodologies and concepts. Informatics must have a prominent place in learning. The AEHR in simulation parallels practice. Soon there will be no other way to document care that is given except in the EHR. Learners must be exposed to the AEHR in simulation and as a simulation itself. When the AEHR is used in simulation, it provides a way to introduce informatics methodologies, concepts, and skills beyond navigation of software. Learners gain an understanding of data and input together with policy, guidelines, and continuous improvement as a by-product of AEHR use in simulation. Learners, while achieving clinical learning objectives, also have the opportunity to learn about and achieve quality, safety, and informatics competencies.

ORGANIZATIONAL AND PEDAGOGICAL FRAMEWORK FOR AEHR

Numerous organizations and workgroups within and outside nursing currently are leading this change to support health professional education reform. Table 16.1 targets some main initiatives directed at developing informatics and technology competencies for practice in the 21st century. Several of these reform initiatives have been the drivers for integrating enhanced technology criteria into revised accreditation standards (e.g., National League for Nursing's Accrediting Commission, Commission on Collegiate Nursing Education), certification programs, and licensure requirements for health professionals. These forces of change are compelling schools of nursing to rethink their curriculum and teaching approaches.

Despite these efforts to reform education, according to the Institute of Medicine's (2010) "The Future of Nursing" (2010) report, faculty reluctance has been cited as the largest barrier to greater integration of technology into the nursing curriculum. Perhaps

TABLE 16.1

Forces for Change

Initiative	Purpose
Technology and Informatics Guiding Education Reform (TIGER)	The TIGER initiative addresses a set of skills that is needed by practicing nurses and nursing students to fully engage in the unfolding digital electronic era in health care.
Quality and Safety in Nursing Education (QSEN)	The QSEN project addresses the challenge of preparing future nurses with the knowledge, skills, and attitudes (KSAs) necessary to continuously improve the quality and safety of the health care systems.
American Medical Informatics Association (AMIA) 10X10	The AMIA 10X10 program uses online courses to address the education and training of a new generation of clinical, public health, research, and translational bioinformatics informaticians to lead the transformation of the American health care system.
Health Resources and Services Administration (HRSA) Integrated Technology into Nursing Education and Practice (ITNEP)	The ITNEP initiative supported nursing collaboratives for faculty development in the use of information and other technologies (informatics, simulation, telehealth, and e-learning) in order to expand the capacity of collegiate schools of nursing to educate students for 21st-century health care practice.
Office of the National Coordinator (ONC) Health IT Workforce Development Program	The Health IT Workforce Development Program was designed to educate and train health IT professionals to help providers implement electronic health records to improve health care quality, safety, and cost-effectiveness. The Health IT Workforce Curriculum consists of 20 components.

this is because faculty are not the only component that has to change—the organization and the pedagogy must change as well to successfully support faculty to integrate technology and actively engage learners. This is an immense challenge for many academic institutions, especially those steeped in a tradition of hierarchical beliefs where research and scholarship are rewarded and educational innovation is not.

Organizational Culture

Each institution has an **organizational culture** that drives much of the organizational structure and individuals' behaviors within the institution. Changing individual behaviors without attention to the culture usually does not accomplish the desired outcome because the behaviors and the culture are in conflict. Integrating technology through innovative teaching strategies in the curriculum requires creating an environment that fosters success with innovative education. To fully integrate a culture of innovation within the organization, key concepts of innovation need to be reflected in the organization's mission, vision, leadership, core values, hiring practices, metrics, rewards, and compensation. Faculty and staff in this environment should feel comfortable and supported to take risks without fear of failure or retribution.

Pedagogical Framework

Pedagogy is a broad term that includes multiple theories of learning. When integrating technology into the curriculum, we should not use the technology just because it is available, but rather because it is a best fit with the pedagogy and enhances the learning outcomes. Many times technology is forced into the curriculum with little attention to the pedagogy. Technology such as the AEHR accommodates a variety of learning styles and when meaningfully used can best support constructivist learning theories (Warren et al., 2010). Many of today's instructional technologies support constructivism principles of learning by creating learning environments that challenge learners to engage in the process and to become more self-directed. For example, the AEHR and other technologies coupled with appropriate teaching strategies built on sound pedagogical principles can create powerful learning experiences and outcomes.

INTEGRATING TECHNOLOGIES WITH SIMULATION

The following examples demonstrate how EHRs and other technologies can be incorporated into learning to simulate real-world documentation and data management. Each exemplar is described along with its purpose and outcomes.

EV1000 Sims with iClickers

In this scenario, the hospital staff development nurses collaborated with the school of nursing clinical learning lab director and staff to develop a simulation integrating multiple forms of technology: iClickers, EV1000 software, and Laerdal's Classic SimMan®. The EV1000 software, developed by Edwards Life Sciences, simulates the use of newer hemodynamic monitors in real-time clinical practice. By integrating this software with Laerdal's Classic SimMan technology, participants are able to replicate hemodynamic values generated by more sophisticated technology in practice. Both software programs run simultaneously during the simulation, controlling the responses of a high-fidelity manikin.

Although literature supporting simulation in health care education is abundant, a recognized limitation is the small number of people who can physically participate in the action. Recent literature (WHO, 2010) suggests that observing other students performing a simulation exercise maximizes the effect of the simulation. Based on this literature, an audience response system (iClickers) was integrated to drive nursing interventions during a real-time simulation.

Objectives

1. Accurately interpret hemodynamic parameters.
2. Implement appropriate nursing interventions based on hemodynamic parameters.
3. Integrate functional hemodynamic measures in managing the patient with shock.

During the simulation, a patient (SimMan) presents with occult hemorrhagic shock. Bedside critical care nurses were elicited to serve as actors caring for the patient with their actions driven by the audience participation. Hemodynamic parameters and basic vital signs were projected onto a large screen for the entire audience to view. Audience members signaled a simulation timeout by ringing a bell when they recognized a clinical situation that required intervention. A PowerPoint slide was then displayed providing a list of several possible interventions that could be implemented, and the participants were asked to identify their desired intervention using the audience response system (iClickers). Results were displayed and the most popular intervention was performed by the actors in the scenario, causing an authentic alteration in the patient's parameters.

Learning About Quality Through EHR Queries

In response to the need for a broader vision of the concept of simulation, faculty from a school of nursing partnered with an informatics specialist to develop a learning activity that incorporated simulation, beyond manikins into a didactic course in a classroom setting. Approximately 100 undergraduate nursing students in a quality improvement course participated in this AEHR simulation. Students performed chart reviews navigating the AEHR for the purpose of assessing whether care provided and documentation met the core measures of heart failure. The activity involved identifying different types of data, structured versus nonstructured, and the power of querying a database. Informatics learning was a by-product of the carefully structured activity that was intentionally designed for the informatics "ah-ha moment" to be achieved at the conclusion of the simulation. Although the task was designed for undergraduate nursing students, the assignment could be generalized for a number of other health care professions for both undergraduate and graduate programs.

Objectives

1. Describe appropriate measurement tools and processes for quality indicators of heart failure.
2. Evaluate data from various information sources that inform the delivery of care.
3. Understand how differences between structured and nonstructured data affect discoverability and knowledge generation.

The simulation setting was in a core curriculum course involving quality improvement content presented to second-semester junior nursing students. This exercise involved students auditing medical records to assess an institution's compliance with core measures. Prior learning activities introduced the concept of core measures and reimbursement structures based on compliance with these measures. The learning activity focused on the quality of care for heart failure patients. Students were provided with an audit tool to record whether the patient documentation met or did not meet each heart failure criterion. The class collectively reviewed four cases in an AEHR. Two patient records contained entirely scanned documents and two patient records were documented as discrete data. The learning activity allowed students to explore the advantages of structured data and the natural link between quality and informatics. The learners discovered the value of using information and technology to communicate, manage knowledge, mitigate error, and support decision making.

The achievement of the stated learning objectives supported the quality, safety, and efficiency goals of the Institute of Medicine and subsequently the quality and safety education for nurses (Leonard, Graham, & Bonacum, 2004) and health care and education accrediting bodies. In today's world, students are increasingly sophisticated in navigating technology; for example, most know how to tweet, social network, text, and play video games. Therefore, instead of needing to instruct learners on "clicking" or navigation of systems, this opportunity lies in taking technology education to the next level. Using the AEHR in the classroom engages students in active learning and reinforces informatics competencies beyond pointing and clicking. Learners gain knowledge many professionals do not have, even after several years of exposure to the EHR system. Students exposed to this broader vision of simulation expressed understanding of why structured data are meaningful and how to appreciate the efficiency that technology can bring to the workplace. Learners are less likely to perform workarounds in practice that could not only compromise patient outcomes and quality initiatives but could also destroy the ability to reuse EHR data.

Learning How to Work in Teams: Using Technology Tools

The Cara Morgan case is an example of an **interprofessional** simulation where **Team-STEPPS®** (Team Strategies and Tools to Enhance Performance and Patient Safety)[1] tools are incorporated with the scenario. The interprofessional team includes undergraduate nursing students, medical and pharmacy students, pediatric residents, and on some occasions respiratory therapy students.

Objectives

1. Describe examples of the impact of team functioning on safety and quality of care.
2. Explain how authority gradients influence teamwork and patient safety.
3. Follow communication styles that diminish the risks associated with authority gradients among team members.
4. Communicate with team members, adapting their own style of communicating to needs of the team and situation.

---

[1] http://teamstepps.ahrq.gov/

Cara Morgan presents to the emergency department with a fever. Upon reviewing her record in the AEHR, students learn Cara has not been immunized due to her parents' religious beliefs. The medical and pharmacy students meet and work together to write admission orders, including medications, for Cara. Nursing students then review the chart and orders placed prior to participation in the simulation. When the simulation occurs, students from all professions meet at a designated time to participate. The team of students works together to provide care for Cara, including a lumbar puncture on the manikin. During the simulation, one of the nursing students documents in the AEHR the assessment and procedures being completed for Cara, creating real-time documentation of the team's actions.

Collaborating to Unfold and Connect

The National League for Nursing (NLN) developed several unfolding cases that evolve over time in an unpredictable manner for the learners. The "Advancing Care Excellence for Seniors" (ACES) cases are currently available for educators to borrow and integrate into simulations. The veterans cases, developed through a partnership with the NLN and the Veterans Administration, are currently being piloted by several universities and eventually will be released for others to use. With all of the unfolding cases, new situations are revealed with each encounter, and each encounter can be integrated in multiple ways within a curriculum. At the University of Kansas, cases have been built into the AEHR. Prior to participating in simulation, students are required to review the AEHR. The electronic chart is available throughout the simulation and used for documentation as required by the scenario. Below is an example of how these cases are used.

Objectives

1. Describe examples of the impact of team functioning on safety and quality of care.

2. Implement holistic, patient-centered care that reflects an understanding of human growth and development, pathophysiology, pharmacology, medical management, and nursing management across the health–illness continuum, across the lifespan, and in all health care settings.

3. Using the TeamSTEPPS format, communicate observations or concerns related to hazards and errors to patients, families, and the health care team.

The NLN ACES case implemented at the University of Kansas contains three scenarios for patient Butch Sampson. The scenarios are simulated back to back over the course of three hours as part of the clinical makeup time for second-semester junior level students. Butch is a Vietnam veteran who had a toe amputated and is dealing with lifestyle issues, including poor diet and smoking. The goal for these three simulations is for students to educate Butch on healthier lifestyle habits while providing both inpatient and home health care.

Root Cause Analysis: Where Simulation Meets Information Management

The patient simulation for Maria Ruiz is an interprofessional simulation between nursing and health information management (HIM) students revolving around completing a root cause analysis of a medication error involving the EHR.

Objectives

1. Use principles of safe medication administration (six rights).
2. Demonstrate understanding of opioid effects and side effects.
3. Implement patient teaching regarding urolithiasis prevention as appropriate.

The simulation begins with second-semester junior nursing students reviewing Maria's chart in the AEHR and then providing care for Maria. The scenario includes an order given electronically via the AEHR during the simulation for an overdose of a pain medication. Instead of giving a verbal order for the pain medication, the provider tells the nursing student over the phone that she will be inputting the order in the chart and to refresh the patient's chart to review the order. Once the chart is refreshed, the order appears. At this point, it is up to the team of nursing students providing care to review the order and either administer or not administer the medication (as it is an overdose). Most teams administer the medication without further thought as the patient is loudly vocalizing her discomfort and her daughter/son, played by another student, is also loudly advocating for the patient to receive the medication; it is an extremely high pressure situation. During the debriefing session, the HIM students are introduced. The nursing students discover that the HIM students observed the simulation and are there to help lead the team through a root cause analysis of either the drug overdose or the near miss.

Teaching Teamwork and Collaboration with Simulation

Teaching the skills of collaboration and teamwork to those who will graduate as collaborative practice–ready professionals is crucial to the future quality of health care. If we are to educate for practice, then interprofessional education (IPE) must be used throughout health care professions education. The World Health Organization describes IPE as follows: "Interprofessional education occurs when students from two or more professions learn about, from and with each other to enable effective collaboration and improve health outcomes" (WHO, 2010, p. 7). The following simulation scenarios are in the planning stage; therefore, objectives have not been established at this time.

Using the NLN's ACES cases, faculty representing many disciplines come together to plan the activities: pharmacy, nurse practitioner, health information management, occupational therapy, physical therapy, nutrition, and health informatics. The group decides on usage of a simulation including synchronous and asynchronous components. Student numbers, availability on campus versus distance learners, and education levels of the students are discussed. From these discussions, decisions are made on the number of simulations and student groups as well as the configuration of each interprofessional group. The technology includes the AEHR and the use of a live meeting functionality. The AEHR has an internal communication function so when a student signs in, a question can pop up somewhat like a sticky note from another profession. This functionality will be used as an asynchronous communication path. The students are given a "group" room in a live meeting software, and each will have the ability to create and schedule meetings with the interprofessional group as he or she negotiates times and schedules for synchronous meetings.

This IPE simulation centers around a patient record in the AEHR based on Red Yoder, an ACES unfolding case. The students are introduced to one another using the AEHR clinical notes functionality. (This is a purely educational use of this functionality; in practice this usage would not exist because only patient data would be entered or merged into the clinical notes tab in the EHR. However, in the academic setting, this functionality can be used to give students an overview of the roles and responsibilities of each profession before the simulation starts.)

The simulation begins with nurse practitioner students examining a standardized patient who matches the case study, and they document the findings and implement an interprofessional plan of care. Each profession completes its documentation based on the case study. Once the documentation is finished, HIM does a chart review and sends questions out to their group in any way they would like to communicate, including sticky notes or synchronous meeting. Health informatics students serve as a resource for navigation and functionality of the AEHR. The health informatics students are instructed to create meetings to meet their needs. They may need a quick meeting with one other professional group or a meeting with everyone involved. As questions come up, it is their call whom they would likely need to meet with to have the issue resolved.

SUMMARY

Health care is information intensive. Management of large amounts of data and information requires automation through the use of technology. The best way to teach health professionals to work in patient-centered, technology-rich environments is to integrate the technology and the competencies into their education. The role of simulation and other technology in nursing education has evolved from the simple use of a simulator to teaching basic skills to the integration of a versatile set of learning tools that change how students learn skills and competencies for 21st-century practice throughout the curriculum and within interprofessional teams. This chapter presented several examples of the use of the AEHR with simulation; however, this is just the tip of the iceberg.

■ Key Concepts

- Educating health professional students today requires the integration of an academic electronic health record and other technologies with simulation to ensure that graduates are using the technology consistently and accurately.
- The utilization of technology is promised to improve the quality, safety, efficiency, and effectiveness of health care.

- The Health Information Technology for Economic and Clinical Health Act provided the framework and financial incentives to drive the vision for the meaningful use of health information technology and to develop a Nationwide Health Information Network and a learning health system.
- A learning health system aligns science, informatics, incentives, and culture for continuous quality improvement and innovations.
- Nursing informatics skills and tools are important components of developing a learning health system to support quality health care.
- To successfully integrate technology into the curriculum, attention must be paid to the organizational culture and the pedagogical principles of learning.
- The AEHR and other technology tools coupled with appropriate teaching strategies built on sound pedagogical principles can create powerful learning experiences and outcomes.
- Learning in interprofessional teams can be done through simulations in addition to the incorporation of EHR and other activities involving informatics.

References

Connors, H. R. (2006). Transforming the nursing curriculum: Going paperless. In C. Weaver & C. Delaney (Eds.), *Nursing and informatics for the 21st century: An international look at the trends, cases, and the future* (pp. 183–194). Chicago, IL: Healthcare Information and Management Systems Society Press.

Connors, H. R., Warren, J. J., & Weaver, C. (2007). HIT plants SEEDS in healthcare education. *Nursing Administration Quarterly, 31*, 129–133.

Grossman, C., & McGinnis, J. M. (2011). *Digital infrastructure for the learning health system: The Foundation for Continuous Improvement in Health and Health Care: Workshop series summary.* Washington, DC: National Academies Press.

Haugen, H. (2102). The advantages of simulation training: how to improve EMR adoption. *Health Management Technology.* Retrieved from http://www.healthmgttech.com/ebook/201204/resources/12.htm

Institute of Medicine. (2010). *The future of nursing leading change, advancing health.* Washington, DC: National Academy of Sciences.

Leonard, M., Graham, S., & Bonacum, D. (2004). The human factor: the critical importance of effective teamwork and communication in providing safe care. *Quality and Safety in Health Care, 13*(Suppl 1), i85–i90.

Patterson, M. D., Blike, G. T., & Nadkarni, V. M. (2008). In situ simulation: Challenges and results. Advances in patient safety: New directions and alternative approaches. Retrieved from http://www.ahrq.gov/downloads/pub/advances2/vol3/advances-patterson_48.pdf

Piwowar, H. A., Becich, M. J., Bilofsky, H., & Crowley, R. S. (2008). Towards a data sharing culture: Recommendations for leadership from academic health centers. *PLoS Medicine, 5*(9), e183.

Smith, M., Saunders, R., Stuckhardt, L., & McGinnis, J. M. (Eds.). (2013). *Best care at lower cost: The path to continuously learning health care in America.* Washington, DC: National Academies Press.

Waitman, L. R., Warren, J. J., Manos, E. L., & Connolly, D. W. (2011, October). Expressing observations from electronic medical record flowsheets in an i2b2 clinical data repository to support research and quality improvement. Paper presented at the American Medical Informatics Association Annual Symposium, Washington, DC.

Warren, J. J., & Connors, H. R. (2007). Health information technology can and will transform nursing education. *Nursing Outlook, 55*(1), 59–60.

Warren, J. J., Manos, E. L., Meyer, M., & Roche, A. (2013). Integrating an academic electronic health record into simulations. In S. Campbell & K. Daley (Eds.), *Simulation scenarios for nursing educators: Making it real* (2nd ed., pp. 519–528). New York, NY: Springer.

Warren, J. J., Meyer, M. N., Thompson, T., & Roche, A. (2010). Transforming nursing education: Integrating informatics and simulations. In C. Weaver, C. Delaney, P. Weber, & R. Carr (Eds.), *Nursing and informatics for the 21st century: An international look at practice, trends and EHR technologies* (2nd ed., pp. 145–161). Chicago, IL: Healthcare Information and Management Systems Society.

World Health Organization (WHO). (2010). *Framework for action on interprofessional education & collaborative practice*. Geneva: Author. Retrieved from http://whqlibdoc.who.int/hq/2010/WHO_HRH_HPN_10.3_eng.pdf

17

Using Simulations to Promote Clinical Decision Making

Janet Willhaus, PhD, RN

Learning Objectives

1. Define terms from the literature that describe how nurses make decisions.
2. Identify valid and reliable instruments from the literature to evaluate learner decision making in simulation.
3. Describe tools and methods to assist learners develop decision-making skills before, during, and after simulation sessions.
4. Identify instruments and methods for measuring decision making in clinical practice.

Key Terms

- Clinical judgment
- Clinical reasoning
- Cognitive flexibility
- Critical thinking
- Situated cognition (also referred to as situated learning)

It is not enough to *know about* health and illness, nor is it enough to *know how* to perform nursing actions. *Knowing about* and *knowing how* must be coupled with *knowing when and which* nursing actions should take place. Simulation pedagogy offers opportunities for both cognitive and psychomotor practice and provides a vehicle to demonstrate **clinical nursing judgment** and **situated cognition**. Simulation scenarios, done with peers and a faculty mentor, followed by facilitated reflections, help students integrate performance, knowledge, and emotion into nursing action (Mariani, Cantrell, Meakim, Prieto, & Dreifurst, 2013).

Students are able to practice the **cognitive flexibility** required in patient-centered health care (Spiro, Feltovich, Jacobson, & Coulson, 1991) in an environment where mistakes can be discussed and corrected and do not result in threats to a real patient. A call for increased use of technology, specifically simulation, to help meet the needs of future nurses with problem-solving and **critical thinking** skills was one of the themes that emerged during the Institute of Medicine's forums on nursing education (IOM, 2011). Guiding students through a simulation to promote decision making requires access to expert practice knowledge and also expert experience in conducting simulations and debriefings.

SIMULATION WORK AND DECISION MAKING

Regardless of what the decision-making process is called, educators must first have a way to identify when it occurs successfully. Faculty who desire to evaluate or score students in decision making during simulations should seek valid and reliable instruments for this purpose.

Although the nursing process of assessment, diagnosis, planning, intervention, and evaluation describes the model for nursing care, it does not reflect the *way* nurses plan and formulate care. The "Thinking Like a Nurse" model by Tanner (2006) is based on four action-oriented activities: noticing, interpreting, responding, and reflecting. These four actions help guide students and nurses in both clinical and simulated settings. In 2007, the Lasater Clinical Judgment Rubric (LCJR) was developed using the "Thinking Like a Nurse" model to identify the level of nursing students' **clinical judgments** in simulations (Lasater, 2007). The LCJR instrument has been used in multiple studies since its release with valid and reliable results (Adamson, Gubrud, Sideras, & Lasater, 2012; Dillard et al., 2009; Jensen, 2013; Mariani, Cantrell, Meakim, Prieto, & Dreifurst, 2013).

Another valid and reliable instrument available with a component to measure critical thinking in simulation is the Creighton Simulation Evulation Instrument© (Adamson et al., 2011; Todd, Manz, Hawkings, Parsons, & Hercinger, 2008). An adaptation of this instrument, the Creighton Competency Evaluation Instrument©, is being used in the National Council of State Boards of Nursing's simulation study to evaluate students in both clinical and simulated settings (NCSBN, 2010).

Other instruments under development can be considered for use with video or computer-based simulation. Weatherspoon and Wyatt (2012) developed the Triage Acuity Instrument for use with computer-based simulations. A self-assessment scale for critical thinking in nursing is also under development and may be useful for simulations (Nair & Stamler, 2013). In a systematic review of simulation studies and **clinical reasoning** skills (Lapkin, Levett-Jones, Bellchambers, & Fernandez, 2010), only eight were found that measured clinical reasoning qualities such as knowledge acquisition, critical thinking, and the ability to identify deterierorating patients. Although faculty understand that decision making is an important skill, tools to measure this process are limited in both the simulated and practice settings.

TOOLS FOR PRACTICING DECISION MAKING

The goal of any simulation activity in nursing should be to promote learning and measure learning outcomes. Students learn nursing in three domains, which can be incorporated into simulations. *Cognitive learning* in nursing education is often obtained by listening to a lecture or reading and is traditionally tested by written or oral questioning.

Psychomotor learning comes from watching and then practicing hands-on skills either in a lab setting or on real patients. The *affective domain* of learning stems from the cultural, ethical, and emotional exposures a student will encounter. When testing any one of these domains independently, a student can readily demonstrate the desired learning; however, when combined, the domains offer a more complicated milieu for decision making. For example, a student may know *what* to do, but not know *how* to do it or may not have attained mastery in a needed skill. A student may have formulated a plan of action and then detoured from the plan when distracted by some emotional trigger such as the sight of bleeding, a loud noise, or a distinctive smell. Simulation allows the student to experience this confusing environment and gives practice in filtering distractions and honing the desired patient-centered actions.

Preparation Sheets

Some faculty believe that by telling the student what to study in advance, they are "giving away the surprise" of a simulation learning activity. Preparing for learning in the clinical environment, however, is a standard practice. Students are asked to review and practice specific skills, study certain medications or disease processes, and consider age and culture prior to most clinical experiences. Using preparation sheets for simulation activity is a similar process. A preparation sheet should give the student a set of objectives and a short summary of the scenario with the age, sex, and symptoms being experienced by the patient. It can include instructions on study of lab values, medications, and specific skills. (See Box 17.1 for a preparation sheet example.)

What we know about student learning in simulation is that the student, despite *knowing* what can happen, may still require several repetitions of practice before being able to coordinate the expected decision-making actions. In a study of nursing student actions during a cardiopulmonary arrest simulation, Linnard-Palmer (1995) found that even after practicing cardiopulmonary recusitation to 100 percent accuracy, approximately one month later, students required 6 to 13 repetitions to regain 100 percent accuracy in a simulation scenario.

Prebriefing

Orienting students to the lab environment is as critical as orienting to the clinical practice setting. A student who is asked to obtain and use supplies, medications, and communication tools during patient care must know where and how to obtain the required items. Allowing students to look at and explore differences in kits and packaging also helps alleviate problems during the patient care portion of the simulation. Using the example from the sample preparation sheet, having students "feel" a simulated boggy and firm fundus before beginning the simulation allows those with limited assessment experiences to note differences.

During prebriefing, it is important to clarify roles students will take during the scenario. Students should verbally identify the scope of each role. If a student is to take the role of the *charge nurse,* for example, it is important to understand what the charge nurse can and might do. This role clarification helps students focus their decision-making ability. The charge nurse may have a major communication role, while a staff nurse may

BOX 17.1 EXAMPLE OF A PREPARATION SHEET

- Postpartum Hemorrhage Simulation Prep Sheet

Objectives
1. The student will be able to identify and respond to signs and symptoms of postpartum bleeding emergencies.
2. The student will be able to demonstrate therapeutic communication techniques.
3. The student will be able to communicate effectively with members of the health care team.

Jenny Smith is a 28-year-old patient of Dr. Meyers who delivered a viable male infant weighing 4.450 kg 90 minutes ago. Jenny has just been transferred to your care on the postpartum unit. She has an IV in her left forearm with an infusion of lactated ringers with 10 units of pitocin added running at 75 mL/hr. Jenny is married to an air force officer who is currently deployed in Afghanistan. She is accompanied by a friend from their military family support unit. She nursed the baby for 20 minutes shortly after delivery. Her last assessment revealed a BP 115/70, pulse 80, resp. 18, temp. 98.6. Her fundus was firm at the umbilicus and she had a moderate rubra vaginal discharge. She had no perineal repair. She has required no pain medication and reports her pain at 2/10. Her epidural is beginning to wear off, but she is still unable to walk to the bathroom to void. Her bladder was emptied by straight catheterization upon delivery.

Skills to practice: Postpartum assessment, catheterization, IV fluid management, medication administration, therapeutic communication, SBAR (Situation-Background-Assessment-Recommendation) communication, fundal massage.

Medications to study: Analgesics, narcotics, medications used to control bleeding in the childbearing setting.

be performing more tasks associated with direct patient care. Roles will be discussed again during the postconference debriefing reflection.

Prebriefing is also a time to prepare students for practicing the intentionality of *noticing* during patient care. Students may assess a patient formally as taught in an assessment course, but what they will *notice* gives them a perceptual grasp of the larger situation. "What will you notice when you enter the room and how will this help you care for the patient?" is a good question to ask during the prebrief. This helps the student develop a mental checklist prior to the beginning of the simulation. The same type of discussion can also occur during the reflective debriefing by asking students to recall what they noticed or did not notice. This helps them to better describe interpretations and responses to the situation. Intentional noticing is also an important task for observers or other role players.

Simulations

The vast majority of compulsory simulations in undergraduate nursing programs as reported by faculty are medical surgical or emergency care scenarios (Kardong-Edgren, Willhaus, Bennett, & Hayden, 2012). There are, however, many scenarios available that promote decision making in other settings such as community health, behavioral health, pediatrics, geriatrics, and obstretrics. Only a few years ago many faculty wrote and developed their own simulation scenarios because very few were otherwise available. These early scenarios were not always piloted or validated, which posed some difficulties for both students and faculty. Now many well-written, validated scenarios are available either for purchase or for free from commercial and nonprofit sources. Scenarios that have been trialed and validated by numerous sources often offer additional faculty and student support materials, such as patient records, moulage, and setup advice; pre- and postbriefing questions; and suggested student preparation assignments. Some commercial packages provide scenario programming for simulators, while others provide only written or electronic materials. Many scenario packages are available to faculty at no charge because generous donors and foundations have supported their development. The National League for Nursing (NLN) scenarios "Aging Care Excellence for Seniors" and "Joining Forces" (about the care of military veterans) are two such examples available for free download from the NLN website. Other packages available for purchase from the NLN include medical/surgical cases, obstetrics, and pediatric cases through the Laerdal SimStore.

Scenarios should be leveled for the learner and ideally mapped to the curriculum to ensure that the student has practiced the skills and been exposed to the content required for successful decision making. Otherwise, students might notice something but not understand its importance if they have not had the appropriate preparation. Faculty review of each scenario prevents this from happening. Faculty should not conduct a scenario before required content is introduced in a semester or quarter. Simulations must also be coordinated with the simulation lab scheduler so as not to create a bottleneck with other faculty who may want to use the simulation lab at the same time during a semester or quarter.

Scenarios that focus solely on the performance of psychomotor tasks do not make good decision-making scenarios unless the students are well accomplished in the expected tasks. For example, a complex scenario involving blood administration requires students to have mastery over a number of psychomotor tasks prior to the scenario. When and if difficulties occur with a single task, students may be blinded to other decision-making cues that require their attention; therefore, deliberate practice of complex psychomotor tasks should not be an objective in a decision-making scenario.

Using scenarios that are unfolding or end in different ways is an excellent method to engage clinical groups of students in decision-making development. For example, the postpartum bleeding scenario from the practice sheet begins the same way each time; however, there is a different cause of the bleeding over three different iterations of the scenario: a boggy fundus from a tired uterus and big baby, a distended bladder keeping a uterus from contracting, and a previously undetected vaginal wall laceration with a firm uterus. Students debrief between each version of the scenario. This allows clinical groups of 8 to 10 students to participate in all three versions with roles being rotated so that all can participate in a scenario and also learn while observing peers.

OBSERVATION AND DECISION MAKING

Using the "Thinking Like a Nurse" model (Tanner, 2006), students who have an observation role can take part in active noticing and may notice more cues than students who are directly engaged in the simulation. Students who are observing will develop their own interpretations and can discuss how they might have responded differently or in the same way as peers during the reflection period. Students who are observing also learn. No differences in written testing knowledge have been found in students who observed versus those who participated in simulations (Kaplan, Abraham, & Gary, 2012). Additionally, studies on video and computer-based simulations that are primarily observational in nature demonstrate that students improve in clinical judgment when participating in screen-based scenarios (Weatherspoon & Wyatt, 2012). Student observers do not need to rate peer performance, only notice, interpret, and devise their own potential reponses to share in the debriefing.

REFLECTION TO PROMOTE FUTURE DECISION MAKING

Other chapters in this book have been devoted to the art and science of debriefing. Some faculty question whether it is necessary for all debriefings to be conducted in the same way at a single institution. For nursing students in a single curriculum, it is helpful for faculty to use the same or similar debriefing format. This consistency helps the students and observers know and understand what type of reflection will be expected of them. However, different levels of learners can benefit from different styles of debriefing. Debriefing for Meaningful Learning© is a method designed specifically for prelicensure students (Dreifuerst, 2012), while other styles of debriefing such as the Plus/Delta are more direct and general in nature and are often used by military, medical, or interprofessional debriefers.

Regardless of the method used, practice is essential to good debriefing. Debriefing is valued as the most important learning component in any simulation activity (Shinnick, Woo, Horwich, & Steadman, 2011). For this reason, it is important that debriefing skills be deliberately practiced. Debriefing in simulation is learner centered and debriefer guided. It can be difficult for a teacher or faculty member who is a practice expert to not immediately point out any errors or give practice advice to students. This turns the debriefing into a lecture rather than a reflective exercise. Observing other expert debriefers, participating in courses and workshops for debriefing, and practicing with peers are excellent ways to improve in this reflective activity. A good debriefer skillfully guides the students to reveal and reflect what they have learned. Generally students will find the answers to their own questions either from their own knowledge or from a peer. A student might be directed to look up a key point of information in a text or drug book available during a debriefing. When the answer is not completely known or is in error, expert practice faculty can add richness with evidence-based information as a member of the group without taking over the experience. The expert debriefer is a questioner and a guide, while the practice expert is an observer and a standby resource.

REPEATING SCENARIOS

Simulation is time-consuming (Shinnick et al., 2011), therefore, using unfolding simulations or simulations with divergent endings as a way to engage an entire clinical group at once can capitalize on time and enhance learning. Unfolding cases also reinforce continuity of care and demonstrate how patients can improve or deteriorate over time. Repeating the same scenario within a group is another option. Students will know what to expect and will have the debriefing experiences to help guide their actions in repeated iterations. Students continue to learn even when the interventions and outcomes are familiar or expected and seldom attain mastery without repeated practice.

MEASURING DECISION MAKING IN CLINICAL PRACTICE

A 2007 survey of nurse executives (Berkow, Virkstis, Stewart, & Conway, 2009) indicated that only 20 percent of new graduates demonstrated satisfactory decision-making skills. The nurse executive survey asked for opinions about new graduate competencies from the 5,700 nurse leaders who responded. Although opinion is important, it may be more prudent to attempt to measure decision-making skills objectively. Tools available to measure critical thinking skills of practicing nurses include scenario-based online competency tests such as the Performance-Based Development Systems, clinical narratives, and the Critical Thinking Diagnostic available through the Nurse Executive Center (Berkow, Virkstis, Stewart, Aronson, & Donohue, 2011). Limited information is available about the validity and reliability of these instruments, therefore, further evaluation may be needed before adopting their use. The Critical Thinking Diagnostic demonstrated valid and reliable results in five hospitals with 128 staff nurses in the areas of problem recognition, clinical decision making, prioritization, clinical implementation, and reflection.

Measuring critical thinking, clinical judgment, and decision making in new and transitioning graduates who have had simulation practice has not been extensively studied; however, new work is emerging as the National Council of State Boards of Nursing (NCSBN, 2010) simulation study enters its third year. Researchers will collect data on nursing graduates from 10 schools across the nation. Students were randomized during their nursing education into three groups receiving 10 percent, 25 percent, and 50 percent, respectively, of their clinical education in a simulated setting. More information about this research can be obtained from the NCSBN website. At the time of this publication, the first year's study results are available.

CONCLUSION

Much of the research in simulation pedagogy to date has focused on student self-efficacy and satisfaction with the learning method. More research is needed to determine how simulation improves the learning of decision-making skills and whether decision-making skills are retained in the practice setting. This chapter provides guidance and reports best practices and research findings to develop simulation strategies to teach decision making among nursing students. In this rapidly evolving pedagogy, it is clear that faculty must continue to measure outcomes of simulation programs and share the responsibility of decision-making evaluation past prelicensure status.

■ Key Concepts

- ■ Decision making is described by various authors as critical thinking, clinical judgment, clinical reasoning, situated cognition, situated learning, and cognitive flexibility.

■ In order to evaluate learner decision making in simulation, educators should select valid and reliable instruments designed to reveal gains or deficits in the process. This allows for identification of problem areas for further remediation.

■ Supports to prepare the learner prior to simulation include preparation sheets and prebriefing techniques. Simulation scenarios selected to promote decision making should be validated and ideally leveled and mapped to the learners' curriculum. Reflection and debriefing are critical to any simulation experience. Debriefing should be learner centered and guided.

■ Instruments to measure simulation's impact on decision making in clinical practice are limited. New data on how simulation learning impacts the decision-making abilities of new graduates are expected to emerge with the culmination of a major multisite study conducted by the NCSBN, which will conclude in 2015.

References

Adamson, K., Gubrud, P., Sideras, S., & Lasater, K. (2012). Assessing the reliability, validity, and use of the Lasater Clinical Judgement Rubric: Three approaches. *Journal of Nursing Education, 51*(2), 66–73.

Adamson, K. A., Parsons, M. E., Hawkings, K., Manz, J. A., Todd, M., & Hercinger, M. (2011). Reliability and internal consistency findings from the C-SEI. *Journal of Nursing Education, 50*(10), 583–586.

Berkow, S., Virkstis, K., Stewart, J., Aronson, S., & Donohue, M. (2011). Assing individual frontline nursing critical thinking. *The Journal of Nursing Administration, 41*(4), 168–171.

Berkow, S., Virkstis, K., Steward, J., & Conway, L. (2009). Assessing new graduate nurse performance. *Nurse Educator, 34*(1), 17–22.

Dillard, N., Sideras, S., Ryan, M., Carton, K. H., Lasater, K., & Siktberg, L. (2009). A collaborative project to apply and evaluate the clinical judgement model through simulation. *Nursing Education Research, 10*(2), 99–104.

Dreifuerst, K. T. (2012). Using debriefing for meaningful learning to foster development of clinical reasoning in simulation. *Journal of Nursing Education, 53*(6), 326–333.

Institute of Medicine (IOM). (2011). *The future of nursing: leading change, advancing health.* Washington, DC: National Academies Press.

Jensen, R. (2013). Clinical reasoning during simulation: comparison of student and faculty ratings. *Nurse Education in Practice, 13*(1), 21–28.

Kaplan, B. G., Abraham, C., & Gary, R. (2012). Effects of participation vs. observation of a simulation experience on testing outcomes: implications for logistical planning for a school of nursing. *International Journal of Nursing Education Scholarship, 9*(1), 1–15.

Kardong-Edgren, S., Willhaus, J., Bennett, D., & Hayden, J. (2012). Results of the National Council of State Boards of Nursing national simulation study: Part II. *Clinical Simulation in Nursing, 8*(4), e117–e123.

Lapkin, S., Levett-Jones, T., Bellchambers, H., & Fernandez, R. (2010). Effectiveness of patient simulation manikins in teaching clinical reasoning skills to undergraduate nursing students: A systematic review. *Clinical Simulation in Nursing, 6*(6), e207–e222.

Lasater, K. (2007). Clinical judgement development: using simulation to create an assessment rubric. *Journal of Nursing Education, 46*(11), 496–503.

Linnard-Palmer, L. (1995). The effects of a skills algorithm on nursing student response rate, skill accuracy and reported attentional management during simulated cardiopulmonary arrests. Unpublished dissertation, University of San Francisco, UMI 972187.

Mariani, B., Cantrell, M. A., Meakim, C., Prieto, P., & Dreifurst, K. T. (2013). Structured debriefing and students' clinical judgement abilities in simulation. *Clinical Simulation in Nursing, 9*(5), e147–e155.

Nair, G. G., & Stamler, L. L. (2013). A conceptual framework for developing a critical thinking self-assessment scale. *Journal of Nursing Education, 52*(3), 131–138.

National Council of State Boards of Nursing (NCSBN). (2010). *Simulation study.* Retrieved from https://www.ncsbn.org/2094.htm

Shinnick, M. A., Woo, M., Horwich, T. B., & Steadman, R. (2011). Debriefing: the most important component in simulation? *Clinical Simulation in Nursing, 7*(3), e105–e111.

Spiro, R., Feltovich, P., Jacobson, M., & Coulson, R. (1991). Cognitive flexibility, constructivism, and hypertext; Random access instruction in ill-structured domains. *Educational Technology, 31*, 24–33.

Tanner, C. A. (2006). Thinking like a nurse: A research-based model of clinical judgement in nursing. *Journal of Nursing Education, 45*(6), 204–211.

Todd, M., Manz, J., Hawkings, K., Parsons, M., & Hercinger, M. (2008). The development of a quantitative evaluation tool for simulations in nursing education. *International Journal of Nursing Scholarship, 5*(1), 1–17.

Weatherspoon, D. L., & Wyatt, T. H. (2012). Testing computer-based simulation to enhance clinical judgment skills in senior nursing students. *Nursing Clinics of North America, 47*, 481–491.

18

Technological Considerations to Run and Manage a Simulation Center

Scott Alan Engum, MD, FACS
Thomas Dongilli, AT

Learning Objectives

1. Identify the best governance structure for your center.
2. Identify and list key stakeholders of your center.
3. Consider the key elements to create your own three-year plan.
4. Describe two possible models of operation for your center.
5. Describe two possible models of fiscal management for your center.

Key Terms

- Budget
- Equipment
- Governance
- Operations
- Personnel
- Scheduling
- Stakeholder
- Strategic planning

Simulation centers have become the centerpiece of teaching institutions, and accrediting bodies are continuing to increase support related to simulation and innovative approaches in healthcare simulation education. The American College of Surgeons and the Accreditation Council for Graduate Medical Education are two that come to mind. Simulation centers replicate the clinical setting and allow the learner the opportunity to integrate theory, practice, and critical thinking in an effort to ensure patient safety. This learning environment is referred to by many names: skills lab, nursing lab, learning resource center, clinical proficiency center, learning center, simulation center, simulation lab, and clinical simulation lab. One primary role of the simulation center is to serve as a resource to faculty, professionals, and learners during development, implementation, and evaluation of simulation activities. This chapter will focus on the physical learning environment and operational functionality of a simulation center. Topics will include collaboration, governance, organization, personnel, technology, space, supplies, resources, and equipment.

This chapter will guide you in setting up your center's three-year plan. A three-year plan should list your potential users for each year, additional courses and service offerings, space requirements, resource requirements, and associated financial calculations for each year. This plan can be used to forecast resource, revenue, and curriculum expansions.

By the end of this chapter, you should have the tools available to identify the best governance structure for your center, identify and list key stakeholders for your center, and create a three-year plan or roadmap that correlates with your end-user needs and governance philosophy and be able to describe two possible operational models and consider various financial models and identify the one that best applies to your center.

Glossary of Terms for This Chapter

Hub and Spoke Model: A model of operation where there is a primary governing body that creates policy, financial, and operational oversight and deliverables for the other facilities that are related to the primary facility.

Stakeholder: An individual, department, or entity that shows or has an interest in participating in the development or utilization of the simulation center.

Three-year plan: A strategic plan for the creation or expansion of a simulation-based training facility or program.

CREATING YOUR CENTER'S ROADMAP

Developing a Partnership

Partnerships involved in a simulation center come in all shapes and sizes in today's health care climate. Outside of university programs, it is not uncommon for a single entity to try and "go it alone" in the development of a new center. This may be a very short-sighted mistake in their long-term mission or vision. When a sole proprietorship is chosen, the simulation lab might be limited in the number of simulation activities, funding, and number of disciplines participating in events, utilization of equipment and staff, and cost-efficiency. There are multiple advantages in a partnership that relate to increasing revenue sources, improved opportunity for collaboration, opportunities for interprofessional activities, justification for specialized equipment (Harvey®, vascular and ultrasound simulators), opportunities for large program offerings, and the ability to knit the mission and vision of the university and health care system. This partnership can develop as a business-type model such as for-profit, not-for-profit, governmental, or trust. The partnership encourages collaboration of administrators, educators,

TABLE 18.1		
Areas of Importance for Simulation Leadership Team		
Organizational	**Individual**	**Team Process**
• Clear purpose • Appropriate culture • Specified task • Distinct roles • Suitable leadership • Relevant members • Adequate resources	• Self-knowledge • Trust • Commitment • Flexibility	• Coordination • Communication • Cohesion • Decision making • Conflict management • Social relationships • Performance feedback

SOURCE: Mickan, S., & Rodger, S. (2000). Characteristics of effective teams: a literature review. *Australian Health Review, 23*(3), 201–208.

technicians, and end users to develop meaningful learning environments and priceless learning opportunities.

Challenges are present when combining multiple disciplines and can increase the complexity of a single shared mission, vision, goals, objectives, budget, established levels of accountability, scheduling priorities, and staffing responsibilities. None of these challenges should ever dissuade the pursuit of a relationship; however, the early acknowledgment of hurdles will keep lines of communication open as the process proceeds.

In the initial planning phases of your center, you should consider the development of a stakeholder analysis. **Stakeholders** are departments, programs, or individuals with an expressed interest in the development of simulation programs. The analysis should focus on the size of programs, types of course requests, and projected equipment needs. This process will allow you to create a center that is based on specific training needs and requirements. It will also aid in the creation of budgets, equipment purchases and allocations and personnel and space planning.

Planning teams are critical to the successful development of simulation centers, and it is recommended that planning teams consist of simulation center leadership, project management (usually from parent organization), facilities planning, business administrative discipline, and the architectural firm. A decision-making process should be agreed upon prior to the start of the program as quality team function will determine the survival of a successful simulation center. The planning stages of any center offer tremendous team-building opportunities, and investing in those skill sets at that time will reap tremendous dividends as the simulation center opens its doors and begins functional operation. Table 18.1 highlights areas of importance when looking at your organizational, individual, and team processes. Leadership should foster these skill sets as these will be the foundation for the viability of your center.

Funding Sources

When beginning to think about the development of a simulation center, funding is a key issue. There are two major components to a simulation center **budget**: operating costs and capital costs. However, during the construction phase of your project, you will also need to manage or be mindful of your construction cost budget. You will want to ensure that the construction costs are independent of the functional simulation center operating and capital costs budgets. Capital purchases should be reflected in the **equipment** and software needed to operate your center and teach. Construction costs should be affiliated with items that are critical to the build-out of your center. In the everyday functional budget, capital costs are usually associated with expenses that exceed a certain dollar amount set by your institution or project and often related to simulators, medical equipment, and furniture. In the center I work at there is a $5,000 threshold for operating fund purchases versus capital account purchases. Anything over $5,000 must be considered a capital purchase and special authorization is required. The operational budget will dictate the operational size of your center. This should not be confused with the physical size. The operational size includes number of employees and available resources.

The initial start-up funding for the simulation center construction and equipment can come from multiple sources, as reflected in Table 18.2. The majority of funding will be spent on the build-out and equipping of the center. If the project can be incorporated into a current building initiative, cost savings can be realized. For example, the purchase and installation of head walls should be considered part of your construction budget and by including such items in the construction budget, you could reallocate those available funds toward other capital purchases. In addition, if your center is one floor of a building being built for multiple purposes (administrative and education), then the simulation center constructions costs are being optimized within the global project because construction personnel are already onsite and savings could be realized. This does pose some timeline pressures to stay on track with the major construction project but benefits the institution upon efficient completion. Further revenue efficiencies can be acquired if a center is able to take advantage of current purchasing agreements (hospital system) among the partners and industry.

Maintaining a consistent streamlined business and operational planning team will ensure continued progress within the project with minimal setbacks and possibly free

TABLE 18.2

Examples of Funding Sources for Simulation Centers

Funding Sources	Examples
Philanthropic support	• Professional organizations • Industry • Individuals
Grant funding	• International • Governmental • Individual foundation/endowment
Institutional/health care system	• School and/or medical center sponsorship • Departmental grant • Endowment • Foundation grant • Gift

up dollars for redistribution. Incorporating current business and development experts from a partnering system can share in the responsibility of project management and can minimize hiring extra staff for the build-out and implementation phases. Lastly, using available and relevant equipment (from hospital storage) within the system can free up capital to address the unexpected cost increase adjustments that are common in construction of a center.

ORGANIZATIONAL STRUCTURE AND GOVERNANCE

It is important to define the position of the simulation center in the hierarchy of the organization. This forethought will be important as a health care system or university grows and develops partnerships with affiliated organizations. Depending on the parent organization and simulation center structure, it may involve **governance** leadership with the deans of the individual schools and high-level administration within a hospital system or board of directors. Although these individuals may be the primary support for the center, they likely report to executive leadership above them such as the vice president or president or chief executive officer (CEO) of a hospital system or university. A clear understanding of who is ultimately responsible for the simulation center is important to gain buy-in, budgetary support, academic appointments, and personnel hiring and assist in strategic planning of the organization's educational mission.

Day-to-day functions within a center will need to be maintained by the simulation center leadership. This often involves the director, coordinator or manager, educators, and information technology (IT) leadership. Frequent and regularly scheduled meetings are beneficial to discuss past, current, and future processes and concerns. A director of operations or operational coordinator may also be of value to manage more integral day-to-day issues that relate to workflow, assignments, schedules, and simulation case concerns. Additional **personnel** for **operations** may include a manager or coordinators, technicians, IT support, administrative assistants, and schedulers. Having routine (weekly, biweekly), standing meetings allows for simulation center activities to be scheduled around these meetings and guarantees that all of the center's individuals have input into process improvement. An example of one hierarchy system would be:

- Executive committee (dean of school, CEO of hospital, etc.)
- Governance committee (appointed leadership determined by the executive committee)
- Leadership committee (members within the simulation center who function in leadership roles and are stakeholders)
- Operational committee (support individuals within the simulation center who ensure daily activity completion)

Open lines of communication among the executive level down through ancillary and operational services will keep the center operating smoothly. Regularly scheduled leadership meetings will be necessary to ensure the center is remaining on target with budgetary, educational, and operational goals and objectives. The operations manager or director coordinator should establish regular meetings with technicians and support staff on a recurring basis. This will promote a sense of belonging within the team and establish clear pathways for problem discovery and resolution. Frequent conversations at all levels will need to occur regarding work assignments, expectations, project deadlines, customer interactions, and active planning for future events, knowledge sharing, team building, and open dialogue.

SIMULATION CENTER LOCATION, CAPABILITIES, AND LIMITATIONS

The allocation of space for a simulation center reflects the institution's commitment, need, and resources. Whether large or small, the simulation center space should accommodate multiple teaching and evaluation strategies that are based on the desired learning objectives and outcomes. Center design and location should be based on the courses identified and learner group sizes determined by the stakeholder analysis. The identification of potential teaching approaches will determine the exact needs of each simulation lab. The explosion of simulations in health care education is broadening and transforming the way these learning spaces are designed and equipped (Hyland & Hawkins, 2009; Kardong-Edgren & Oermann, 2009).

With the teaching strategies identified, the design phase of the simulation center development begins by assembling an interprofessional planning and design team. Depending on the environment, the team should consist of senior administration, facilities management, faculty, key educators, a learner representative, simulation specialists, an architect, a technology consultant, an audiovisual consultant, and business management personnel. The design team will need to keep several concerns in mind as they develop the plan for the new space. With so many people involved in the design process, a team leader and final decision maker will need to be identified. This person (or committee) will need to make final decisions on any conflict resolutions that involve design, equipment, locations, budget, and other areas that can plague the timeline of any construction project.

Location of a simulation center is critical to ensure convenient use. Many institutions will have a broad set of users that are geographically separated but institutionally hardwired for similar needs and education. The options are to develop a single, centrally located center in the area of concentrated learners or multiple key sites operating under a common administration. This is called the Hub and Spoke Model (NASSCOM® 2012 "Hub and Spoke Operating Model," from www.nasscom.in/hub-and-spoke-operating-model), where the main center or governing body should be considered the hub and any offsite location should be considered the spoke. Sizes of the hub or spokes can vary, with some spokes being nothing more than a simulator on a stretcher stored at an offsite location, while some are more elaborate with multibed simulation facilities. Training needs, geographic location, and group sizes should reflect the model that may work best for your organization, with each philosophy carrying positives and negatives.

If a multiple site model is chosen, this can afford lower-scale renovations, customized equipment that fits that health care environment, and 24-hour access to the center by local users driving higher utilization. The downside relates to the inability for future expansion as it relates to the size and scope of center, duplication of services, travel for staff, as well as equipment location and IT and personnel, all adding operational costs to the program.

If a single central site is chosen, this allows for all resources to be maximized and cost savings to be gained, with efficiency of workforce and equipment; however, utilization by peripheral partners will be less as this mandates travel, increased personnel time away from clinical site, and associated costs.

One of the first decisions is whether the space will be onsite or offsite. Each health care system or university will need to determine where their learners and customer base are coming from as this will allow you to determine the most efficient location to create a new center. A second major issue relates to whether to use existing space with renovations or new construction. Since I have been involved in many of these projects, my experience has been that there are times where the total costs may be higher when attempting to renovate existing structures instead of creating new ones. Examples of this include existing limitations of space (pillars, elevators, etc.), asbestos or containment removal, and the adaption of existing services like heating, ventilation, air-conditioning, and electrical and plumbing systems. The closer a system can place a simulation center to its customers and learners, the better the opportunity would be to carry out educational programs and reduce travel time for instructors and staff, as well as allow the learner flexibility to do independent activities. Maintaining a simulation center within the main teaching facilities limits transportation concerns for both learners and educators; however, it may also limit both parties from remaining fully immersed in the simulation center activity as they attempt to balance two worlds (real and simulated). Being offsite prevents parties from feeling torn between two necessities and helps them remain focused in the educational experience.

When a location is chosen, the group may be faced with the decision whether to build an independent structure or to combine with another project. This decision is often made at a level above the design team; however, construction costs can be optimized if the parent organization incorporates the new simulation center space into an existing project as all construction entities are already onsite. This does pose some concerns about logistics and maintaining timelines that may not be in the simulation center's best interests but the overall project's best interests. If the decision is made to combine projects, this may ensure construction efficiencies are maximized. Also, if the combination project is incorporating educational space into their footprint, this may lessen some of the floor plan requirements the simulation center had initially scripted and will free up space for another purpose.

Renovation of existing space will always have limitations due to structural supports, ceiling height, established footprint, and facilities infrastructure; however, each design team will need to work with the footprint allowed by the parent organization.

Center Mission, Vision, and Strategic Planning

A mission statement, simply stated, is the fundamental purpose of your simulation organization and its reason for existence. This statement guides the organization's direction and decision making. To be effective, it must show the aim of the organization, which includes its primary stakeholders and customers, and clearly state what products it has to share and their core purpose. The vision outlines what the simulation center wants to be along with its long-term view and primarily looks to the future.

Strategic planning is an organization's process of defining its direction and how to make decisions and allocate resources in an effort to accomplish the vision and mission (Armstrong, 1986; Gantt, 2010). In order to implement a strategy, the organization must know the direction or end vision it is working toward. There are two primary approaches to strategic planning: the Situation-Target-Proposal and Draw-See-Think-Plan methods (Phillips & Bergquist, 1987):

1. Situation-Target-Proposal
   - Situation: Evaluate the current situation and how it came about
   - Target: Define goals and/or objectives (for ideal state)
   - Proposal/Path: Map a possible route to the goals/objectives
2. Draw-See-Think-Plan
   - Draw: What is the ideal desired end state?
   - See: What is today's situation? What is the gap from the ideal state desired, and why?
   - Think: What specific actions must be taken to close the gap between today's situation and the ideal state desired?
   - Plan: What resources are required to execute the activities?

When doing strategic planning, there are a number of tools an organization can use, but the SWOT (strengths, weaknesses, opportunities, and threats) analysis is one of the most widely used. By looking at the internal strategic factors (strength/weaknesses), the organization can then take into account the external factors (opportunities/threats) in a constructive manner. Other tools include:

- Balanced scorecards: creates a systematic framework for strategic planning (Kaplan, 2000).
- Scenario planning: analyzes future scenarios (Schoemaker, 1995).
- PEST analysis: looking at political, economic, social, and technological factors.
- STEER analysis: looking at sociocultural, technological, economic, ecological, and regulatory factors.
- EPISTEL: evaluating environmental, political, informatics, social, technological, economic, and legal factors.
- ATM approach: using antecedent conditions, target strategies, and measuring progress and impact. Once the desired end state is defined, one can use a root cause analysis to understand the threats, barriers, and challenges to achieving the end state (Renger & Titcomb, 2002).
- Stakeholder analysis approach: involves the project leadership team completing a detailed assessment of current and future simulation and educational activities with each of the simulation center stakeholders.

Stakeholders usually include hospital leadership, chairpersons, risk management, educators, and patient safety officers. On the academic side, the stakeholders are usually deans, professors, instructors, and program coordinators. The goal of the meetings should be

BOX 18.1 STRATEGIC OUTLINE AREAS

- Education and training of students and residents
- Health care system improvement (care delivery/operational outcomes)
- Assessment and testing
- Research
- Simulation learning for existing health care professionals
- Community service
- Leadership and advocacy
- Faculty development
- Sustainability
- Management
- Facilities
- Innovation

to identify who is currently doing simulation, who would like to do simulation, and where there are opportunities for simulation that may not be identified yet. You should also identify sizes of groups and frequency of training. This will allow you to predict the size of the center, number of rooms, types of rooms and equipment, and personnel to be allocated.

When any organization initiates strategic planning, it is important to outline the areas of interest your group wants to concentrate on. There are no hard or fast rules to the development of the strategic outline; however, it is always easier to develop a wide scope list that can be strategically narrowed down at the time of any organizational retreat. Box 18.1 lists areas to consider. An organization can then follow a cycle of management, which includes strategic planning, budgeting, program implementation, performance monitoring and reporting, and program evaluation. This cycle of activity then promotes customer-focused services while emphasizing employee involvement and teamwork. It utilizes performance measurements that are focused on results that lead to efficient and effective resource allocation and utilization (Amasaka, 2002; Collins, Cordon, & Julien, 1996).

FINANCIAL MODEL

Budgetary

Rigorous attention to cost containment and new revenue streams can keep the simulation center within budget. The simulation center administration will be responsible for developing the business plan and budget and provide a systematic process of review to ensure adherence. All centers should maintain consistent records and transparent communication with schools and hospital administrative leadership who are responsible for center oversight. When assessing the need for spending, always consider whether the expenditure will support the educational mission, goals, and objectives of the center without creating an imbalance. Centers can use a simple model for purchases that looks at the number of courses offered and trainee types that may benefit from a purchase. This model allows many users to have access to a single purchase and may be beneficial to those who are starting a new program.

Some centers find additional funding sources by attracting external partners and customers who will pay fair market value to use available spaces. These external users can consist of other hospitals, emergency medical services, schools or universities, and possibly commercial programs. These external relationships can generate revenue; however, you should consult with your parent organization on the utilization of your center by commercial entities prior to engaging in commercial conversations.

Revenue streams can come from multiple sources such as grant agencies, private donors, and research organizations and include invoicing all customers, invoicing some customers, and sharing the budgetary responsibilities among the partners. Most centers follow a collective business model where the organization is composed of a relatively large number of professionals in the same or related fields of endeavor, which pools resources, shares information, and provides benefits for their members. Another option is to charge a user fee, which then allows full access to services and no expense on the way out the door for any specific event or learner.

Depending on the predetermined partnership, some programs have an annual budget where each partner pays a percentage of the annual operating budget upfront. In this type of situation, all services are provided to that partner at no cost to the educator or learner groups as all expenses are a fixed cost within the system. This takes tremendous pressure off the simulation center staff and educators to carry out curricular objectives and does not ration center usage due to budgetary reasons.

Other centers might adopt a model that requires the center to be self-sustaining and all customers are invoiced for services. With a self-sustaining model, the majority of program decisions may be determined upon budget and revenue sources. Tensions can mount in the fee-for-service environment and development of curriculum will need to be strategically planned and implemented based on budgetary approvals.

Some have used a hybrid model where partners pay an annual fee, affiliate facilities pay a percentage of their use costs or a fixed per-learner use fee, and external nonaffiliated customers pay full service expenses at fair market value.

Another method of charging is to have a fee schedule that is graduated over time. In this type of arrangement, the user may have a set fee (three-year commitment) for year one that will increase in year two and peak in year three. This allows the user to gain experience and confidence in the simulation center and work to a known budget of expenses while maintaining the simulation center's financial responsibility to cover expenses. This method of billing allows a center to charge a percentage of the actual cost to a user, and as time goes on, the percentage increases to 100 percent. This allows for users to create initial programs and generate data for future utilization and expansion. It also allows programs to start using the center and to plan for increased expenses over an agreed upon timeframe. Most centers that use this model have a multiyear agreement with the end user.

Lastly, grants and donations can be invaluable to a center as these can subsidize your budget. Grants and donations are not a guaranteed source of revenue and cannot be the cornerstone around which to build your center. Long-term strategic development is the best foundation to ensure a simulation center's viability and sustainability.

BOX 18.2 SIMULATION LAB OPERATIONS BUDGETARY CONSIDERATIONS

1. Standardized patients
2. Specialized equipment needs
3. New equipment warranties
4. Transitioned (donated to center) equipment warranties
5. In situ simulation support by simulation center staff
6. Disposable supplies
7. Service life of equipment
8. Software and hardware advances
9. Server storage space
10. Inflationary expenses
11. Economic downturn or recession
12. Hiring freeze or budgetary cuts
13. Catering
14. Replacement of outdated equipment
15. Replacement parts (bulbs for projectors)

There are major budgetary concerns that develop as a center matures and curriculum offerings expand. This is not a tremendous problem in a center where the costs are covered by the system; however, consumable expenditures can challenge a center. The sections that follow list identified items that can challenge a budget if funding sources for these items are not anticipated and planned for in advance. Usage and associated costs of these items have many variables, including, but not limited to, faculty orientation to the equipment, student volume, frequency of use, and conditions of use. For a list of additional budgetary considerations, see Box 18.2.

Capital Expenditures

Capital expenditures are often mentioned at the time of opening a new simulation center; however, after all the excitement and glamour of opening a new center is gone, leadership soon realizes that an operational budget does not afford the center the ability to purchase capital expenditures. After a few years, equipment starts to break and wear down, and new equipment will be required so a capital expenditure account will be necessary. The creation of a capital expenditure account should be discussed at the time the simulation center opens. This could be a yearly amount (use it or lose it) or a fund that remains intact with a decreasing balance.

Each piece of capital equipment should have a life expectancy (the amount of time the equipment will last or is expected to last), and you can usually get this information from the vendor. As an example, if you purchase a $30,000 piece of equipment that has a life expectancy of five years, then you should be allocating $6,000 per year toward the replacement of that. In your three-year budgetary plan, you will need to explain these increases in certain years as they relate to depreciation of equipment.

Cost and Billing Structure

Unfortunately, the best business model for a simulation center has not been discovered, and, often, what will work in one individual's environment will not benefit another's. Each center should know its annual budget and costs, because this will allow you to properly identify costs associated with each program offered. Annual operational costs should reflect your three-year plan. Each year, as you increase course offerings, you will need to demonstrate the increase in operational costs. This can be best explained if you share your three-year plan with your parent organization or those who control your funds.

Establishing a cost value for every function and service a simulation center offers carries a few benefits. First, it establishes a starting point as to what something costs and how much a customer will be charged. Profit can be built into any calculation in an effort to have future funds to advance education, increase personnel, and repair or replace equipment. If the cost structure is not used for billing a customer, then these data can be used to show return on investment for the services offered within the simulation center. Often, administrative leadership will ask how the simulation center is benefiting the health care environment and whether the system is getting its money's worth.

In these cases, return on investment (ROI) can be demonstrated in various ways. You may want to work with your parent organization (risk management, patient safety) to discover the impact of simulation-based courses as it relates to patient safety initiatives. Most of the time, the ROI involves reductions in patient safety concerns like infections and reduction of medical errors or training time of staff. You may also reflect cost saving in reduction of training times, orientation requirements, or testing of system issues. Unfortunately, it is difficult to trace single simulation events directly back to the patient bedside and a specific outcome, but the cost can be shown and education services provided in relation to the budget that was expended to make that occur. In most centers, it would be expected that this is a net positive for services rendered.

Fee Schedule

Once a center has determined its internal and external relationships, budgetary commitments by programs, and actual operating and capital costs, the next part of the process is to decide how you are going to bill for services (create a fee schedule).

As stated earlier in the chapter, the fee schedule can be predetermined or done on a case-by-case basis. Centers affiliated with hospitals or health systems will need to create models for internal billing and transfer of funds as some departments will want to pay the center directly for employee courses. This is usually done through an internal transfer process. If your center plans on offering external courses for fee, then you will need to create a model where you can process payment from internal and external users. Some centers rely on the infrastructure of their parent organization to handle this, and some centers need to create model and process billing and payment independently.

Many centers have a blended model where they offer courses both internally and externally and will need to manage both payment methods. This can become confusing in the health care system as hospital systems join forces to provide global patient services. This may involve internal customers (parent organization that pays the bills), affiliates (partnering hospitals that share relationship but no financial responsibilities), and external customers. Affiliates may be offered a reduced fee (50 percent of the cost) because of their relationship or carry some variation of full-cost expectations, and each system will need to determine the best working relationship for local progress in education.

OPERATIONAL COSTS

Personnel

Following the center's opening, a successful and thriving organization will need to integrate all personnel into the center's mission and vision. It is important to incorporate not only the educational, but also the clinical and research missions of the entity or partners into the simulation center fabric as many initiatives occurring within the simulation center will directly impact these processes. Because health care systems are held responsible for improving patient safety and clinical outcomes, these items will undoubtedly be tied to the simulation center's educational initiatives to bring about improved communication and safer bedside care. The goal is to translate learning from the simulation center to the point of care, and the center's staff play a vital role in that learning.

Appropriate staffing a simulation center is critical to success. Depending on a simulation center's size, organizational structure, technological capabilities, and offerings, staffing can be quite variable, however, this aspect of simulation center management can be your Achilles' heel. Most hospital-based centers function with a medical director who is typically part time and not uncommonly a practicing health care professional (physician) and commonly maintains a faculty position in an academic system. In addition, the director should understand the curriculum and how the simulation center can help faculty meet the curricular goals. In many cases, this individual is a member of the health care system or school's curriculum committee. The director can also serve on other appropriate committees that assist in advancing education as they will be able to assist educators with integrating simulation into a curriculum. It is common to see 50 percent of the director's time devoted to the administrative functions of the simulation center.

In addition, it is critical to have a full-time director of operations, manager, or coordinator who is designated to manage the day-to-day operations of the simulation center. This individual must not only have the administrative skill set to manage employees, provide mentoring, and coaching, but also possess an advanced working knowledge of medicine, simulation planning, programming, education, debriefing, equipment function, and IT framework.

Personnel requirements and qualifications will vary by facility. Simulation technicians, coordinators, IT support, and faculty will make up the core of your team. Job descriptions for each will simplify both hiring and the management of personnel. The simulation center operational personnel will assist in all aspects of the center's operations. These include instructor training, room set up, repair, maintenance of equipment, and scenario programming among many other tasks. Operational personnel will need some key skills such as the ability to understand medical terminology, interact with and program technology, interpersonal skills, computer skills, prioritizing, and organizational skills. The qualifications of these individuals can come from many backgrounds, such as emergency medical technician, paramedic, nursing, anesthesia technologist, or those out of college with degrees in media, audio, video, or even engineering. They must possess the skills to flexibly perform all tasks needed to operate and maintain a simulation center. A center that follows a single-site model with multiple rooms and various course offerings may need several technicians and a coordinator to assist with handling the larger volume of customers. The staffing model for centers that function as a multisite model will often function with a director and a number of technicians who support both the local and offsite training.

The number of technicians relates to the number of events a facility wants to conduct, with some models referring to a single technician for each room running. However, most centers cannot afford nor need this luxury. In this model, with a single high-fidelity room, the minimum number of support individuals is typically an educator and a simulation technician. Thus, the example of an emergency room interprofessional event running three rooms simultaneously would require three technicians and three educators. In a similar event involving an interprofessional virtual hospital ward with medical and nursing students, five rooms are running simultaneously and would necessitate 10 individuals involved. This is a major resource requirement for any simulation center, and careful planning is necessary as any other activities in the center must be self-sufficient and need minimal operational support to happen simultaneously. So, even in a large center, the coordination of support alongside lower-level events allows for simultaneous events to occur with high customer satisfaction and center staff maintaining emotional sanity.

Sufficient training of instructors combined with simulation session design and support technology can contribute to the reduction of operational personnel needed to support a simulation session. Some models have the operational personnel teach instructors to operate their own equipment. This model allows for one operations person to support multiple rooms.

School- or university-based centers typically have lab coordinators manage the center and report directly to the dean of the parent organization. These academic models are based on integration of existing curriculum and typically rely on existing staff to run sessions with the lab coordinator supporting the operational needs.

A multisite system will typically pull all educators, the simulation center director, and coordinator/manager/director of operations into the picture for large-scale events to support requirements. When not running a simulation session, the operational personnel and coordinator/manager/director of operations could assist with course creation and coordination, as well as facilitate all other events along with scheduling and public relations in addition to their administrative duties.

The majority of faculty for a simulation center will come from the clinical units, divisions, departments, or schools that use the center for training. Typically, the faculty are employed or appointed from their home institution and their salary and benefits are already addressed. The vast majority of faculty will be fulfilling their teaching mission and requirements for promotion and tenure and will be the driving force for new initiatives. It is common that these new users will need education about the simulation process, how to develop quality simulation-based programs, equipment selection, manikin selection, scenario programming, the use of manikins and the process of how to run a scenario, and debriefing techniques. When instructed and mentored properly, these individuals will be the future champions in the simulation process.

All centers will need to determine their core workforce, and this can be a mix of volunteers, full-time, part-time, and supplemental employees. Full-time employees usually carry a 40-hour workweek and full benefits package, which can be anywhere from 25 percent to 40 percent of the salary costs, depending on the environment. Providing a comprehensive orientation program will require less supplemental training for each event, allowing them to gain experience and confidence and become a loyal and dependable staff member who supports the mission, vision, and goals of the center. The average training time for a new hire simulation operations person is 6 to 12 months. This is a substantial time and resource commitment and this should be well documented and planned.

Employment costs should be built into the annual budget with a supporting job description. Careful tracking of center statistics will help to justify adding or releasing full-time staff. As center usage volumes change, these statistics can be invaluable when trying to justify additional staff, especially during a hiring freeze. With economic downturns and health care budgetary cuts, it has become increasingly difficult to receive permission from oversight committees for the addition of new staff. The creation of your three-year plan will also assist with the development of future hires to the center. You should be able to demonstrate your growth plan, which includes courses, personnel, and equipment.

When considering full-time, part-time, and supplemental staff, a few items are important to keep in mind. Part-time employees typically work 20 hours per week, have partial benefits, and, after experience is gained, can be very valuable during flex times as many of them have flexible hours and can adjust to center volume changes. A significant downside to part-time and supplemental employees is that each event will require planning, physical setup, implementation, and teardown. Many of these functions occur around other scheduled events and sometimes a day or two ahead of the scheduled event, which can put additional workload on full-time staff if the part-time staff does not have flexible hours. Some centers use active supplemental employees. These individuals work on an as-needed basis and are not benefits eligible. If the simulation center is fully staffed with operational personnel, supplemental employees can be invaluable to fill in during high service times and carry lower financial compensation because they do not carry a benefits package. However, a center should not rely upon this type of individual as the backbone of services rendered. If you have a set budget but have the need for multiple employees, you may want to consider purchasing a percentage of people's time from various departments. As an example, you could purchase 50 percent of IT support from your IT department and 50 percent secretary support from your own department in an effort to have two services for one full-time employee salary amount.

There are times within all organizations when a specific type of expertise is required that may not be available within the simulation team and a "contracted employee" may be needed to fill this requirement. Information technology is one of those specialty areas in which the search for the proper individual may take time, but the services these individuals are responsible for are needed today. A simulation center should be able to contract with an outside company to provide temporary expertise, and the contracting company will carry all the benefits and employer requirements. You need to understand that this method of coverage does come at a premium and may cost the simulation system 40 to 50 percent more over time; however, within the right area, this may be an excellent short-term solution until a long-term solution is determined or someone is trained.

If a simulation center is going to provide objective structured clinical examination (Harden, Stevenson, Downie, & Wilson, 1975) with standardized patients who portray the role of human patients, then the vital role of standardized patient educator or coordinator needs to be established. This individual spends a significant amount of time working with customers who utilize standardized patients to plan the events, create proper scripts, evaluate checklists, and train the standardized patient for consistent role performance. Depending on the volume of learner encounters your system projects, this will likely be a full-time position.

Further staffing of the simulation center can take many forms, and some individuals may have multiple duties depending on the resources, funding sources, center size, and capabilities. As simulation centers become busier, it is not uncommon for a receptionist to be required to direct educators and learners where they are scheduled and to greet guests and welcome tour groups. The receptionist can also assist in administrative functions to optimize efficiencies.

Larger simulation centers may have business development and project management oversight support staff within the center. This revenue-producing position is a valuable asset for systems to use with strategic planning and budgetary oversight. If a center is unable to afford or maintain this type of person on the payroll, investigate using the school's or hospital system's business department. Asking the business department for a specific person to be designated to the simulation center will allow for a relationship to be established. There are few simulation center business models available for review, so a resource person with business expertise can assist in developing appropriate guidance in this maturing area.

Volunteers are a valuable resource for all centers, both large and small. These can be individuals who come from the community or even students from the undergraduate or graduate level. All of these individuals provide valuable man hours to assist in carrying out the mission of the simulation center. It is not uncommon to have a graduate or undergraduate student develop innovative curriculum plans while doing volunteer or elective rotation work. In addition, college and high school students can assist simulation technicians in setup, implementation, and teardown after education. Volunteers can also be trained to provide routine maintenance of equipment and assist with inventory management.

Simulation centers offer a rich environment for data collection and research. A research assistant can come from many locations. If you are in an academic environment, each of the academic divisions typically have research personnel who can assist in carrying out projects; however, their simulation knowledge may be limited and selecting an individual with an educational background may be beneficial. Educators might also have a research background that can be used to initiate new opportunities. If a primary researcher is funded, this could be part time or full time depending on the funding source. In either situation, the simulation center could fund the initiative under a global budget or share the cost burden with other educational systems to keep the center's budgetary funds intact.

Administrative support is necessary for record keeping, ordering, invoicing, employee timekeeping, assistance with scheduling of instructors and students, catering, and scheduling of meetings. This positions' skill set will also depend on the center's size, capabilities, and organizational partners. A moderately busy simulation center is capable of keeping an administrative assistant engaged with full-time assignments. Department-based centers typically use a percentage of the existing department administrative staff to support the center.

Very often individuals who support the physical plant such as maintenance, janitorial, and facilities are overlooked. Simulation activities cannot occur without proper support from all of these entities and, often, these expenses can be shared with other occupants of a building or campus.

One critical concern relates to protected time for all simulation center employees and liaisons to carry out their functions. If an employee is full or part time and simulation center–based, his or her functions will be focused on center objectives. Managers and educators can have dual roles that mandate job sharing, with dedicated time between multiple department and health care system or university environments. Success of a center will be determined by these individuals having adequate protected time to ensure the quality of currently developed programs as well as advance the growth and program offerings of the simulation center. These times will need to be negotiated with their primary department.

SCHEDULING

The day-to-day functions of the simulation center strongly depend on an organized **scheduling** system that can account for center rooms, equipment resources, learner data, and personnel availability. An organized scheduling system will prevent a learner group from arriving unexpectedly and minimize the occurrences of multiple groups not having appropriate space for their number of learners.

A block time schedule may work well for some customers, while open access with flexibility works better for others. The manner in which a center's time is allotted depends on the customer and uses. A goal of a simulation center is to project the schedule prior to the start of a fiscal or academic year. Unfortunately, there is no ideal world in the simulation center as new classes are added, customers are recruited, learner needs change, and tours and presentations with the community can occur with no or little warning. Although there is always an unpredictable aspect to the simulation center, one can work to establish a calendar of "big events" to avoid major conflicts.

Simulation center scheduling of all activities and durable equipment, supplies, personnel, and other information will always be a challenge when trying to meet the requests of customers. There are some software systems on the market and they vary in price and functionality. You should explore in detail your center's needs and requirements and compare that to what is commercially available. Many systems have developed local, homegrown software systems or are using less sophisticated processes. These less sophisticated processes have been tolerated in the past due to the relative small size of most simulation centers and the predictable number of learner groups for that system. However, with new simulation centers being built throughout the world, few of them have the small footprint of past centers. With the increased size, complexity, and number of personnel and the fact that all of these centers are now run as a sophisticated business, software solutions are critical.

One can approach scheduling through a coordinator or operational personnel (manually), but this will require one or two key personnel to schedule all aspects of the center's use. This would be recorded on some form of calendar. Another method is to use an electronic or web-based system that allows real-time scheduling that is visible to the user. This will allow for an electronic copy of the request to be saved and housed within the system in the event of lost or mistaken data. This also will allow for confirmation notices to be sent alerting the educator of all specific reservation data for his or her event. Some centers will use multiple scheduling systems before they find the best fit for their environment.

Centers should have an individual or team that manages the schedule request process. These individuals would be responsible for the approval or denial of schedule requests and it is typically within the job description of the center coordinator or manager to orchestrate this process. There should be a process in place where those requesting use of the center understand that requesting use does not mean approval. You should develop a "Request and Approval" process prior to implementing your scheduling system. Most centers function on a first-come, first-served basis; however, a priority system may be required when dealing with large combination health care and university systems. Some areas of prioritization are shown in Box 18.3. Box 18.4 includes items that might be important to consider when selecting a software system. Examples of a simulation center reservation form's items, whether submitted online, via e-mail, or in writing, can be seen in Box 18.5.

It is critical for any system to have the ability to recognize and resolve conflicts. These conflicts might be rooms, equipment, supplies, and staff availability, to name only a few. One example that may occur is when a customer requests two ventilators for use in a simulation and the center only has one available. The software should alert scheduling staff of the equipment conflict, which will then allow the system to locate a second ventilator, or work with the customer to adjust the simulation event to stagger the use of the ventilator so all aspects of the scenario can be maintained.

BOX 18.3 AREAS OF PRIORITIZATION

Simulation Event
- Interprofessional
- Multidisciplinary
- Single discipline
- Research
- Task training
- Didactic

Standardized Patient Event
- Summative exam
- Interprofessional
- Single discipline
- Video recording mandatory
- Research
- Practice exam
- Task training
- Didactic

Grants
- Large external funding
- Local/regional funding
- Internal funding
- In-kind donation of center

Tours
- High-level administration
- Student/resident applicants
- Outside health care systems
- Industry
- Inside health care system
- Community
- Youth

BOX 18.4 SELECTING A SOFTWARE SYSTEM

- Online capabilities for customer registration, the ability to request time and place, and for an event request to be placed into the scheduling software
- Multiple status levels for request order (preliminary, reviewed, active, cancelled, invoiced)
- Ability to schedule all rooms associated
- Ability to schedule equipment
- Ability to schedule supplies
- Have journaling entries to follow communication thread
- Allow for invoicing
- Allow for complete reporting
- Allow for online payments of services
- Project management software to assign tasks and communicate needs
- Maintain full customer database and contact information
- Provide database for statistical tracking of customer base, research, and competencies evaluation
- Provide online calendar and room availability for customers
- Have multiuser platform
- Self-registration for courses
- External view of calendar

SUPPLIES, INVENTORY, RESTOCKING

The volume of equipment, supplies, and transactions that are needed for the day-to-day operations of a simulation center necessitate a structured record-keeping program. The inventory system can be written or automated (e.g., barcode or spreadsheet). A planned system will save time and increase accuracy in supply distribution and acquisition. Ideally, a system would provide cross-referencing, automatic notification of low inventory items, notification of routine equipment maintenance or calibration, and generation of reports. Periodic automatic replenishment (PAR) levels and the current level of supplies should be noted in the system as well. No matter what format is selected, you must be able to retrieve information about equipment, manikins, task trainers, special equipment, clinical simulators, and supplies needed, used, or available.

BOX 18.5 SAMPLE RESERVATION FORM ITEMS

1. Name, contact information, affiliation
2. Event title, purpose, objectives
3. Learner group and numbers of participants
4. Date requested, times, and other optional dates
5. Rooms requested
6. Equipment desired
7. Personnel required
8. Supplies desired

Keeping track of disposable supplies to be used and those actually used can be one of the most difficult and time-consuming aspects of the functioning simulation center. The inventory of the equipment can either be formatted by skill (e.g., tracheotomy care), by the type of equipment (e.g., gauze pads, 4 × 4s), or cross-references that allow you to change the format based on the need at the time (e.g., lab setup or review of total equipment available per category).

In addition, some programs base equipment lists on course type or instructor preference. Whatever system you employ, accurate documentation of equipment as it relates to courses should be created. A detailed equipment list and a photo of the setup may also be beneficial for future use. An inventory system spreadsheet contains the item name, description, location in the simulation center, cost, how it is supplied (single, box, case), where to order the supply, how to order the supply (hospital central supply, supply vendor), and an accurate inventory of supplies on hand.

Some inventory management options that simulation centers have elected to use to maintain records include simple paper and pencil, electronic spreadsheet, bar code system with database, database proper, or a complete scheduling system that incorporates all aspects into a single software system. No matter the system the center employs to maintain records and efficiency, there are multiple departments involved in maintaining adequate supplies in any simulation center. Establishing contacts within the local hospital system can assist in locating expired equipment, consumables, disposables, drug containers, and instruments.

We have noted in our environment that the operating room is a good example of discarded supplies due to the large number of cases; many stock supplies are pulled for each case in preparation and never used or have become nonsterile and subsequently discarded as trash. When the supplies have not had any patient or operative field exposure, they can be collected and subsequently recycled to your simulation center for use, allowing the center and health care system to save on supply costs. It is not uncommon to have a representative at each of the hospital facility operating room units who is looking for and collecting these supplies and alerting simulation center leadership when a bag is ready to be picked up. Commonly, there are individuals who donate supplies that have expired or they no longer have any use for, and these items can be incorporated into all educational events. Vendors commonly will have a set amount of supplies they can donate for educational purposes (e.g., suture, tubing, lines), which helps in maximizing curricular opportunities. Lastly, many hospital systems have a warehouse of expired and outdated supplies and furniture that could still have value. Take advantage of this and learn where the system maintains this warehouse so you can schedule a visit as it may contain some treasures for your center.

Restocking is a critical and time-consuming component of simulation center staff. Once supply orders have been filled, they need to be placed in storage locations depending on your environment. This takes vital time away from the staff's day and limits their ability to service customers either running, developing, or programming simulations. Look within your system to determine if you have the ability to automate this process. If allowed, take advantage of the hospital system supply chain and all of its amenities. Using the standard hospital restocking system with PAR levels for all supplies, self-stocking of the simulation center shelves by hospital personnel, and automated billing for the supplies consumed is most convenient.

By establishing PAR levels, the center will never have more supplies than the storage system can tolerate. When an event requires a large volume of a set of supplies, an order can be placed in advance, specifically for that event, and delivered via the hospital system. This pulls all simulation center staff from maintaining any supplies considered standard and allows them to dedicate time to higher priority tasks. If your center is not affiliated with a system, allocating a person with time to manage supplies is critical. Some programs have elected to organize supplies by course and create bins for each course. Whatever model works best for your facility should be implemented and, more importantly, documented. Creation of PAR levels based on course use should be one of your first tasks. Routine review of your center's calendar (looking ahead one week to one month) may afford you the ability to predict supply use.

Another area of efficiency is using volunteers within your system to assist with supply-related activities. There are many volunteer systems within the medical community that can regularly schedule one or more volunteers, but keep in mind they will need guidance and supervision.

Plan to recycle as much as possible. Many disposable items can be reused in the simulation environment before they become fatigued and unusable. Recycling and reusing will require some ingenuity and engineering, but the cost savings are worth the effort. Items to reuse multiple times over include endotracheal tubes, oral and nasal airways, nasogastric tubes, urinary catheters, defibrillation pads, refilled intravenous fluid bags, intravenous fluid tubing and connectors, central venous catheters, oxygen adjuncts, drug vials, and injection devices, to name only a few. Before disposing of equipment, always ask the questions: Can this item be repurposed? Will this work for another purpose? Customers will frequently request a piece of commonly utilized medical equipment (in real clinical practice) in their simulation scenario and to make it function properly in the simulation, but it may require creative challenges for incorporation.

SUMMARY

Simulation centers are dynamic by nature and require a special skill set in the planning and operations of them. Once your center has been created, many components will contribute to successful management. It is recommended that any system contemplating expansion of their current facility or establishing a new simulation center should consider visiting other centers that have structurally similar needs prior to the planning phase of your facility. Creation of a three-year plan is essential to keep your organization's focus in an effort to design a facility that is based on your mission and educational needs today, tomorrow, and into the future.

■ Key Concepts

- ■ A three-year plan will allow you to accurately forecast planning and budgetary needs to minimize setbacks in future implementation.
- ■ Ensuring your center has a structured hierarchy, integration plan with the parent institution, and a robust operational infrastructure is critical for success.

- New centers may want to initially rely on existing departmental structures (billing, payment processing, human resources, etc.) until they have created their own methodology.
- Creating documentation and processes for the operational side of the center will contribute to its final success.

References

Amasaka, K. (2002). New JIT: A new management technology principle at Toyota. *International Journal of Production Economics, 80*(2), 135–144.

Armstrong, J. S. (1986). The value of formal planning for strategic decisions: A reply. *Strategic Management Journal, 7,* 183–185.

Collins, R., Cordon, C., & Julien, D. (1996). Lessons from the "Made in Switzerland" study: What makes a world-class manufacturer? *European Management Journal, 14*(6), 576–589.

Gantt, L. T. (2010). Strategic planning for skills and simulation labs in colleges of nursing. *Nursing Economics, 28*(5), 308–313.

Harden, R. M., Stevenson, M., Downie, W. W., & Wilson, G. M. (1975). Assessment of clinical competence using objective structured examination. *British Medical Journal, 22*(1), 447–451.

Humphrey, A. (2005, December). History corner. SWOT analysis for management consulting. *SRI Alumni Newsletter.* Retrieved from http://www.sri.com/sites/default/files/brochures/dec-05.pdf

Hyland, J. R., & Hawkins, M. C. (2009). High fidelity human simulation in nursing education: A review of the literature and guide for implementation. *Teaching and Learning in Nursing, 4*(1), 4–21.

Kaplan, R. S., & Norton, D. P. (2000). *The strategy-focused organization: How balanced scorecard companies thrive in the new business environment.* Boston, MA: Harvard Business School Press.

Kardong-Edgren, S., & Oermann, M. (2009). A letter to nursing program administrators about simulation. *Clinical Simulations in Nursing, 5*(5), e161–e162.

Mickan, S., & Rodger, S. (2000). Characteristics of effective teams: a literature review. *Australian Health Review, 23*(3), 201–208.

Phillips, S. R., & Bergquist, W. H. (1987, March). Focusing problem management. *Training and Development Journal, 41*(3), 87.

Renger, R., & Titcomb, A. (2002). A three step approach to teaching logic models. *American Journal of Evaluation, 23*(4), 493–503.

Schoemaker, P. J. H. (1995). Scenario planning: A tool for strategic thinking. *Sloan Management Review, 36*(2), 25–40.

19

Using a Consortium Model to Develop a Simulation Center

Jim Battin, BS
Rhonda Savage, MPH
Jennifer W. Geers, MHA
Pamela R. Jeffries, PhD, RN, FAAN, ANEF

▮ Learning Objectives

1. Articulate the benefits of working in a consortium versus working in isolation.
2. Construct the nine steps of the Consortium Model and interpret the purpose, benefits, and challenges of each step.
3. Identify the roles and responsibilities of the leadership structure that are required in the start up of a consortium.
4. Explain the value of having a strategic plan.
5. Examine lessons learned from a case study of the Consortium Model that are relevant for replication of the Model.
6. Assess how the implementation of the Consortium Model through two cycles over a four year period generated improved results and commitment.
7. Describe the importance of aligning goals with regional and national metrics and organizational priorities as they related to sustaining a Consortium.

▮ Key Terms

- Area Health Education Centers
- Consortium
- Santayana Review
- Standards of excellence

Today in health care, with the creation of new cost and reimbursement models, the transformation of care delivery, the implications of the Affordable Care Act, and the evolution of higher education, health care organizations, including academic and practice institutions, can no longer afford to or should work in silos.

With the insurmountable changes, working in consortiums is becoming necessary to develop new clinical models of practice and care delivery approaches, to participate in cost sharing, and to embark on collaborative professional development. Working in consortiums can be cost-effective and provide the efficiency of care through teams now warranted by health care professionals, and it is realistic with practice and the needs of patients today.

A **consortium** as defined by *Merriam-Webster's Dictionary* is "an agreement, combination, or group formed to undertake an enterprise beyond the resources of any one member." It often starts with a single individual, grows to a small group, and eventually becomes a broader group of stakeholders. As personal visions and thoughts are shared, common themes and possibilities emerge. Although each individual's vision and perceived needs and benefits may be slightly different, a common ground and vision comes forth that will enable each party to become more committed to a move toward expanding, shaping, and eventually formalizing a concerted effort into a structured arrangement.

This chapter discusses a consortium model used to assist different academic institutions, hospitals, and other organizations with the mission of embarking on and adopting the simulation pedagogy within their organizations, utilizing a collaborative approach. Using the Consortium Model, the structure helps to guide the development, implementation, and evaluation of the collaborative work around simulations. Leaders within the collaboration discuss the elements of the Consortium Model that facilitate the achievement of adopting simulations within their institutions, building simulation centers, facilitating faculty development in simulations, and creating a plan of excellence to measure and document outcomes and achievements of the collaborative work.

THE CONSORTIUM MODEL

In developing the model, information was gathered through working directly with several long-term (three- to five-year) projects, observing other projects, and interviewing leaders of simulation center consortiums throughout the United States. From this research and experiences emerged a consistent set of elements present in the initiatives.

We have captured the elements in the Consortium Model and use a clock metaphor to describe them in more detail for practical application (Figure 19.1). There are nine elements in this model. The three foundational elements are Building the Consortium, Leading and Managing the Consortium, and Collaborating with Others. As the clock diagram in Figure 19.1 shows, the remaining elements rest upon this solid base.

To understand the sequence of the six remaining elements, begin at 12 o'clock and go in clockwise fashion. From beginning to end, these include: Developing a Strategy, Evaluating the Strategic Plan, Planning for Professional Development, Implementing the Strategy, Reflection and Renewal, and Planning for Sustainability. Upon completion of the first cycle, the model becomes self-sustaining by repeating the sequence of elements over and over.

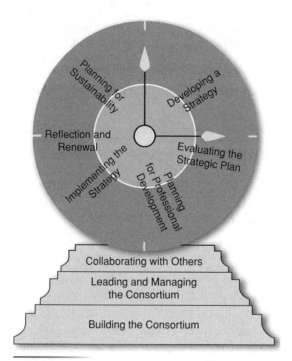

FIGURE 19.1 The Consortium Model schematic.

Well-known quality expert Joseph Juran (1989) calls the phenomenon of learning from repetitive cycles of prior activity "the **Santayana Review**," named after the philosopher George Santayana. This concept is relevant to the Consortium Model in that it promotes continuous improvement and repetitive analysis of low-frequency cycles of activity. This chapter describes two such cycles of activity spanning over a seven-year period. The advantage of being able to document such long cycles and learn from them is that we can repeat those practices that work well, while adjusting and eliminating those that do not. Table 19.1 takes a deeper look into the application of the model and describes key activities for each step.

With each subsequent cycle of the model, less time is required in planning because the foundation has been laid and the process is familiar. This allows time for creative exploration and reinforces continuous improvement to achieve more aggressive goals.

Although the Consortium Model is shown as a sequential process, it is important to acknowledge that during applications, it often takes on characteristics of an iterative and dynamic process, where specific elements are temporarily bypassed and others are explored out of sequence as the need arises. The value of the model is that over time and at a general level, it represents the key elements of most large projects involving collaboration of key stakeholder groups.

After this introduction of the model and a brief overview of each element, the next section will provide a more detailed description of each element, its purpose, benefits, challenges, and lessons learned.

TABLE 19.1

The Consortium Model: Key Activities for Each Step

Step of Model	Key Activities
Building the Consortium	Building relationships and finding common ground among key stakeholders
Leading and Managing the Consortium	Establishing a structure of three key groups— (1) steering committee, (2) simulation user group, and (3) staff support team
Collaborating with Others	Learning to work together through both advocacy and dialogue
Developing the Strategy	Evaluating factors that impact the environment of simulation initiatives in a region; defining the current state; defining the future desired state; analyzing strengths, weaknesses, opportunities, and threats to the consortium; developing goals, resources, milestones, and a project plan for implementation
Evaluating the Strategic Plan	Defining standards of excellence that provide operational direction through each cycle of performance
Planning for Professional Development	Defining the knowledge and skills that support excellence
Implementation	Removing barriers, maintaining motivation, and reporting progress
Reflection and Renewal	Taking pause, identifying successes and areas for improvement for the next cycle
Sustainability	Transferring the momentum of success into a sustainable model that utilizes consortium assets effectively for the long term

Building the Consortium

A consortium is a group of individuals and organizations that come together to discuss and find common ground around an opportunity or a threat. It often starts with a single individual and grows from there to a small group and eventually to a broader group of stakeholders. As personal visions and thoughts are shared, common themes and possibilities emerge. Although each individual's vision and perceived needs and benefits may be slightly different, a common ground and vision comes forth that will enable each party to become more committed to move toward expanding, shaping, and eventually formalizing a concerted effort into a structured arrangement. The work in this initial step involves some of the following activities:

- Defining the need, the potential benefits, and the potential challenges
- Identifying the scope, the available assets, and the key stakeholders
- Defining the resources required (leadership, knowledge, skills, etc.)

If the energy continues to build, the consortium develops a sense of urgency and agrees to take the next action step.

Leading and Managing the Consortium

There are three leadership groups to consider in the design of an effective simulation consortium: the steering committee, the simulation user group, and the support team. The roles and responsibilities of each group are described in Table 19.2.

All key stakeholders must be represented in the structure. Each team member has leadership potential and opportunity consistent with his or her roles, responsibilities, knowledge, skills, and abilities. Generally each group meets as a standalone committee, but there are times when groups meet jointly to clarify and advance common goals.

TABLE 19.2

The Consortium Model: Leadership Groups' Roles and Responsibilities

Leadership Groups	Roles and Responsibilities
Steering committee	<ul><li>Develop the vision, mission, and values of the consortium</li><li>Become lead advocates for the simulation initiative</li><li>Monitor and review project status</li><li>Help manage the scope of the project</li><li>Provide resources and organizational support</li></ul>
Simulation user group	<ul><li>Provide data and input on simulation needs</li><li>Provide operational input to the strategic plan</li><li>Implement the strategic plan</li><li>Share practices and innovations with other partners</li></ul>
Support team	<ul><li>Design agendas</li><li>Facilitate meetings</li><li>Provide technical assistance and expertise</li><li>Design the strategic planning process</li><li>Ensure regular communication between and across all three leadership groups</li></ul>

Collaborating with Others

Collaboration is a core value in the Consortium Model. Stakeholders benefit in each element of the model if they come together focused on a common goal. Collaboration builds community and ownership as plans are developed, decisions are made, and resources are shared to implement the plan. Finally, sharing rewards is the payoff for all.

An excellent resource book, *Collaboration: What Makes It Work* (Mattessich, Murray-Close, & Monsey, 2001), provides information on key factors that have been demonstrated to be effective practices in forming collaborative initiatives. Consortiums can benefit from taking an initial baseline inventory and measuring progress periodically as they take action on factors that may need strengthening and reinforcement.

DEVELOPING THE STRATEGY

Stephen Haines's (1995) *Successful Strategic Planning* is a brief but powerful book that lays out the steps to develop the strategy for the consortium. Haines covers the following steps:

1. Plan to plan
2. Your ideal future vision
3. Key success factors
4. Current state assessment
5. Core strategy development
6. Three-year business planning
7. Annual plans and strategic budgets
8. Plan to implement
9. Strategy implementation and change

Following the process outlined above provides the consortium with a significant amount of data and direction to develop a specific strategy. When applied to developing simulation centers, it can include completing a needs assessment of the current state (simulation equipment, applications currently being used, resources available, technical needs, and facility requirements). In addition, a SWOT (strengths, weaknesses, opportunities, and threats) analysis helps the consortium evaluate its current state in even more detail. As the future state is defined and the top four to six goals are established, the process enables defining the implementation plan with a high degree of confidence and direction.

Evaluating the Strategic Plan

Most strategic plans are considered a onetime event to be completed in three to five years. The Consortium Model takes a different view in that as each cycle occurs, planning, implementing, checking, and improving become a continuous process flowing into the next cycle. As a result, it is important to document the core simulation processes in place so each of the partners define their roles and responsibilities through **standards of excellence**.

Based on our research, there are several criteria used by health care organizations to evaluate their simulation work processes. For example, the Malcolm Baldridge National Quality Award, the Magnet Model, and Studer's (2003) principles of service and operating excellence, as outlined in *Hardwiring Excellence,* were frequently noted as models used by academic institutions and hospitals to measure nursing performance. Regardless of the system used, they have several common threads:

- A description of the criteria for excellence
- Descriptions of principles or processes on how excellence will be achieved
- Coverage of several functions of operating excellence: leadership, planning, customer focus, process management, professional practices and training, measurements, quality and results, people focus, and continuous improvement
- A measurement and review process
- A reward and recognition process

An annual review of the standards of excellence takes into account new changes that are required to maintain and improve previous standards set.

Professional Development Plan

A well-designed professional development plan answers the question, What knowledge, skills, and abilities are required for achieving and sustaining simulation excellence? Members of the steering committee, the simulation user group, and staff support can analyze their standards of excellence and identify important knowledge, skills, and abilities required of their roles and positions. Sources of training and development activity include:

- On-the-job training and experience through practice of simulation, design, debriefing, and evaluation
- Research articles and studies
- National League of Nursing website and others
- Simulation workshops and conferences
- Online training modules
- Degree programs and studies
- Mentoring
- Sharing of best practices with consortium members through committee meetings

Measuring professional development activities against goals and then correlating them with results can provide evidence of the value of simulation professional development.

Implementing the Strategy

Up to this point in the process, there has been a great deal of planning using the Consortium Model. Future cycles will require less planning time and more implementation of new goals as the previous foundational steps have been standardized as part of the normal work cycle.

The major goals of implementation are to remove barriers, build capacity ahead of demand, avoid project creep by staying focused on the project plan, and maintain motivation through the design and celebration of short-term wins that are relevant to meeting the goals that have been established. These actions help avoid burnout because implementation can be a long and tiresome process. Reporting progress and outcomes and providing feedback and recognition on a regular and earned basis are important steps to keep implementation on track against the strategic plan.

Reflection and Renewal

The reflection and renewal step in the model is oftentimes underrated in importance. The question is often asked, Why spend time doing this? By taking time to stop and reflect at the end of an extended period of work, the consortium can review and reflect on all phases of the model. The best way to do that is through an annual standards of excellence audit. By reflecting on the consortium's performance against planning goals, standards of excellence, completion of the training and development plan, and the results themselves, the consortium can appreciate its achievements and more objectively see areas for improvement. In addition, the reflection may reveal new standards of excellence that need to be developed for the next cycle. The reflection and renewal period is a precursor to the next planning cycle.

Sustainability

What is the process of developing a plan? Box 19.1 lists eight critical steps for developing a plan of sustainability. Without focusing on these steps, the consortium runs the risk of losing value among members and losing organizational support.

BOX 19.1 CRITICAL STEPS FOR SUSTAINABILITY

1. Evaluate the benefits that have been received from the simulation project.
2. Identify the activities that have had the greatest impact on the results.
3. Eliminate or reduce activities that are not adding value.
4. Add additional activities that have been identified through the learning process.
5. Rearticulate the vision and mission of the consortium and reinforce the level of commitment to sustain the consortium.
6. Review the assets that are available: in-kind services, grants, leverage of resources among partners, membership fees, endowments, cash contributions, fees for service, etc.
7. Develop funding options (ideally a blending approach) that will reinforce a successful continuation.
8. Consider change of the structure or transferring to another organization that may be better suited to carry on the initiative.

This completes the description of the Consortium Model. The remainder of the chapter demonstrates how one consortium made a transition of sustainability and developed the next cycle of improvement.

BUILDING THE CONSORTIUM

An example of successful implementation of the Consortium Model can be seen with the Southeast Indiana Simulation Consortium (hereafter the Consortium). Roots of this Consortium grew out of efforts and interests of groups focused on health care quality and nursing workforce in a 10-county area of Southeast Indiana. As these health care groups aligned with other economic sectors in the region, a large grant application was submitted and funded.

For the health care sector, the main goal of the grant was to build a simulation coalition. The initial thought was that one mobile simulation unit would be purchased for the region. The mobile lab would travel among the 14 consortium member sites. As steering committee and users group members were identified and consulted, it became clear that their idea to create a successful model involved dividing the funding so each site would have its own lab. Members agreed that the size and capacity of each member's facility would be fair measures to determine the size and resources contributed to each lab. This ongoing process of group decision making contributed to a level of trust and respect that remained strong within the Consortium.

At the end of the second year of the three-year grant, the Consortium support team began holding interviews with members of the steering committee to discuss sustainability. Connections and aligned goals with the East Indiana **Area Health Education Center** (AHEC) were frequently mentioned. At the close of the three-year grant, the Consortium steering committee agreed to transition the oversight of the Consortium to the East Indiana AHEC. This was the beginning of cycle II of the Consortium Model.

Although implementation was the emphasis of the initial cycle of the Consortium Model, growth and sustainability have become emphases of the subsequent cycle. Over time, the Consortium has solidified as it advances through the elements of the Consortium Model. The Consortium Model sets up a sharing relationship that builds on everyone's strengths. This, in turn, strengthens the foundational elements of the Consortium Model.

The relationship between the Consortium and AHEC is synergetic, with each supporting the other's goals. AHEC offers critical administrative and facilitation support and embraces Consortium participation in overall sustainability efforts. Similarly, the Consortium is an effective way to foster AHEC's goals to identify, train, and retain a primary care workforce for Southeast Indiana.

LEADING AND MANAGING THE CONSORTIUM

When AHEC assumed responsibility for the sustainability of the Consortium, a change in leadership structure was needed. The steering committee that was dominant in cycle I assumed more of a directional, rather than managerial, role. This group of regional leaders meets periodically to ensure alignment of program goals with organizational and regional priorities. It is this regional leadership group that maintains the value proposition for the

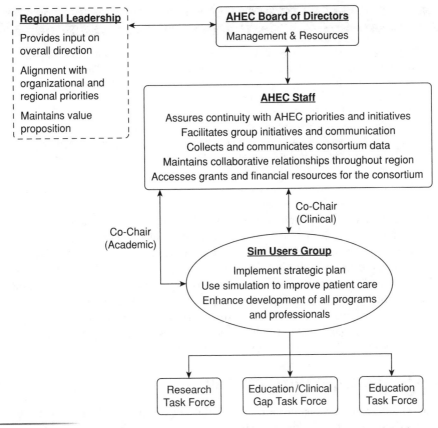

FIGURE 19.2 The Area Health Education Center board of directors leadership structure.

Consortium by making sure its work progresses and stays relevant to the region. This group is updated on Consortium data and projects through a quarterly newsletter.

The AHEC board of directors has assumed oversight of the Consortium. Many of the existing AHEC board members, stakeholders, and contacts are familiar with the regional simulation effort and were involved with the project in cycle I. This has paved the way for a smooth transition. Figure 19.2 presents the current leadership structure.

East Indiana AHEC staff provides day-to-day management and support to this structure. AHEC's executive director provides access to certain financial resources and ensures continuity with AHEC priorities. The AHEC simulation coordinator facilitates group initiatives and meetings, represents simulation in AHEC initiatives, and analyzes quarterly simulation data. In addition, AHEC's outreach coordinator provides technical support and data management as needed.

The simulation users group, which includes representatives of all member organizations, is the main working body of the Consortium. It is facilitated jointly by co-chairs, one representing the academic setting and one representing the clinical setting. The main function of this group is to guide the Consortium through mission-driven priorities.

BOX 19.2 GUIDING PRINCIPLES

- Prioritize consortium, regional, and organizational needs together in a way that maximizes collaboration and trust and minimizes competition.
- Assist all members to grow professionally and develop quality simulation programs within their own organizations.
- Align work with regional and national metrics, such as the Robert Wood Johnson Foundation's Institute of Medicine report (2010), the Centers for Medicare & Medicaid Services (n.d.) quality measures, Hospital Consumer Assessment of Healthcare Providers and Systems, and other quality and safety measures.

High priorities include developing and tracking data, enhancing program development, and working collaboratively to show the benefits of simulation as they relate to patient care. All work is sifted through the Guiding Principles (shown in Box 19.2), which were articulated by the group at the end of cycle I.

Keeping work relevant and engaging for Consortium members are important parts of the Consortium Model. Several task groups have been set up to advance priorities between quarterly meetings. Task force groups are focused on research, bridging the education–practice gap, and continuing education. This subcommittee structure keeps work manageable and more meaningful for members.

COLLABORATING WITH OTHERS

Collaborating with others is the core value of the Consortium Model, and the Consortium has focused on this continually. Simulation users group meetings are centered on creating opportunities for partnership and sharing. Each agenda outlines time for sharing, brainstorming, and creative problem solving. Allowing for task force updates during meetings provides opportunities for all members to contribute feedback and direction. During meetings, all successes, even small ones, are celebrated. Creating a group communication forum, where members can post information, exchange ideas, and dialogue, is a key component to supporting the ongoing sharing critical to true collaboration.

Networking outside the group and its 10-county region is important for the Consortium's long-term growth. The Consortium has established and enjoyed collegial relationships with Fairbanks Simulation Center, Indiana Hospital Association, Indiana Center for Nursing, and Indiana University School of Medicine, among others.

DEVELOPING THE STRATEGY

Once the transition to AHEC had occurred and support staff were in place, the Consortium went through a needs assessment process to provide specifics to its vision and strategic plan. The simulation coordinator met with each member organization to determine individual program needs and direction. This information was used to complete an overall SWOT analysis for the Consortium. The analysis was shared with AHEC board members and users group leaders and members. These discussions helped design priorities

TABLE 19.3

Consortium Strategic Plan

Consortium Priority	Action Steps
Establish forum for member communication	• Develop a Google Group to share information and dialogue
Provide funds to foster individual program needs	• Develop mini-grant program to support program development • Borrow equipment for short-term use
Provide technical support for growing programs	• Dialogue with manufacturer • Share technical expertise among group members
Address the nursing education/practice gap in our region	• Develop task force to begin a conversation about using simulation to prepare graduates for the clinical environment
Assist members with limited staffing and develop a case for dedicated staffing for simulation	• Share scenarios and other simulation tools among members • Track data to prove progress • Conduct a time study to support staffing and budget decisions
Prove impact of simulation on regional health care	• Conduct simulation research • Provide a test site for various simulation research • Foster dialogue between academic and clinical professionals • Develop an efficient means to collect/report data to stakeholders
Provide opportunities for continued professional development	• Establish a professional network • Post learning opportunities on communication forum • Introduce education/problem solving to simulation users group meetings; offer group education as needed

for the next level of simulation innovation. The Consortium's strategic plan, shown in Table 19.3, has been unfolding quickly.

Great progress has been made in designing and implementing simulations throughout the region that are consistent with accepted standards in medical simulation. Learning together allowed for standardization throughout the region around the ideas and processes from leaders in the field, including Pamela R. Jeffries (Jeffries, 2007), the Center for Medical Simulation (2009), and Laerdal Medical (2010). Tracking participants since January 2011 shows a total of 9,081 participants in the two-year period from 2011 to 2012 for the region. This is well above the original planning goal of 2,400 simulation participants per year.

Over the past few months, the Consortium has developed a web-based reporting mechanism. The Consortium is now able to collect desired group data and all data requested by AHEC in an easy and meaningful format. This tool, implemented in June 2013, tracks simulation contact hours, simulation development and execution time, fidelity, objectives, and interprofessional simulations.

Information from this database shows 54 percent of simulations are based in academic centers, while 46 percent are in the clinical setting. Roughly 67 percent are scenario-based simulations as opposed to less complex skills-based simulations. Fifty percent of simulations meet the definition of high fidelity and 28 percent of the simulations have elements of interprofessional education. All simulation objectives are recorded and show an interesting emergence of scenarios related to clinical handoff, communication, customer satisfaction, and training for nonclinical personnel. In addition, communication with area leadership has increased through an annual meeting and the development of a consortium newsletter, *Sim News*. Two research projects are in various stages of development.

EVALUATING THE STRATEGIC PLAN

The strategic plan is continuously evaluated through ongoing assessment of action steps and formal or informal feedback at each simulation users group meeting. The Consortium also administers a member feedback survey annually to ensure it is still aligned with group priorities and still helping individual simulation programs grow. Regularly asking if Consortium goals are relevant and activities are aligned with these goals allows for continuous improvement over time.

PLANNING FOR PROFESSIONAL DEVELOPMENT

Cycle I allowed for comprehensive and targeted educational opportunities, which formed the foundation of simulation knowledge for Consortium partners. Cycle II has shifted its focus from learning together to learning from one another. Building professional relationships and trust among members and allowing for professional development to occur through collaboration and sharing are some of the most important parts of all simulation users group meetings. Educational workshops are convened as needed and information about upcoming educational opportunities sponsored by outside organizations is promoted to all group members.

IMPLEMENTATION

Table 19.4 describes the activities related to both cycles of the implementation phase. Many factors from the implementation phase of cycle I are also relevant in cycle II. Relationship building and trust will always be important to the Consortium Model. There will always be a high need to bring people together to experience challenges, remove barriers to success, and define priorities.

Surprisingly, the development of a user-friendly database for the Consortium has proven to be a critical factor for implementation in cycle II. Capturing data that are

TABLE 19.4

Cycles I and II of the Consortium

Key Activities	Cycle I	Cycle II
Building the consortium	• Form the consortium of seven hospitals, three community colleges, two four-year universities, and two career technical education centers	• Transition to Area Health Education Center (AHEC) • Earn stakeholder buy-in
Leading and managing the consortium	• Form the steering committee, simulation users group, and staff support team • Hold regular meetings	• AHEC board: day-to-day management • Regional leadership: provide direction • Recruit academia and hospital liaisons for simulation users group • Develop guiding principles
Collaborating with others	• Collaborate with partners in each element of the Consortium Model	• Continue quarterly simulation users group meetings • Ongoing sharing among members • Create group communication forum
Developing the strategy	• Develop strategic simulation plan • Vision, mission, values • Needs assessment • Current and future states • Project plan; budget, metrics	• Simulation coordinator conducted needs assessment, visiting each partner
Evaluating the strategic plan	• Standards of excellence • Measure progress against standards	• Ongoing assessment of action step progress and relevance to regional initiatives • Evaluation forms at end of meetings • Annual feedback survey • Evaluate adherence to guiding principles
Planning for professional development	• Professional development plan for 30+ simulation educators • Workshops, online training modules, webinars, research articles, studies, scenario development, and debriefing	• Simulation users group meeting topics are identified by user request • Conference information is shared among users • Periodic educational workshops convened

(continued)

TABLE 19.4

Cycles I and II of the Consortium (*Continued*)

Key Activities	Cycle I	Cycle II
Implementation	• Build capacity ahead of demand • Remove barriers • Create short-term wins • Report and recognize progress • Balanced scorecard	• Facilitate data reporting to be user friendly • Collect data that are meaningful to group and others • Share data to motivate users, leadership, stakeholders • User-to-user sharing to help overcome barriers
Sustainability	• Sustainability committee • Funding for transition to AHEC	• Grant opportunities • Exploring membership program • Social enterprise

useful to the group and also demonstrate growth to leadership and key stakeholders has become an important priority that supports implementation. The Consortium's goal is 100 percent participation in data reporting, improving the percentage of scenario-based and interprofessional education simulations, and capturing the total time required for impactful simulations.

SUSTAINABILITY

The transition of the Consortium to the East Indiana AHEC has been beneficial for both parties and has allowed for the sustainability of the Consortium for at least two to three years. The fact that AHEC is a neutral nonprofit focused on the health care sector has been a positive when discussions around ownership of the Consortium initiatives is concerned. Ownership is an important aspect to group work. The openness of the group allows for participation to remain authentic.

To be sure, sustainability is an ongoing endeavor. Currently, AHEC addresses funding through grant opportunities and sponsorships, particularly for simulation research activities. East Indiana AHEC has included simulation as a key component of its social enterprise initiative and is exploring a membership program that would offer organizations benefits for financially supporting the Consortium.

SUMMARY OF KEY CONCEPTS

The Consortium Model is a tool to help groups work toward shared goals. Working through the nine elements of the model creates an on-going process for the group to grow and build. In this chapter, an example of a Simulation Consortium is provided to illustrate how a group has gone through the first and second cycles of the model.

In summary, there have been lessons learned about successful use of the model. Experience has demonstrated that constant reflection leads to constant improvement. It has also been apparent that alignment with regional goals and national metrics has been important for the Consortium to stay relevant. Additionally, greater impact has been seen through combining shared efforts of the group. By working together, skills and knowledge have increased in ways that may not have been possible for solo organizations. As the Consortium continues to advance, it will rely on the model to help it remain relevant and valuable to members.

References

Center for Medical Simulation. (2009). Debriefing Assessment for Simulation in Healthcare (DASH). Retrieved from www.harvardmedsim.org/debriefing-assessment-simulation-healthcare.php

Centers for Medicare & Medicaid Services. (n.d.). *Home.* Retrieved from www.cms.gov

Haines, S. G. (1995). *Successful strategic planning.* Menlo Park, CA: Crisp Publications.

Institute of Medicine. (2010). *The future of nursing: Leading change, advancing health.* Retrieved from www.iom.edu/reports/2010/The-Future-of-Nursing-Leading-Change-Advancing-Health

Jeffries, P. R. (2007). *Simulation in nursing education from conceptualization to evaluation.* New York: National League for Nursing.

Jeffries, P. R., & Battin, J. (2011). *Developing simulation successful health education simulation centers.* New York, NY: Springer.

Juran, J. M. (1989). *Juran on leadership for quality.* New York, NY: Free Press.

Kaye, D. (2013). *Red thread thinking.* New York, NY: McGraw-Hill.

Laerdal Medical. (2010). *Scenario validation checklist.* Retrieved from http://simulation.laerdal.com/forum/files/folders/checklists_worksheets/downloads

Mattessich, P. W., Murray-Close, M., & Monsey, B. R. (2001). *Collaboration: What makes it work,* 2nd ed. St. Paul, MN: Amherst H. Wilder Foundation.

Studer, Q. (2003). *Hardwiring excellence.* Gulf Breeze, FL: Fire Starter Publishing.

20

Clinical Simulation Gone Global: The Use of Simulation in International Settings

Nicole Ann Shilkofski, MD, MEd
Juriah Abdullah, MBBS, MEd

■ Learning Objectives

1. To understand patterns and trends of simulation-based medical education (SBME) use in developing countries and resource-limited settings.
2. To compare the potential utility of SBME in developing countries to that of developed countries.
3. To describe priority areas for application of SBME in the global setting, including patient safety, medical decision making, technical skills, teamwork and communication development, and resource allocation.

■ Key Terms

- Fidelity
- Hybrid simulation
- Simulated or standardized patients (SP)
- Simulation-based medical education (SBME)
- Underresourced setting

RATIONALE FOR USE OF SIMULATION IN THE GLOBAL SETTING

The aphorism coined by William Halsted in the early 1900s that summarized clinical training in medicine and nursing—"see one, do one, teach one"—has been largely supplanted in this era of technology and advances in medical and nursing education to "see one, then simulate before doing one or teaching one." This idea of formative "practice on plastic" has also seen an increase in the developing world, with many applications of different types of simulations being implemented in international settings. The need to

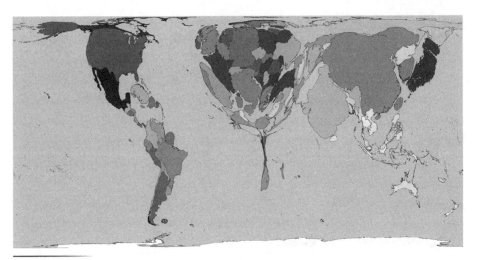

FIGURE 20.1 Physician Workforce Worldwide. Territory size shows the proportion of all physicians that work in that area. The most concentrated 50 percent of physicians live in territories with less than a fifth of the world population. The worst-off fifth are served by only 2 percent of the world's physicians. (From www.worldmapper.org © Copyright SASI Group [University of Sheffield] and Mark Newman [University of Michigan].)

deliver context-sensitive content in medicine and nursing has been a primary driver for pedagogical change throughout the world. The promotion of curricular change, development of educational infrastructure, and integration of resources (such as simulation) in education and training across multiprofessional groups becomes even more salient in the developing world. This is due to a mismatch of supply and demand; developing countries often have higher morbidity and mortality rates with the highest burden of disease globally, while being underresourced in the number of practicing clinicians and equipment within the country. Figures 20.1 through 20.3 demonstrate this mismatch pictorially in regard to a major worldwide problem, early neonatal mortality, compared with the number of health care workers worldwide.

There is an encouraging trend toward the globalization of education, which has resulted in partnerships between developed and developing countries that are generating effective solutions for today's global health challenges. A World Health Organization (WHO) patient safety study identified 10 key health areas where developed countries have the most to learn from the developing world; low-technology simulation training was one of these key areas (Syed et al., 2012).

This chapter describes the use of various forms of simulation (being broadly defined) for education in underresourced settings, including the use of manikin-based simulation, partial task trainer models, animal models, **standardized or simulated patients (SP)**, virtual reality simulation, and screen-based or computer simulation. The chapter will highlight **simulation-based medical education** (SBME) programs that have been implemented in multiple sites internationally as an example of attempts to target the Millennium Development Goals (MDGs) established by the United Nations (United Nations, 2013).

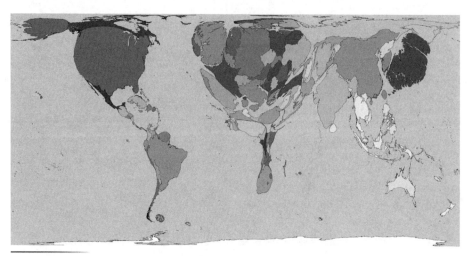

FIGURE 20.2 Nursing Workforce Worldwide. The highest numbers of nurses per person can be found in Western Europe. The fewest nurses working per person in the population are in Haiti, Bangladesh, and Bhutan, territories where there is much more need for nurses than is found in many other places. (From www.worldmapper. org © Copyright SASI Group [University of Sheffield] and Mark Newman [University of Michigan].)

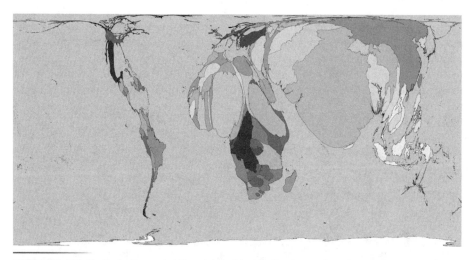

FIGURE 20.3 Early Neonatal Death Worldwide. Territory size shows the proportion of early neonatal deaths worldwide that occurred there in 2000. An early neonatal death is when a child dies during the first week of life. In 2000 there were 3 million such deaths. Worldwide, 2.3 percent of children who were born alive died during the following week. The three main causes of neonatal deaths around the world are asphyxia at birth, low birth weight including prematurity, and infections. Access to health care can reduce these deaths. (From www.worldmapper.org © Copyright SASI Group [University of Sheffield] and Mark Newman [University of Michigan].)

OVERVIEW OF SBME IMPLEMENTATION IN GLOBAL SETTINGS

SBME has been documented repeatedly in the literature as a method to assess quality of care provided by health care practitioners in a multitude of settings. The examples provided here focus on the use of simulation in rural and **underresourced settings** throughout the world. Existing assessment methods in medical education may be inaccurate, costly, or not feasible in many developing country settings. Therefore, creative approaches are necessary when implementing new assessment methods in these settings. Simulation is one creative approach that can be used in education and assessment of practicing clinicians in urban and rural settings, including community health workers and traditional birth attendants functioning in underresourced areas. In many of these settings, a country's lack of available trained medical and nursing staff is a major obstacle that impedes progress toward improving health care outcomes. The use of simulation in the creation of a sustainable system to manage emergencies can help to negate this obstacle.

A systematic review of the literature on resuscitation training in developing countries concluded that this type of training was well received and viewed as valuable (Meaney et al., 2010). The review concluded that training in trauma and newborn resuscitation in developing countries has been shown to reduce mortality, but this has not been demonstrated with other training programs. However, few studies in the review examined both educational and patient outcomes. Other investigators have examined models for the design of training programs in fields beyond resuscitation and acute care, such as surgical training programs (Mutabdzic, Bedada, Bakanisi, Motsumi, & Azzie, 2012). Studies by Moldovanu et al. (2009), Okrainec, Henao, and Azzie (2010), and Okrainec, Smith, and Azzie (2009) have documented the use of simulation to teach fundamentals of laparoscopic surgery courses in rural locations in Romania and Botswana. Okrainec et al. (2009) demonstrated feasibility of conducting this type of surgical skills course in a resource-restricted country and were able to show significant improvement in technical skills in this setting. Bench-top surgical simulation with objective structured assessment of technical skills has also been used in Ethiopia. This study used task-trainer simulation in surgery to focus on skills such as knot tying and closure of skin lacerations, and was able to demonstrate a feasible, safe, and cost-effective approach to train a multitude of health care professionals in technical skills. The authors concluded that this type of training program could help to address the human resources deficit in Africa (Dorman et al., 2009).

Other simulation studies have described the creation of innovative models for use in developing countries and low-resource settings. Many of these models were designed with the tenets of cost-effectiveness, portability, and sustainability in mind. Kalechstein et al. (2012) described the use within a trauma course in Guyana of a reusable tool to introduce a standard hollow needle for pediatric intraosseous (IO) infusion designed for use in developing countries, where standard IO needles are often not available for emergency use. Another study by Perosky et al. (2011) described the development and evaluation of a low-cost simulator for learning to manage postpartum hemorrhage (PPH) in Africa. This low-cost, portable simulator was designed to train traditional birth attendants and nurse midwives in the use of bimanual compression to manage PPH. The assessment of this simulator's efficacy included its use to train illiterate learners, because some traditional birth attendants living in rural areas may not be literate.

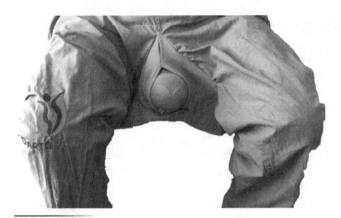

FIGURE 20.4 PartoPants Birthing Simulator.
(Reprinted with permission from Pronto International [http:
//prontointernational.org/partopantstm-birth-simulator.])

Within the field of surgery, investigators have shown that laparoscopic box trainers can be built using a high-definition webcam with a computer that provides image quality comparable to commercially available laparoscopic simulators (Kiely, Stephanson, & Ross, 2011). Kigozi et al. (2011) described the use in Uganda of a low-cost penile model to simulate the procedure of male medical circumcision. Investigators in orthopedic surgery in Thailand developed a simple and affordable knee model for intra-articular injection and arthrocentesis training made from plastic, rubber, and silicone (Waikakul et al., 2003). Within the field of obstetrics, Cohen, Cragin, Rizk, Hanberg, and Walker (2011) described the creation of an inexpensive and accessible low-tech birth simulator known as PartoPants™ (Figure 20.4). It was created by adaptation of a pair of scrub pants fitted with simulated pelvic organs and has been successfully used in Mexico for obstetrical emergency training. It can be used with standardized patients to enhance the realism of the learning experience (Walker et al., 2012). All of these models represent creative thinking to overcome cost and access limitations in the use of simulation in resource-poor areas. Diffusion of these innovations has the potential to benefit health care in both the developed and developing worlds.

Yet another technological innovation that has advanced the field of international simulation is the phenomenon of telesimulation. This novel concept combines the principles of simulation with remote Internet access to teach procedural skills, conduct simulated resuscitation sessions, or teach other concepts remotely to a target audience within rural or underresourced areas, provided there is a stable Internet connection. This technology has been used successfully in the field of surgery to teach laparoscopic skills as well as the procedure of IO needle insertion by a group in Canada to remote locations in Botswana (Mikrogianakis et al., 2011; Okrainec et al., 2010). New research by Yang, Hunt, Shilkofski, Dudas, and Schwartz (2012) demonstrated the use of telesimulation to conduct pediatric resuscitation training and debriefing sessions between consulting and remote hospitals, with a trend toward improved quality cardiopulmonary resuscitation endpoints by practitioners in target hospitals. Telesimulation can be a way to overcome the lack of specialty expertise within resource-challenged areas of the world, through remote teaching by facilitators in developed nations.

CULTURAL AND LINGUISTIC CONSIDERATIONS IN GLOBAL SIMULATION

Leadership and Teamwork: Cultural Differences in Hierarchy

The examples above show that simulation is feasible and effective in global settings throughout the world. However, conducting simulation sessions and debriefing sessions in international settings requires consideration of the culture and language of the region in order to be maximally effective. Culture can be conceptualized as shared motives, values, beliefs, identities, and interpretations or meanings of significant events that result from common experiences of members of collectives that are transmitted across generations (Yamazaki, 2005). It has been well documented in the literature that a dichotomy exists between Western and non-Western cultures in the ways of learning and conceptualizing entities such as the team construct and learning within teams (Joy & Kolb, 2009). Culture and nationality of origin have an impact on conceptualization of different team dynamics, including hierarchy, leadership and followership models, and role delineation within teams during emergency situations. This may be influenced by different cultural interpretation of values, such as the more stereotypically Western "individualism" as compared with a more Eastern "collectivistic" approach to team dynamics and learning (Joy & Kolb, 2009). Similarly, there are some cultures that value communal learning and others in which learning is an individual enterprise (Yamazaki, 2005). In ad hoc teams with members from different cultures and nations, this dichotomy can create barriers to communication and effective patient care.

Simulation itself can help improve communication and create a shared mental model that reaches beyond cultural bounds for these types of teams (Shilkofski & Hunt, 2009). These shared mental models can improve the functionality of medical teams in the care of patients (Hunt, Shilkofski, Nelson, & Stavroudis, 2007). As a form of experiential learning, simulation can appeal to diverse types of learners within a team. In addition, simulation can improve several areas of team functionality, including membership, role, context, process, and action taking by focusing intentional learning effort and debriefing on each of these areas (Shilkofski & Hunt, 2009).

Fahey et al. (2013) described the curricular adaptations made in a curriculum for obstetric and neonatal emergencies in Guatemala to account for cultural issues deemed important by Guatemalan health authorities. The adaptations included design and refinement of new activities and simulations for training in cultural humility and humanized birth, taking into account the issues mentioned above. Another study describes the importance of taking into account local sociocultural constraints and local epidemiology when designing vignettes for use in computerized patient simulation for decision support in district hospitals of Sub-Saharan Africa (Bediang, Bagayoko, Raetzo, & Geissbuhler, 2011). Investigators in Romania attempted in their study to examine the impact of language and cultural differences as limiting factors for international exchange of virtual patients (Muntean, Calinici, Tigan, & Fors, 2013). These are examples of the importance of incorporating these considerations into wide-scale simulation and educational programs.

Impact of Culture and Language on Patient Safety: Implications for Simulation

Any educational intervention in an international setting must take into account cultural norms and the impact of culture on preferred learning style and communication style in order to be effective. It has been recognized that cognitive processes are embedded in a nested, culturally determined set of factors. Therefore, to influence cognitive processes and habits of thought, cultural differences are monumental factors whose impact must be accounted for in the design of interventions in simulation. The influence of culture on assertiveness and leadership styles, uncertainty avoidance, reflective capacity, and the individual degree of introversion or extroversion must also be considered in the design of the debriefing process of simulations for interprofessional teams in global settings.

Multiple barriers exist that impact the effective functioning of both individuals and teams that can be identified through the use of in situ simulations within a practice setting. These barriers include cultural impact on communication, leadership and organizational norms and team efficacy, language barriers that result in miscommunication and potential patient harm, and latent threats to patient safety in a resource-limited setting (including appropriate equipment and medication availability and lack of systematic emergency procedures). In a study conducted across medical professionals in different countries in Asia, Africa, and South America, physicians and nurses identified language as a major component for misunderstanding during the conduct of simulation debriefings (Shilkofski & Hunt, 2009). Accented speech, methods of pronunciation, differing colloquialisms, and frank language barriers were identified as the origin of misunderstandings and lack of awareness by team members. In situ simulation can be an effective educational tool that can identify and address these barriers as a target for remediation and improvement within the context of patient care, thereby serving as a patient safety tool.

MANIKIN AND TASK TRAINER SIMULATION IN UNDERRESOURCED SETTINGS AND DEVELOPING COUNTRIES: EXAMPLES OF PROGRAM IMPLEMENTATION

Technology Versus Fidelity: Their Roles in Creating Sustainability in Underresourced Settings

In the field of simulation, **fidelity** has been used to describe how well a simulation replicates or represents "reality." The concept is sometimes further defined in the subdimensions of physical fidelity, environmental fidelity, equipment fidelity, and psychological fidelity (Dieckmann, Gaba, & Rall, 2007). Some investigators have tried to understand the relationship between fidelity and the degree of learning achieved through simulation. Although the results of these studies are inconclusive, several investigators support the idea that fidelity is not the key ingredient in a simulation to produce transfer of learning (de Giovanni, Roberts, & Norman, 2009; Hoadley, 2009; Norman, Dore, & Grierson, 2012; Tan et al., 2012). Because the process of using simulation is a "social practice," it may be that the conduct of the simulation, debriefing of the learners, and ongoing feedback are the more critical ingredients to a successful simulation. A systematic review of the evidence in educational science regarding the features of simulations that lead to the most effective learning strategies identified educational feedback as the most commonly mentioned "important feature" (Issenberg et al., 2005).

The concepts of fidelity and transfer of learning are salient in the developing world when considering sustainability of a simulation program in resource-poor settings. It is often assumed that "high-tech" manikins or equipment translate to "high-fidelity" environments and transfer of learning to clinical settings. However, this is not always the case, nor is it feasible and sustainable in areas of the world where the technology is not affordable or the resources do not exist for this type of training. These resources can include physical resources (e.g., computers to run high-tech manikins or something as simple as a consistent electrical power source) as well as human resources (because high-tech manikins require some degree of training to operate). The example in the next section demonstrates a large-scale and widespread simulation program initiative in the developing world that uses low- to medium-fidelity equipment to create a sustainable educational framework.

Example of a Large-Scale Simulation Program Design and Implementation in Global Settings

Helping Babies Breathe (HBB) is an initiative of the American Academy of Pediatrics in collaboration with other partners, with curriculum development input from the World Health Organization (WHO). It is a neonatal resuscitation curriculum for resource-limited circumstances and was developed on the premise that assessment at birth and simple newborn care are things that every baby deserves (Helping Babies Breathe, 2013).

The prior curricula, Essential Newborn Care and Neonatal Resuscitation Programs, for birth attendants in rural communities demonstrated mixed outcomes (Bhutta et al., 2011; Carlo, Goudar et al., 2010; Carlo, McClure et al., 2010). Evidence from several observational studies has shown that a range of community health workers can perform basic resuscitation skills that have the potential to substantially reduce intrapartum-related neonatal deaths, but that a major gap exists in terms of strategies to address home births and births in rural, underresourced areas far from referral facilities (Wall et al., 2009). The HBB program was developed to address these gaps.

The program was piloted in Kenya and Pakistan, where participants expressed high satisfaction with the program and high self-efficacy with respect to neonatal resuscitation after participation. Assessment of participant knowledge and skills pre- and post-program demonstrated significant gains. Bag valve mask ventilation was identified as a skill that required more active practice, continued learning, and mentoring in order to be mastered by some participants (Singhal et al., 2012). The program has subsequently been implemented in many developing countries and studies of its efficacy in these settings are ongoing. In India, a train-the-trainer cascade model has been used to train almost 600 birth attendants from rural primary health centers and district and urban hospitals. Investigators examined over 4,000 births before and after implementation of training and were able to demonstrate a significant reduction in stillbirths in the area where training had been integrated. However, neonatal mortality rates remained unchanged (Goudar et al., 2013).

The HBB strategy was used to train master instructors in Tanzania, who then delivered the program to regional instructors, who in turn trained health providers in smaller facilities. In the two years after intervention, there was a 24 percent reduction in the rate of stillbirths and a 47 percent reduction in early neonatal mortality, defined as death within the first 24 hours. This program was focused on the grassroots birth attendants, many of whom practice in rural facilities, rather than on hospital-based physicians (Msemo et al., 2013).

HBB program implementation has also been subsequently formally studied in Ethiopia, Rwanda, and Nepal, with promising preliminary results toward the objective of addressing Millenium Development Goals 4 (MDG 4), to reduce child mortality (Ashish et al., 2012; Hoban et al., 2013; Musafili, Essén, Baribwira, Rukundo, & Persson, 2013). The preliminary successes of this type of program demonstrate the feasibility of an evidence-based curriculum using a low-cost simulator in the developing world.

USE OF SIMULATED OR STANDARDIZED PATIENTS IN GLOBAL SETTINGS

Standardized Patients and Online Virtual Patients

Simulated or standardized patients (SPs) have been used in resource-challenged areas to teach and assess practicing clinicians and students. In settings far from tertiary care facilities that may not have access to specialty care patients, SPs can supplement the learner experience by providing a standardized presentation of specific disease processes for both formative and summative learning. In some instances, they can also provide a safe environment for novice learners to practice sensitive or intimate examinations that may be difficult to gain practice with in certain cultural contexts.

Researchers in Myanmar assessed the ability of providers to diagnose and treat pediatric malaria using trained actors playing the role of the patient's mother and a trained observer (Aung, Montagu, Schlein, Khine, & McFarland, 2012). In Iran, researchers in a department of psychiatry created SP scenarios for assessment of primary care providers' management of depression disorders (Shirazi et al., 2011). Studies by Taghva et al. (2010) and Sadeghi, Taghva, Mirsepassi, and Hassanzadeh (2007) demonstrated the use of SPs within objective standardized clinical examinations (OSCEs) for psychiatric board certification exams in Iran. Another development has been in the use of online virtual patients for technological skills instruction and capacity building for health care educators in Malawi (Dewhurst, Borgstein, Grant, & Begg, 2009). These "virtual patients" are designed by teams of health care professionals to be contextualized for in-country medical and health care education.

The Role of Hybrid Simulation in a Global Setting

When initially learning to perform sensitive examinations such as breast, rectal, or pelvic examinations, students and novice learners often have difficulty finding willing patients. In addition, other factors such as religious and sociocultural preferences come into play. In some conservative societies, female patients often prefer female health professionals, especially when it involves such sensitive examinations. In such a setting where there are limited resources, the opportunity for patient contact in basic clinical skills for students becomes inadequate or restricted. Students depend on opportunities to perform these examinations on ward patients and do so hastily so as to minimize the discomfort and embarrassment of the patients, but this is not optimal for training.

SPs provide a degree of realism that is not possible when using manikins alone. Partial task trainers and manikins provide students with the ability to perform invasive procedures such as venous cannulation, catheterizations, and sensitive examinations to which SPs may not wish to be subjected. When a partial task trainer (such as a pelvic examination model or rectal model) and an SP are combined, as in the case of a **hybrid simulation**, students are able to participate in a realistic human interaction and practice communication skills while performing basic clinical skills, including invasive procedures, in a single simulation (Figures 20.5 and 20.6).

A high-tech, high-fidelity simulator can also be used in conjunction with an SP, depending on the learning objectives or competencies to be addressed within a scenario (and of course local resource availability). Feedback from faculty and SPs can be given on skill performance of a procedure as well as verbal communication and nonverbal

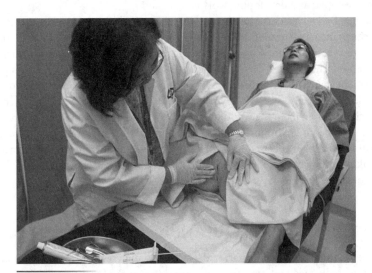

FIGURE 20.5 Pelvic examination using hybrid simulation. A standardized patient is combined with a plastic pelvic model to focus on technical and nontechnical skill development, with a focus on interpersonal communication during sensitive examinations. (Photo courtesy of Perdana University Graduate School of Medicine Simulation Centre Standardized Patient Program.)

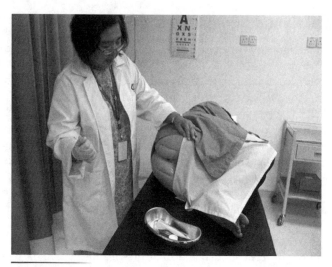

FIGURE 20.6 Rectal examination using a task trainer rectal model and a standardized patient at a medical school in Malaysia. (Photo courtesy of Perdana University Graduate School of Medicine Simulation Centre Standardized Patient Program.)

body language. In short, hybrid simulation provides many educational advantages in both the developed and developing worlds (Box 20.1).

Kneebone, Bello, Nestel, Yadollahi, and Darzi (2007) developed an "Integrated Procedural Performance Instrument" to be used in scenarios that combine SPs with inanimate models to re-create realistic scenarios that address a combination of technical and nontechnical clinical challenges. This was one of the first uses of hybrid simulation to implement a patient-centered and learner-focused approach to both procedural and communication skills (Moulton et al., 2009). Hybrid simulation has also been used in medical and nursing school curricula in the Middle East, where gender and religious preference often limit student exposure to opposite-sex, gender-specific examinations (Sole & Sawan, 2012). Investigators have been able to demonstrate improved student confidence in basic sexual history taking and breast and pelvic examination skills after participation in hybrid simulations for these skills.

FUTURE OF GLOBAL SIMULATION

The future of simulation in international arenas will depend largely on anticipating and overcoming challenges that are inherent in underresourced settings. Partnerships with in-country practitioners or stakeholders, Ministries of Health, and nongovernmental organizations can help to facilitate overcoming barriers of competing priorities and potential diversion of resources. Implementation of any new simulation programs internationally will require consideration of cultural sensitivity and linguistic factors if a program is to be successful longitudinally. Local epidemiology of disease burden should

BOX 20.1 ADVANTAGES OF HYBRID SIMULATION

The advantages to using hybrid simulation include:

1. Allows for the practice of a range of skills similar to those required in clinical practice in a manner that provides a realistic experience for students.
2. Combines technical skills training with behavioral interaction and interpersonal communication.
3. Incorporates elements of patient safety. Faculty can intervene and redirect inappropriate responses in order to preserve patient's safety and comfort.
4. Students can practice with minimal supervision. Well-trained standardized patients may guide students through the examination with a prepared checklist.
5. Various practical skills can be incorporated such as the practice of draping and other physical examination patient preparation.
6. Feedback on performance can be given immediately by faculty supervisor, standardized patients, or both. Self-assessment and reflection on performance can also be facilitated.
7. The session can be repeated in a standardized manner.
8. Provides a safe and nonthreatening environment that supports experiential learning.
9. Ability to record a session for viewing and debriefing with students or for future training of other standardized patients.

be closely examined in order to address pertinent medical issues that are relevant to a particular country or area. All of these factors need to be taken into account to create sustainability of a program or intervention on a large scale that can create meaningful change. Models for program delivery and dissemination should consider train-the-trainer paradigms that can also encourage program sustainability.

Any individual, team, or organization that endeavors to undertake simulation in under-resourced settings should be willing to invest in system strengthening and capacity building within that setting. A plan to demonstrate and measure both the short- and long-term impacts is key to obtaining or sustaining funding for educational projects in these settings. The establishment of attainable and realistic educational goals and rigorous research methodology to measure the impact are the basis for effecting change. Achievement of pragmatic goals will require interprofessional input from local health care providers as partners to incorporate diversity of perspectives and experience. Opportunities for collaborative international projects should be considered in order to form "simulation communities of practice" (Hovancsek et al., 2009). With consideration of all of these factors, simulation has the potential to profoundly impact health care education in the global setting.

■ Key Concepts

- ■ Simulation is relevant and feasible in the developing world, where there is a mismatch between numbers of health care providers and burden of worldwide disease.
- ■ Current educational efforts in health care in developing countries are often impacted by a lack of both physical and human resources.

■ Consideration of cultural and linguistic factors is essential to successful implementation when designing simulation programs for use in international settings.

■ Manikin-based simulation and standardized patient simulation have been used effectively in underresourced settings in the developing world.

■ Hybrid simulation can be used as a method to overcome cultural and religious constraints when novice learners are practicing sensitive examinations.

References

Ashish, K., Målqvist, M., Wrammert, J., Verma, S., Aryal, D. R., Clark, R., . . . Ewald, U. (2012). Implementing a simplified neonatal resuscitation protocol-helping babies breathe at birth (HBB) at a tertiary level hospital in Nepal for an increased perinatal survival. *BMC Pediatrics, 12*, 159.

Aung, T., Montagu, D., Schlein, K., Khine, T. M., & McFarland, W. (2012). Validation of a new method for testing provider clinical quality in rural settings in low- and middle-income countries: The observed simulated patient. *Public Library of Science One, 7*(1), e30196.

Bediang, G., Bagayoko, C. O., Raetzo, M. A., & Geissbuhler, A. (2011). Relevance and usability of a computerized patient simulator for continuous medical education of isolated care professionals in Sub-Saharan Africa. *Studies in Health Technology and Informatics, 169*, 666–670.

Bhutta, Z. A., Soofi, S., Cousens, S., Mohammad, S., Memon, Z. A., Ali, I., . . . Martines, J. (2011). Improvement of perinatal and newborn care in rural Pakistan through community-based strategies: A cluster-randomised effectiveness trial. *Lancet, 77*(9763), 403–412.

Carlo, W. A., Goudar, S. S., Jehan, I., Chomba, E., Tshefu, A., Garces, A., . . . Wright, L. L. (2010). High mortality rates for very low birth weight infants in developing countries despite training. *Pediatrics, 126*(5), e1072–e1080.

Carlo, W. A., McClure, E. M., Chomba, E., Chakraborty, H., Hartwell, T., Harris, H., . . . Wright, L. L. (2010). Newborn care training of midwives and neonatal and perinatal mortality rates in a developing country. *Pediatrics, 126*(5), e1064–e1071.

Cohen, S., Cragin, L., Rizk, M., Hanberg, A., & Walker, D. (2011). PartoPants: The high-fidelity, low-tech birth simulator. *Clinical Simulation in Nursing, 7*(1), e11–e18.

de Giovanni, D., Roberts, T., & Norman, G. (2009). Relative effectiveness of high- versus low-fidelity simulation in learning heart sounds. *Medical Education, 43*(7), 661–668.

Dewhurst, D., Borgstein, E., Grant, M. E., & Begg, M. (2009). Online virtual patients—A driver for change in medical and healthcare professional education in developing countries? *Medical Teacher, 31*(8), 721–724.

Dieckmann, P., Gaba, D., & Rall, M. (2007). Deepening the theoretical foundations of patient simulation as social practice. *Simulation in Healthcare, 2*(3), 183–193.

Dorman, K., Satterthwaite, L., Howard, A., Woodrow, S., Derbew, M., Reznick, R., & Dubrowski, A. (2009). Addressing the severe shortage of health care providers in Ethiopia: Bench model teaching of technical skills. *Medical Education, 43*(7), 621–627.

Fahey, J. O., Cohen, S. R., Holme, F., Buttrick, E. S., Dettinger, J. C., Kestler, E., & Walker, D. M. (2013). Promoting cultural humility during labor and birth: Putting theory into action during PRONTO obstetric and neonatal emergency training. *Journal of Perinatal and Neonatal Nursing, 27*(1), 36–42.

Goudar, S. S., Somannavar, M. S., Clark, R., Lockyer, J. M., Revankar, A. P., Fidler, H. M., . . . Singhal, N. (2013). Stillbirth and newborn mortality in India after helping babies breathe training. *Pediatrics, 131*(2), e344–e352.

Helping Babies Breathe. (2013). *Helping Babies Breathe curriculum: The golden hour.* Retrieved from http://www.helpingbabiesbreathe.org

Hoadley, T. A. (2009). Learning advanced cardiac life support: a comparison study of the effects of low- and high-fidelity simulation. *Nursing Education Perspectives, 30*(2), 91–95.

Hoban, R., Bucher, S., Neuman. I., Chen, M., Tesfaye, N., & Spector, J. M. (2013). Helping Babies Breathe training in Sub-Saharan Africa: Educational impact and learner impressions. *Journal of Tropical Pediatrics, 59*(3), 180–186.

Hovancsek, M., Jeffries, P., Escudero, E., Foulds, B., Husebo, S.E., Iwamoto, Y., . . . Wang, A. (2009). Creating simulation communities of practice: An international perspective. *Nursing Education Perspectives, 30*(2), 121–125.

Hunt, E. A., Shilkofski, N. A., Nelson, K., & Stavroudis, L. (2007). Simulation: Translation to improved team performance. *Anesthesiology Clinics of North America, 25*(2), 301–319.

Issenberg, S. B., McGaghie, W. C., Petrusa, E. R., Lee Gordon, D., & Scalese, R. J. (2005). Features and uses of high-fidelity medical simulations that lead to effective learning: A BEME systematic review. *Medical Teacher, 27*(1), 10–28.

Joy, S., & Kolb, D. (2009). Are there cultural differences in learning style? *International Journal of Intercultural Relations, 33*, 69–85.

Kalechstein, S., Permual, A., Cameron, B. M., Pemberton, J., Hollaar, G., Duffy, D., & Cameron, B. H. (2012). Evaluation of a new pediatric intraosseous needle insertion device for low-resource settings. *Journal of Pediatric Surgery, 47*(5), 974–979.

Kiely, D. J., Stephanson, K., & Ross, S. (2011). Assessing image quality of low-cost laparoscopic box trainers: Options for residents training at home. *Journal of the Society for Simulation in Healthcare, 6*(5), 292–298.

Kigozi, G., Nkale, J., Wawer, M., Anyokorit, M., Watya, S., Nalugoda, F., . . . Gray, R. H. (2011). Design and usage of a low-cost penile model for male medical circumcision skills training in Rakai, Uganda. *Urology, 77*(6), 1495–1497.

Kneebone, R., Bello, F., Nestel, D., Yadollahi, F., & Darzi, A. (2007). Training and assess-

ment of procedural skills in context using an Integrated Procedural Performance Instrument (IPPI). *Studies in Health Technology and Informatics, 125*, 229–231.

Meaney, P. A., Topjian, A. A., Chandler, H. K., Botha, M., Soar, J., Berg, R. A., & Nadkarni, V. M. (2010). Resuscitation training in developing countries: A systematic review. *Resuscitation, 81*(11), 1462–1472.

Mikrogianakis, A., Kam, A., Silver, S., Bakanisi, B., Henao, O., Okrainec, A., & Azzie, G. (2011). Telesimulation: An innovative and effective tool for teaching novel intraosseous insertion techniques in developing countries. *Academic Emergency Medicine, 18*(4), 420–427.

Moldovanu, R., Tarcoveanu, E., Lupascu, C., Dimofte, G., Filip, V., Vlad, N., & Vasilescu, A. (2009). Training on a virtual reality simulator—is it really possible a correct evaluation of the surgeons' experience? *Revista medico-chirurgicală a Societăţii de Medici şi Naturalişti din Iaşi, 113*(3), 780–787.

Moulton, C. A., Tabak, D., Kneebone, R., Nestel, D., MacRae, H., & LeBlanc, V. R. (2009). Teaching communication skills using the Integrated Procedural Performance Instrument (IPPI): A randomized controlled trial. *American Journal of Surgery, 197*(1), 113–118.

Msemo, G., Massawe, A., Mmbando, D., Rusibamayila, N., Manji, K., Kidanto, H. L., . . . Perlman, J. (2013). Newborn mortality and fresh stillbirth rates in Tanzania after Helping Babies Breathe training. *Pediatrics, 131*(2), e353–e360.

Muntean, V., Calinici, T., Tigan, S., & Fors, U. G. (2013). Language, culture and international exchange of virtual patients. *BMC Medical Education, 13*, 21.

Musafili, A., Essén, B., Baribwira, C., Rukundo, A., & Persson, L. Å. (2013). Evaluating Helping Babies Breathe: Training for healthcare workers at hospitals in Rwanda. *Acta Paediatrica, 102*(1), e34–e38.

Mutabdzic, D., Bedada, A. G., Bakanisi, B., Motsumi, J., & Azzie, G. (2012). Designing a contextually appropriate surgical training program in low-resource settings:

The Botswana experience. *World Journal of Surgery, 37*(7), 1486–1491.

Norman, G., Dore, K., & Grierson, L. (2012). The minimal relationship between simulation fidelity and transfer of learning. *Medical Education, 46*(7), 636–647.

Okrainec, A., Henao, O., & Azzie, G. (2010). Telesimulation: An effective method for teaching the fundamentals of laparoscopic surgery in resource-restricted countries. *Surgical Endoscopy, 24*(2), 417–422.

Okrainec, A., Smith, L., & Azzie, G. (2009). Surgical simulation in Africa: The feasibility and impact of a 3-day fundamentals of laparoscopic surgery course. *Surgical Endoscopy, 23*(11), 2493–2498.

Perosky, J., Richter, R., Rybak, O., Gans-Larty, F., Mensah, M. A., Danguah, A, . . . Andreatta, P. (2011). A low-cost simulator for learning to manage postpartum hemorrhage in rural Africa. *Simulation in Healthcare, 6*(1), 42–47.

Sadeghi, M., Taghva, A., Mirsepassi, G., & Hassanzadeh, M. (2007). How do examiners and examinees think about role-playing of standardized patients in an OSCE setting? *Academic Psychiatry, 31*(5), 358–362.

Shilkofski, N. A., & Hunt, E. A. (2009). Use of In situ simulation to identify barriers to patient care by ad hoc multicultural and interprofessional teams in resource-limited settings. *Simulation in Healthcare, 4*(4), 238–239.

Shirazi, M., Sadeghi, M., Emami, A., Kashani, A. S., Parikh, S., Alaeddini, F., . . . Wahlstrom, R. (2011). Training and validation of standardized patients for unannounced assessment of physicians' management of depression. *Academic Psychiatry, 35*(6), 382–387.

Singhal, N., Lockyer, J., Fidler, H., Keenan, W., Little, G., Bucher, S., . . . Niermeyer, S. (2012). Helping Babies Breathe: Global neonatal resuscitation program development and formative educational evaluation. *Resuscitation, 83*(1), 90–96.

Sole, K., & Sawan, L. (2012). Fostering student clinical skills confidence using obstetric and gynecology hybrid simulation. Presented at 15th Ottawa Conference: Assessment of Competence in Medicine and Healthcare Professions, March 10, 2012; Kuala Lumpur, Malaysia.

Syed, S. B., Dadwal, V., Rutter, P., Storr, J., Hightower, J. D., Gooden, R., . . . Pittet, D. (2012). Developed-developing country partnerships: Benefits to developed countries? *Global Health, 8,* 17.

Taghva, A., Panaghi, L., Rasoulian, M., Bolhari, J., Zarghami, M., & Esfahani, M. N. (2010). Evaluation of reliability and validity of the psychiatry OSCE in Iran. *American Journal of Academic Psychiatry, 34*(2), 154–157.

Tan, S. C., Marlow, N., Field, J., Altree, M., Babidge, W., Hewett, P., & Maddern, G. J. (2012). A randomized crossover trial examining low- versus high-fidelity simulation in basic laparoscopic skills training. *Surgical Endoscopy, 26*(11), 3207–3214.

United Nations. (2013). Millennium Development Goals. Retrieved from http://www.un.org/millenniumgoals/.

Waikakul, S., Vanadurongwan, B., Chumtup, W., Assawamongkolgul, A., Chotivichit, A., & Rojanawanich, V. (2003). A knee model for arthrocentesis simulation. *Journal of the Medical Association in Thailand, 86*(3), 282–287.

Walker, D., Cohen, S., Estrada, F., Monterroso, M., Jenny, A., Fritz, J., & Fahey, J. (2012). PRONTO training for obstetric and neonatal emergencies in Mexico. *International Journal of Gynecology & Obstetrics, 116*(2), 128–133.

Wall, S. N., Lee, A. C., Niermeyer, S., English, M., Keenan, W. J., Carlo, W., . . . Lawn, J. E. (2009). Neonatal resuscitation in low-resource settings: what, who, and how to overcome challenges to scale up? *International Journal of Gynaecology and Obstetrics, 107,* S47–S64.

Yamazaki, Y. (2005). Learning styles and typologies of cultural differences: A theoretical and empirical comparison. *International Journal of Intercultural Relations, 29,* 521–548.

Yang, C., Hunt, E., Shilkofski, N., Dudas, R., & Schwartz, J. (2012). Can telemedicine improve adherence to resuscitation guidelines for critically ill children at community hospitals: A randomized controlled trial using high fidelity simulation. *Critical Care Medicine, 40*(12), 328.